Biogenic Monoamines and their Metabolites

in the

Urine, Plasma, and Cerebrospinal Fluid

of

Normal, Psychiatric, and Neurological Subjects

Author

Bruce A. Davis
Neuropsychiatric Research Unit
Cancer and Medical Research Building
University of Saskatchewan
Saskatoon, Saskatchewan
Canada

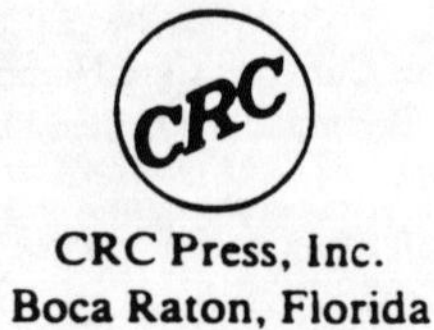

CRC Press, Inc.
Boca Raton, Florida

Library of Congress Cataloging in Publication Data

Davis, Bruce A., 1941—
    Biogenic monoamines and their metabolites in the urine, plasma,
and cerebrospinal fluid of normal, psychiatric, and neurological
subjects / Bruce A. Davis
        p.   cm.
    Includes bibliographical references.
    ISBN 0-8493-4611-8
    1. Mental illness—Physiological aspects—Tables. 2. Nervous
system—Diseases—Tables. 3. Biogenic amines—Tables. 4. Blood—
Analysis—Tables. I. Title.
    [DNLM: 1. Biogenic Monoamines—blood—tables. 2. Biogenic
Monoamines—cerebrospinal fluid—tables. 3. Biogenic Monoamines—
urine—tables. 4. Brain Diseases—tables. 5. Mental Disorders—
tables. WM 100 D258b]
RC455.4.B5D38   1990
616.8'047—dc20
DNLM/DLC
for Library of Congress   89-25470
                                                               CIP

PREFACE

In the last 40 years, the results of hundreds of investigations into the relationships between psychiatric and neurological disorders and the concentrations of biogenic monoamines and their metabolites in biological fluids have been published. A number of reviews have been published on these subjects, but each has been narrowly focused on a particular disorder and only a few amines and metabolites. This report is the most comprehensive tabulation to date of the results of studies on the concentrations of the monoamines and their metabolites in the urine, plasma, and cerebrospinal fluid (CSF) in normal, psychiatric, and neurological subjects.

This report is divided into two main parts: the tables of values and the references. For each amine or metabolite there is a table for concentrations in each of the biological fluids, with separate tables for the unconjugated and conjugated forms in most cases, and for each class of subject: normal, depressed, schizophrenic, aggressive, Parkinson's disease, and Alzheimer's disease. In each table for each reference cited, the concentration of the amine or metabolite, the number of subjects participating in the study, and the analytical method employed (with an indication of whether or not full experimental details are provided) are given. Within each table the references are listed in chronological order of publication (and alphabetically by first author for papers published in the same year), allowing the reader to see at a glance whether the reported values have changed over time. Usually, as analytical methods become more specific and sensitive over the years, the reported values decrease and appear to reach a more or less constant value which may be considered the true value for subjects of a given type and under a specified set of conditions. These should be useful as benchmark values for the purposes of comparison with new results and may also assist researchers in the choice of a suitable method of analysis. It should be noted here that these tables do not represent a comprehensive listing of all references to methods of analysis of the biogenic monoamines and their metabolites, because those papers describing methods which have been applied only to standard solutions or to human or animal tissue are excluded. For ease of comparison, the data from all the references cited have been converted to common units wherever possible (as indicated at the top of the "values" column in the tables). Where a conversion was not possible the units are indicated with the value in the body of the table. Unless otherwise indicated, the subjects were physically healthy and drug free. For the psychiatic subjects, the diagnosis as reported in the paper is given with the number of subjects. All the subjects in the studies cited were adults; this is important since the concentrations of many of the biogenic monoamines and their metabolites in children are highly dependent on age.

The references, which follow the tables, are listed in alphabetical order of the last name of the first author and are also numbered. For different authors with the same last name, alphabetization is by their initials. Where an author has more than one paper cited, alphabetization continues with the last name of subsequent co-authors. For the sake of clarity in the tables, only the reference number and the last name of the first author and the year of publication are cited. Each reference is complete in the sense that all the authors (with all their initials), the journal, year of publication (if a book, also the editors and publishers), volume, first page of the paper, and the full title of the paper are given.

The biogenic monoamines and their metabolites are of interest not only in psychiatry and neurology, but also in toxicology, food science, and nutrition and have been proposed and used as markers in clinical practice and basic research of errors of metabolism (e.g., phenylketonuria), Huntington's chorea, various types of cancer, hypertension, diabetes, and several other physical disorders. The normal values presented in this report should prove useful for comparative purposes to researchers and clinicians in these fields.

THE EDITOR

Bruce A Davis, Ph.D., has been a research scientist and Adjunct Professor with the Neuropsychiatry Research Unit, Department of Psychiatry, University of Saskatchewan, since 1987, and from 1972 to 1987 was a laboratory scientist with the Psychiatric Research Division, Saskatchewan Department of Health, and Adjunct Professor, Department of Psychiatry, University of Saskatchewan. He obtained his B.A. degree in 1963 and his Ph.D. (organic chemistry) in 1966 from the University of Saskatchewan, spent 2 years as a Fellow of the Alexander von Humboldt Foundation at the University of Munich, West Germany, doing research on reaction mechanisms, spent another 2 years (1968 to 1970) at the University of Cambridge, England, as a Fellow of the National Research Council of Canada in research on various aspects of mass spectrometry, and then spent 2 years in teaching and research in the Chemistry Department, University of Saskatchewan.

For the past 17 years, his research interests have been predominantly in the area of analytical chemistry, particularly the development and application of mass spectrometric methods for the quantitative analysis of biogenic amines and their metabolites in human biological fluids. The results of these analyses have been used in the search for biological markers in various psychiatric and neurological disorders, including schizophrenia, depression, Parkinson's disease, and aggression. Other research activities include the development of methods for the synthesis of deuterium-labeled analogues of biogenic amines and their metabolites for use as internal standards in quantitative mass spectrometry and as metabolic tracers.

TABLE OF CONTENTS

Section 1

Abbreviations and Structures

ABBREVIATIONS

Fl   =   fluorometric or spectrophotometric analysis

REA   =   radioenzymatic assay

RIA   =   radioimmuno assay

GC   =   gas chromatography

ECD   =   electron-capture detection

GC-N   =   gas chromatography with nitrogen detection

FID   =   flame ionization detection

GC-MS   =   gas chromatography-mass spectrometry (with selected ion monitoring)

MS-SIM =   mass spectrometry with selected ion monitoring (TLC purification)

TLC   =   thin-layer chromatography

HPLC   =   high-pressure liquid chromatography

EC   =   electrochemical detection

F   =   female

M   =   male

P.D.   =   Parkinson's Disease

A.D.   =   Alzheimer's Disease

Cr.   =   creatinine

Conj.   =   conjugated

†   =   This symbol (following the abbreviation for the method of analysis) indicates that full experimental details for the analytical procedure are given.

STRUCTURES

AMINES

p-Octopamine   (pOA)
   MW = 153

p-Synephrine   (pSYN)
   MW = 167

Noradrenaline   (NA)
MW = 169

Adrenaline   (A)   MW = 183

Normetanephrine   (NMN)
MW = 183

Metanephrine   (MN)   MW = 197

3-Methoxytyramine   (3MeOTA)
MW = 167

**3,4-Dimethoxyphenylethylamine
(DMPEA)   MW = 181**

AMINES

—CH$_2$CH$_2$NHCH$_3$

N-Methyltryptamine (NMT)
MW = 174

—CH$_2$CH$_2$N(CH$_3$)$_2$

N,N-Dimethyltryptamine
(DMT)   MW = 188

HO— —CH$_2$CH$_2$NH$_2$

5-Hydroxytryptamine (5HT)
(Serotonin)   MW = 176

HO— —CH$_2$CH$_2$N(CH$_3$)$_2$

Bufotenin (DM-5HT)
MW = 204

CH$_3$O— —CH$_2$CH$_2$NHCOCH$_3$

Melatonin (MEL)   MW = 232

CH$_3$O— HO— —CH$_2$CH$_2$NHCOCH$_3$

6-Hydroxymelatonin (6OH-MEL)
MW = 248

ACIDS

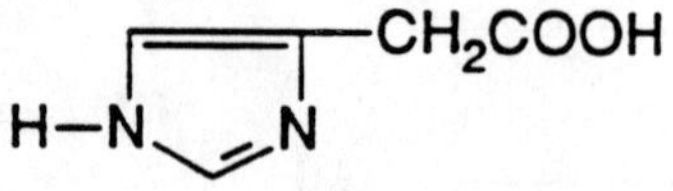

Imidazoleacetic Acid
(ImAA)   MW = 126

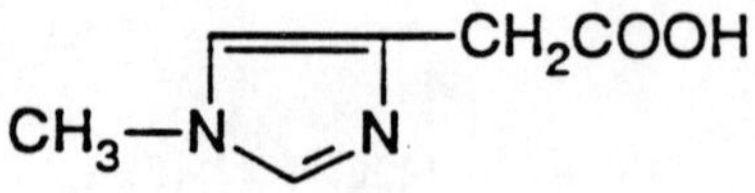

N^τ -Imidazoleacetic Acid
(N^τ -MeImAA)   MW = 140

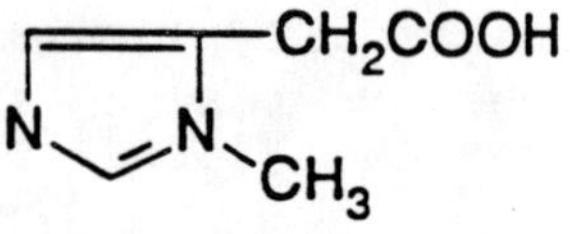

N^π -Methylimidazoleacetic
Acid (N^π -MeImAA)
MW = 140

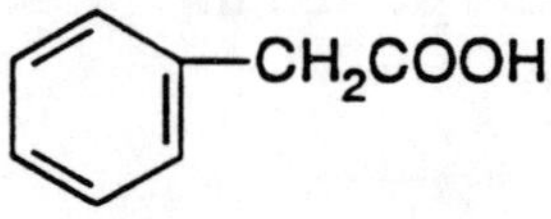

Phenylacetic Acid (PAA)
MW = 136

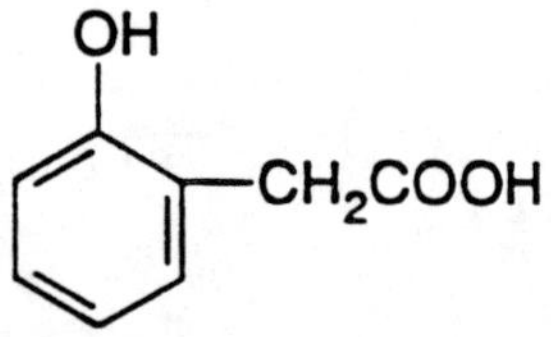

o -Hydroxyphenylacetic Acid
(oHPA)   MW = 152

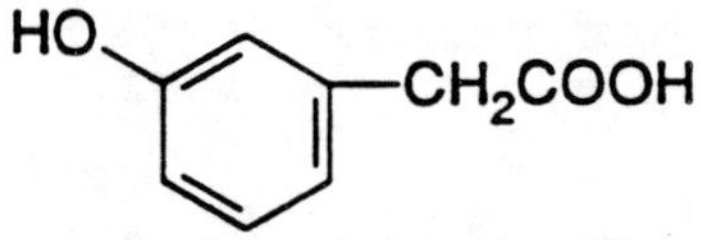

m -Hydroxyphenylacetic Acid
(mHPA)   MW = 152

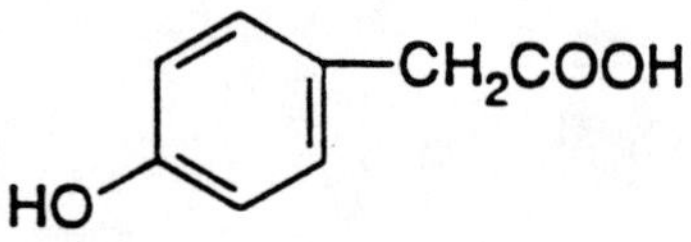

p -Hydroxyphenylacetic Acid
(pHPA)   MW = 152

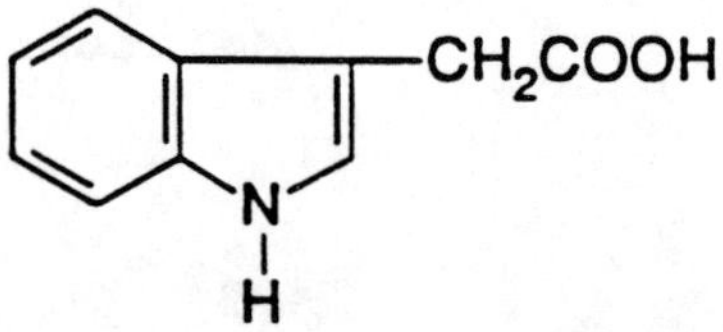

Indole-3-acetic Acid
(IAA)   MW = 175

ACIDS

o –Hydroxymandelic Acid
(oHMA)   MW = 168

m –Hydroxymandelic Acid
(mHMA)   MW = 168

p –Hydroxymandelic Acid
(pHMA)   MW = 168

Mandelic Acid (MA)
MW = 152

Homovanillic Acid (HVA)
MW = 182

Iso-Homovanillic Acid
(iso-HVA)   MW = 182

ACIDS

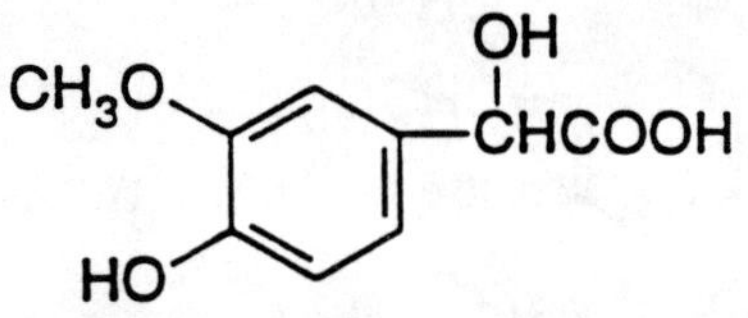

Vanilmandelic Acid (VMA)
MW = 198

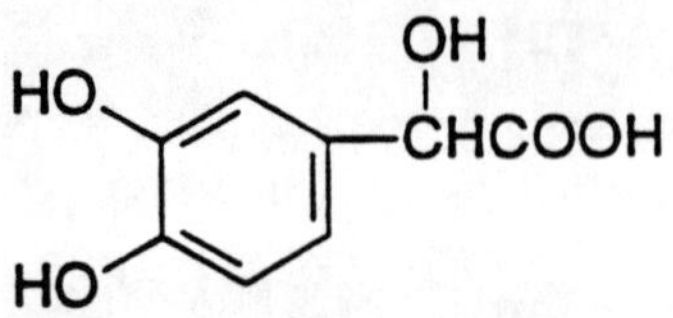

3,4-Dihydroxymandelic Acid (DOMA)   MW = 184

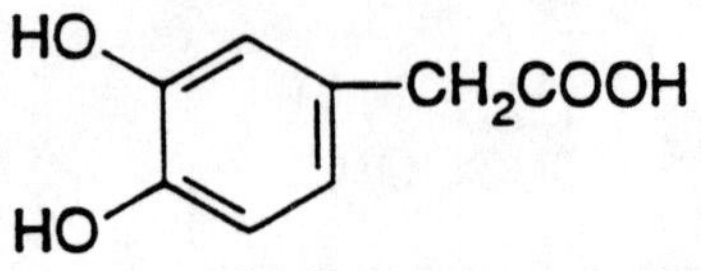

3,4-Dihydroxyphenyl-acetic Acid (DOPAC)
MW = 168

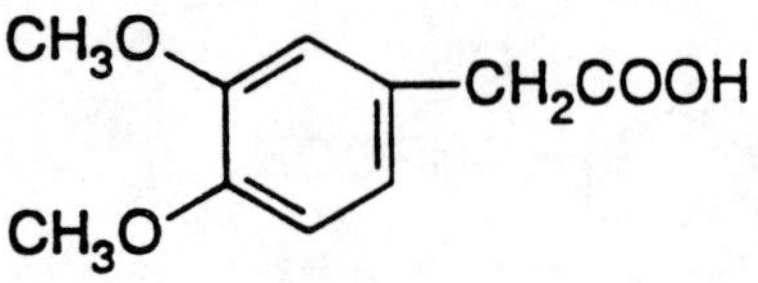

3,4-Dimethoxyphenylacetic Acid (DMPAA)   MW = 196

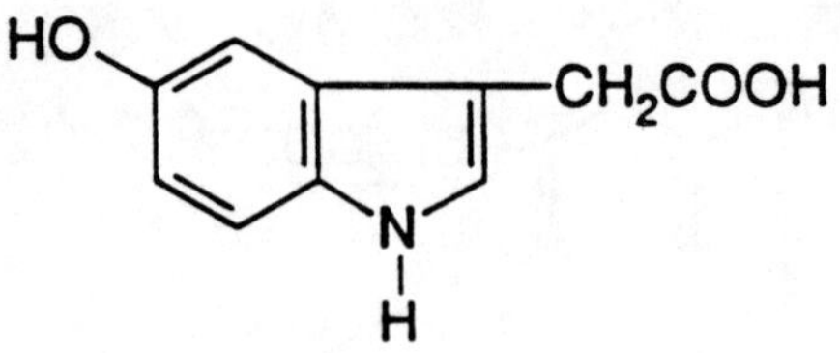

5-Hydroxyindole-3-acetic Acid (5HIAA)   MW 191

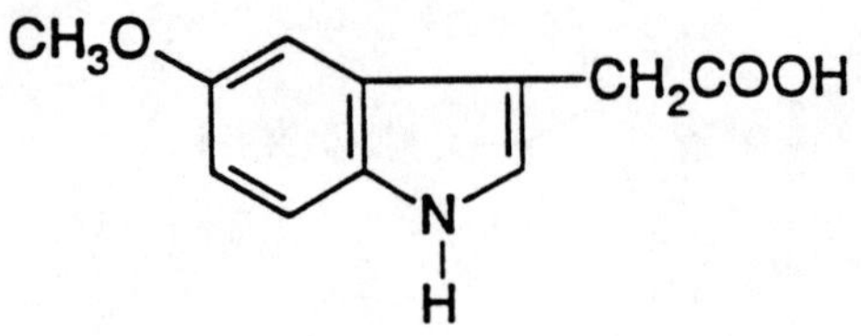

5-Methoxyindole-3-acetic Acid (5MeOHIAA)   MW = 205

ALCOLHOLS AND GLYCOLS

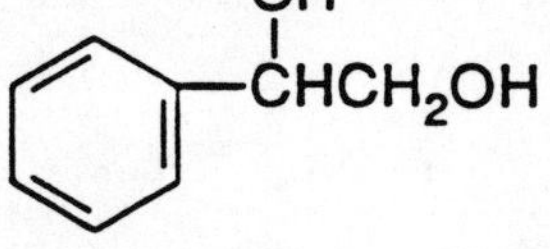

**Phenylethylglycol
(PEG)   MW = 138**

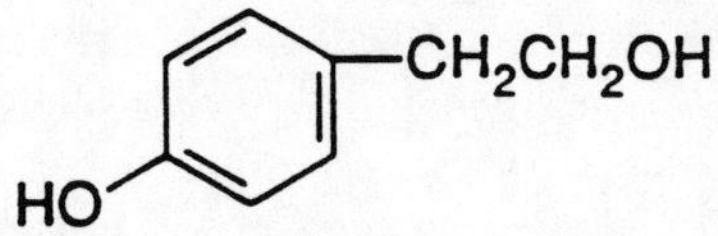

**p-Hydroxyphenylethanol
(pHPE)   MW = 138**

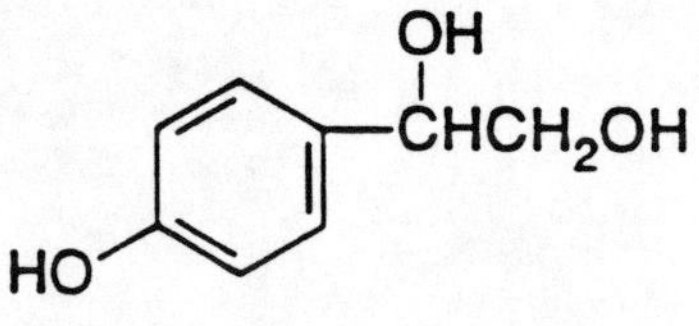

**p -Hydroxyphenylethyl-
glycol (pHPG)   MW = 154**

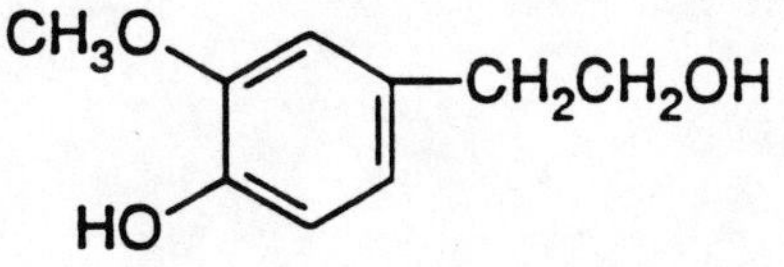

**3-Methoxy-4-hydroxyphenyl-
ethanol (MHPE)   MW = 168**

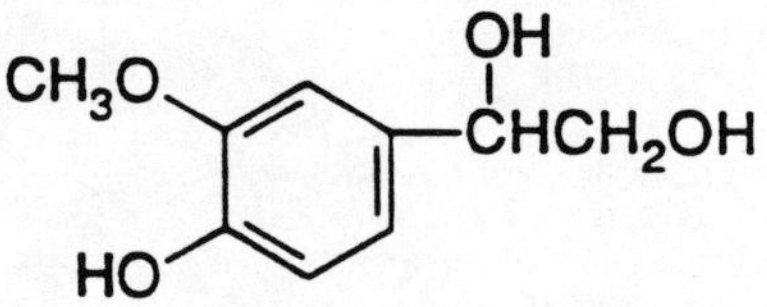

**3-Methoxy-4-hydroxyphenyl-
ethylglycol (MHPG)
MW = 184**

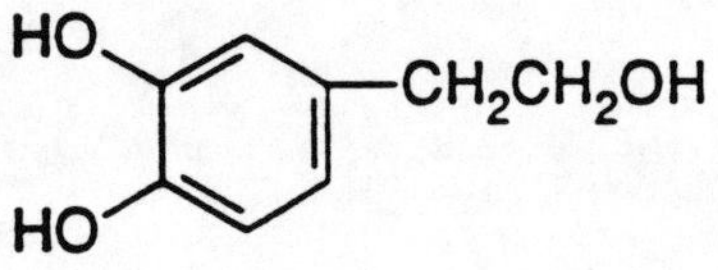

**3,4-Dihydroxyphenylethanol
(DHPE)   MW = 154**

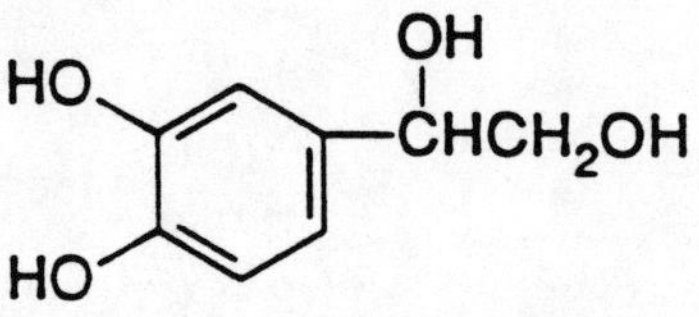

**3,4-Dihydroxyphenylethyl-
glycol (DHPG)   MW = 170**

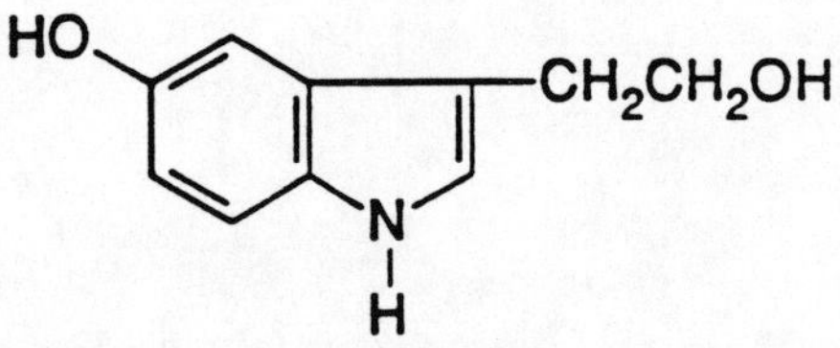

**5-Hydroxytryptophol
(5OH-TRPOH)   MW = 177**

Section 2

Locator Tables

AMINES

Normals - Table No.

Amine	Urine		Plasma		CSF	
	Unconjugated	Conjugated	Unconjugated	Conjugated	Unconjugated	Conjugated
HA	1	2	4	–	6	–
N$^\tau$-MeHA	3	–	5	–	6	–
PEA	11	12	13	–	14	–
oTA	–	–	–	–	–	–
mTA	20	20	22	–	–	–
pTA	23	24	25	–	25	–
TRA	29	29	30	–	30	–
pOA	34	–	35	–	–	–
pSYN	36	–	–	–	–	–
NA	76	77	78	79	80	80
A	87	88	89	90	91	91
DA	97	98	99	100	101	101
5HT	109	110	111	–	112	–
NMN	116	117	120	120	121	–
MN	122	123	120	120	121	–
3-MeOTA	125	–	126	126	126	–
DMPEA	127	–	–	–	–	–
NMT	129	–	–	–	–	–
DMT	128	–	133	–	135	–
DM-5HT	130	130	133	–	–	–
MEL	131	–	134	–	135	–
6OH-MEL	132	132	–	134	–	–

AMINES

Depression – Table No.

Amine	Urine		Plasma		CSF	
	Unconjugated	Conjugated	Unconjugated	Conjugated	Unconjugated	Conjugated
HA	–	–	–	–	–	–
N^{τ}-MeHA	–	–	–	–	–	–
PEA	15	15	16	–	–	–
oTA	–	–	–	–	–	–
mTA	21	–	–	–	–	–
pTA	27	–	–	–	–	–
TRA	33	–	–	–	–	–
pOA	–	–	–	–	–	–
pSYN	–	–	–	–	–	–
NA	81	81	83	–	85	–
A	92	–	95	–	95	–
DA	102	102	106	–	106	106
5HT	113	–	114	–	–	–
NMN	118	118	–	–	–	–
MN	124	–	–	–	–	–
3-MeOTA	125	–	–	–	–	–
DMPEA	–	–	–	–	–	–
NMT	129	–	–	–	–	–
DMT	128	–	133	–	–	–
DM-5HT	–	–	–	–	–	–
MEL	131	–	134	–	–	–
6OH-MEL	132	–	–	–	–	–

AMINES

Schizophrenia - Table No.

Amine	Urine Unconjugated	Urine Conjugated	Plasma Unconjugated	Plasma Conjugated	CSF Unconjugated	CSF Conjugated
HA	-	-	-	-	-	-
N^τ-MeHA	-	-	-	-	-	-
PEA	17	-	18	-	18	-
oTA	-	-	-	-	-	-
mTA	21	-	-	-	-	-
pTA	26	-	-	-	-	-
TRA	32	-	-	-	-	-
pOA	-	-	-	-	-	-
pSYN	-	-	-	-	-	-
NA	82	82	84	-	86	-
A	93	-	94	-	96	-
DA	103	103	104	-	105	105
5HT	113	-	114	-	114	-
NMN	119	119	-	-	121	-
MN	119	119	-	-	-	-
3-MeOTA	-	-	-	-	126	-
DMPEA	127	-	-	-	-	-
NMT	129	-	-	-	-	-
DMT	128	-	133	-	135	-
DM-5HT	130	-	-	-	-	-
MEL	-	-	134	-	-	-
6OH-MEL	-	-	-	-	-	-

AMINES

<u>Parkinson's Disease and Alzheimer's Disease - Table No.</u>

Amine	Urine (P.D. only)		Plasma (A.D. and P.D.)		CSF (A.D. only)*	
	Unconjugated	Conjugated	Unconjugated	Conjugated	Unconjugated	Conjugated
HA	-	-	-	-	-	-
N$^\tau$-MeHA	-	-	-	-	-	-
PEA	19	-	-	-	-	-
oTA	-	-	-	-	-	-
mTA	21	-	-	-	-	-
pTA	28	28	-	-	-	-
TRA	31	-	-	-	-	-
pOA	-	-	-	-	-	-
pSYN	-	-	-	-	-	-
NA	107	-	-	-	108	-
A	107	-	-	-	-	-
DA	107	107	-	-	108	-
5HT	-	-	-	-	115	-
NMN	-	-	-	-	121	-
MN	-	-	-	-	-	-
3-MeOTA	-	-	-	-	126	-
DMPEA	-	-	-	-	-	-
NMT	-	-	-	-	-	-
DMT	-	-	-	-	-	-
DM-5HT	-	-	-	-	-	-
MEL	-	-	-	-	-	-
6OH-MEL	-	-	-	-	-	-

* Table 115 also contains values for P.D.
Note: There are no values for biogenic amines in any of the biological fluids for aggressive subjects.

ACIDS

Normals - Table No.

Acids	Urine		Plasma		CSF	
	Unconjugated	Conjugated	Unconjugated	Conjugated	Unconjugated	Conjugated
ImAA	7	7	9	9	-	-
N^τ-MeImAA	8	-	9	-	10	-
N^π-MeImAA	8	-	9	-	10	-
PAA	37	38	39	40	41	42
oHPA	52	-	-	-	-	-
mHPA	52	52	53	54	55	-
pHPA	58	58	59	60	61	-
IAA	66	66	67	-	68	-
oHMA	73	-	-	-	-	-
mHMA	73	-	74	-	-	-
pHMA	73	-	74	-	75	-
MA	73	73	74	-	-	-
5HIAA	136	136	137	-	138	-
HVA	147	147	148	-	149	149
VMA	180	-	181	-	182	-
DOPAC	187	187	188	-	189	189
DOMA	203	203	204	204	204	-
DMPAA	205	-	-	-	-	-
5MeO-IAA	206	-	206	-	-	-

ACIDS

Depression – Table No.

Acids	Urine		Plasma		CSF	
	Unconjugated	Conjugated	Unconjugated	Conjugated	Unconjugated	Conjugated
ImAA	–	–	–	–	–	–
N^{τ}–MeImAA	–	–	–	–	–	–
N^{π}–MeImAA	–	–	–	–	–	–
PAA	–	43	44	–	44	–
oHPA	56	–	–	–	–	–
mHPA	56	–	57	–	–	–
pHPA	62	–	64	–	65	–
IAA	69	–	71	–	71	–
oHMA	–	–	–	–	–	–
mHMA	–	–	–	–	–	–
pHMA	73	–	–	–	–	–
MA	–	–	–	–	–	–
5HIAA	139	–	137	–	140	–
HVA	150	–	151	–	152	152
VMA	183	–	–	–	185	–
DOPAC	191	–	–	–	192	192
DOMA	202	–	–	–	–	–
DMPAA	–	–	–	–	–	–
5MeO-IAA	–	–	–	–	–	–

ACIDS

Schizophrenics – Table No.

Acids	Urine		Plasma		CSF	
	Unconjugated	Conjugated	Unconjugated	Conjugated	Unconjugated	Conjugated

ImAA	-	-	-	-	-	-
N^τ-MeImAA	-	-	-	-	10	-
N^π-MeImAA	-	-	-	-	-	-
PAA	45	46	47	47	48	48
oHPA	-	-	-	-	-	-
mHPA	-	-	57	57	-	-
pHPA	-	-	64	64	65	-
IAA	70	70	-	-	71	-
oHMA	-	-	-	-	-	-
mHMA	-	-	-	-	-	-
pHMA	-	-	-	-	75	-
MA	-	-	-	-	-	-
5HIAA	141	-	142	-	142	-
HVA	153	-	154	-	155	155
VMA	184	-	-	-	185	-
DOPAC	193	-	193	-	193	193
DOMA	-	-	-	-	-	-
DMPAA	205	-	-	-	-	-
5MeO-IAA	-	-	-	-	-	-

ACIDS

Parkinson's Disease – Table No.

Acids	Urine Unconjugated	Conjugated	Plasma Unconjugated	Conjugated	CSF Unconjugated	Conjugated
ImAA	–	–	–	–	–	–
N^{τ}-MeImAA	–	–	–	–	–	–
N^{π}-MeImAA	–	–	–	–	–	–
PAA	–	–	49	49	49	49
oHPA	–	–	–	–	–	–
mHPA	63	–	–	–	–	–
pHPA	63	–	–	–	–	–
IAA	–	–	–	–	–	–
oHMA	–	–	–	–	–	–
mHMA	–	–	–	–	–	–
pHMA	–	–	–	–	–	–
MA	–	–	–	–	–	–
5HIAA	143	–	–	–	144	–
HVA	156	–	–	–	158	–
VMA	186	–	–	–	–	–
DOPAC	190	–	–	–	194	–
DOMA	–	–	–	–	–	–
DMPAA	–	–	–	–	–	–
5MeO-IAA	–	–	–	–	–	–

ACIDS

<u>Alzheimer's Disease - Table No.</u>

Acids	Urine		Plasma		CSF	
	Unconjugated	Conjugated	Unconjugated	Conjugated	Unconjugated	Conjugated
ImAA	-	-	-	-	-	-
N^{τ}-MeImAA	-	-	-	-	-	-
N^{π}-MeImAA	-	-	-	-	-	-
PAA	-	-	-	-	-	-
oHPA	-	-	-	-	-	-
mHPA	-	-	-	-	-	-
pHPA	-	-	-	-	-	-
IAA	-	-	-	-	-	-
oHMA	-	-	-	-	-	-
mHMA	-	-	-	-	-	-
pHMA	-	-	-	-	-	-
MA	-	-	-	-	-	-
5HIAA	-	-	-	-	145	-
HVA	-	-	-	-	159	-
VMA	-	-	-	-	186	-
DOPAC	-	-	-	-	194	-
DOMA	-	-	-	-	-	-
DMPAA	-	-	-	-	-	-
5MeO-IAA	-	-	-	-	-	-

ACIDS

<u>Aggression and Suicide Attempts – Table No.</u>

Acids	Urine		Plasma		CSF	
	Unconjugated	Conjugated	Unconjugated	Conjugated	Unconjugated	Conjugated
ImAA	–	–	–	–	–	–
N^τ-MeImAA	–	–	–	–	–	–
N^π-MeImAA	–	–	–	–	–	–
PAA	–	–	50	51	–	–
oHPA	–	–	–	–	–	–
mHPA	–	–	57	57	–	–
pHPA	–	–	64	64	–	–
IAA	–	–	71	–	–	–
oHMA	–	–	–	–	–	–
mHMA	–	–	–	–	–	–
pHMA	–	–	74	–	–	–
MA	–	–	–	–	–	–
5HIAA	–	–	–	–	146	–
HVA	–	–	157	–	160	–
VMA	–	–	186	–	–	–
DOPAC	–	–	–	–	194	–
DOMA	–	–	–	–	–	–
DMPAA	–	–	–	–	–	–
5MeO-IAA	–	–	–	–	–	–

ALCOHOLS

<u>Normals - Table No.</u>

Alcohols and Glycols	Urine		Plasma		CSF	
	Unconjugated	Conjugated	Unconjugated	Conjugated	Unconjugated	Conjugated
PEG	72	-	-	-	-	-
PHPE	72	72	-	-	75	-
PHPG	72	72	-	-	-	-
MHPE	195	195	-	-	200	200
MHPG	161	162	163	164	165	166
DHPE	196	-	198	-	201	-
DHPG	196	196	199	199	201	201
5-OH-TRP-OH	-	-	-	-	207	-

<u>Parkinson's Disease - Table No.</u>

Alcohols and Glycols	Urine		Plasma		CSF	
	Unconjugated	Conjugated	Unconjugated	Conjugated	Unconjugated	Conjugated
PEG	-	-	-	-	-	-
PHPE	-	-	-	-	-	-
PHPG	-	-	-	-	-	-
MHPE	-	-	-	-	200	200
MHPG	-	176	-	-	177	177
DHPE	-	-	-	-	-	-
DHPG	-	-	-	-	-	-
5-OH-TRP-OH	-	-	-	-	-	-

ALCOHOLS

<u>Depression - Table No.</u>

Alcohols and Glycols	Urine		Plasma		CSF	
	Unconjugated	Conjugated	Unconjugated	Conjugated	Unconjugated	Conjugated
PEG	−	−	−	−	−	−
PHPE	−	−	−	−	−	−
PHPG	−	−	−	−	−	−
MHPE	−	−	−	−	−	−
MHPG	167	168	169	170	171	172
DHPE	−	−	−	−	−	−
DHPG	−	196	197	197	−	−
5-OH-TRP-OH	−	−	−	−	−	−

<u>Alzheimer's Disease - Table No.</u>

Alcohols and Glycols	Urine		Plasma		CSF	
	Unconjugated	Conjugated	Unconjugated	Conjugated	Unconjugated	Conjugated
PEG	−	−	−	−	−	−
PHPE	−	−	−	−	−	−
PHPG	−	−	−	−	−	−
MHPE	−	−	−	−	200	−
MHPG	−	−	176	−	178	178
DHPE	−	−	−	−	−	−
DHPG	−	−	−	−	−	−
5-OH-TRP-OH	−	−	−	−	−	−

ALCOHOLS

Schizophrenics - Table No.

Alcohols and Glycols	Urine		Plasma		CSF	
	Unconjugated	Conjugated	Unconjugated	Conjugated	Unconjugated	Conjugated
PEG	-	-	-	-	-	-
PHPE	-	-	-	-	-	-
PHPG	-	-	-	-	-	-
MHPE	-	-	-	-	200	-
MHPG	-	173	174	-	175	175
DHPE	-	-	-	-	-	-
DHPG	-	-	-	-	-	-
5-OH-TRP-OH	-	-	-	-	-	-

Aggression (including suicide attempts) - Table No.

Alcohols and Glycols	Urine		Plasma		CSF	
	Unconjugated	Conjugated	Unconjugated	Conjugated	Unconjugated	Conjugated
PEG	-	-	-	-	-	-
PHPE	-	-	-	-	-	-
PHPG	-	-	-	-	-	-
MHPE	-	-	-	-	-	-
MHPG	-	-	-	-	179	-
DHPE	-	-	-	-	-	-
DHPG	-	-	-	-	-	-
5-OH-TRP-OH	-	-	-	-	-	-

Section 3

Histamine and Metabolites

Tables 1 to 10

Table 1. Unconjugated Histamine in Urine of Normal Subjects

Reference First Author, Year	Number of Subjects	Method of Analysis	Values (μg/24h ± S.E.M.)
703. Roberts, 1950	5	Bio-assay[†]	21.6 ± 2.3
578. Mitchell, 1954	5	Bio-assay	14.8 ± 2.4
243. Dunér, 1956	17	Bio-assay[†]	11.9 ± 0.8
242. Dunér, 1961	4	Fl[†]	6.4 – 19
622. Oates, 1962	15 (M) 9 (F)	Fl[†] Fl[†]	42 49
65. Beall, 1965	15	Fl[†]	46.4 ± 4.5
288. Fram, 1965	10	GC, Fl[†]	34.4 ± 4.4
318. Gilbert, 1966	19	Fl	42
795. Sjaastad, 1966	53 32 (M) 21 (F)	Bio-assay[†] Bio-assay Bio-assay	12.6 ± 0.9 14.3 ± 1.7 11.5 ± 1.0
871. Turnbull, 1971	21	–	4.6 ± 0.5
66. Beaven, 1972	16	REA[†]	16 ± 3.7
121. Bruce, 1976	16	REA[†]	23.8 ± 4.5
388. Horakova, 1977	31	REA	19 ± 2
601. Myers, 1981	41	Fl[†]	14 ± 1.4
869. Tsuruta, 1981	18	HPLC–Fl[†]	50.0 ± 6.6
466. Khandelwal, 1982	9	REA[†]	20.2 ± 4.7 μg/g Cr.
462. Keyzer, 1983	10	GC–MS[†]	35.6
951. Wollin, 1985	12 (M) 19 (F)	GC–ECD[†] GC–ECD	33.3 μg/L 44.4 μg/L

Table 2. Conjugated Histamine in Urine of Normal Subjects

Reference First Author, Year	Number of Subjects	Method of Analysis	Values (μg/24h $\pm$ S.E.M.)
703. Roberts, 1950	5	Bio-assay[†]	124.8 $\pm$ 38.5
578. Mitchell, 1954	5	Bio-assay	177.4 $\pm$ 101.5
243. Dunér, 1956	17	Bio-assay[†]	22.0 $\pm$ 3.1
242. Dunér, 1961	4	Fl[†]	6 – 32
795. Sjaastad, 1966	37	Bio-assay[†]	30.0 $\pm$ 5.9

Table 3. Unconjugated N^τ-Methylhistamine in Urine of Normal Subjects

Reference First Author, Year	Number of Subjects	Method of Analysis	Values (μg/24h $\pm$ S.E.M.)
288. Fram, 1965	10	GC, Fl[†]	308 $\pm$ 34
465. Keyzer, 1981	20	GC-MS	60 – 280
869. Tsuruta, 1981	18	HPLC-Fl[†]	258 $\pm$ 21
466. Khandelwal, 1982	9	GC-MS[†]	118 $\pm$ 25 μg/g Cr.
951. Wollin, 1985	12 (M)	GC-ECD[†]	250 μg/L
	19 (F)	GC-ECD	163 μg/L

Table 4. Unconjugated Histamine in Plasma of Normal Subjects

Reference First Author, Year	Number of Subjects	Method of Analysis	Values (pg/mL ± S.E.M.)
618. Noah, 1963	10	Fl[†]	2090
302. Garden, 1966	18	Fl	5400 ± 120
345. Graham, 1968	46	Fl[†]	620 ± 44
574. Miller, 1970	11	REA[†]	610 ± 60
66. Beaven, 1972	7	REA[†]	<500
121. Bruce, 1976	29	REA[†]	444 ± 70
388. Horakova, 1977	31	REA	<1000
868. Tsuruta, 1978	10	HPLC-Fl[†]	610 ± 50
776. Shaff, 1979	13	REA[†]	1000 ± 300 (serum)
	19	REA	600 ± 100 (plasma)
120. Brown, 1980	17	REA[†]	377 ± 78
577. Mita, 1980	5	GC-MS[†]	830 ± 165
350. Guilloux, 1981	50	REA[†]	770 ± 86
	20 (M)	REA	790 ± 180
	30 (F)	REA	760 ± 82
63. Barnes, 1982	26	REA	269 ± 19
246. Dyer, 1982	51	REA[†]	318 ± 25
466. Khandelwal, 1982	5	REA[†]	4350 ±2240
404. Ind, 1983	31	REA	210 ± 20
893. Verburg, 1983	8	REA[†]	303 ± 29
464. Keyzer, 1984	7	GC-MS[†]	311 ± 54 (plasma)
	7	GC-MS	1210 ± 214 (serum)
	25	GC-MS	230 ± 17 (plasma)
26. Arakawa, 1986	5	HPLC-Fl[†]	900 ± 223
367. Harsing, 1986	88	HPLC-EC[†]	800 ± 31

Table 5.   Unconjugated N^τ-Methylhistamine in Plasma of Normal Subjects

Reference First Author, Year	Number of Subjects	Method of Analysis	Values (pg/mL ± S.E.M.)
577. Mita, 1980	5	GC-MS[†]	400
465. Keyzer, 1981	10	GC-MS	1400 ± 125
466. Khandelwal, 1982	5	GC-MS[†]	1675 ± 250

Table 6.   Unconjugated Histamine and N^τ-Methylhistamine in CSF of Normal

Subjects

Reference First Author, Year	Number of Subjects	Method of Analysis	Values (ng/mL ± S.E.M.)
840. Swahn, 1981	5	GC-MS[†]	2.0 ± 0.1 (N^τ-MeH)
466. Khandelwal, 1982	11	REA[†]	43.1 ± 5.7 (H)
	45 (pooled)	GC-MS	0.28± 0.06 (N^τ-MeH)

Table 7.   Unconjugated Imidazoleacetic Acid in Urine of Normal Subjects

Reference First Author, Year	Number of Subjects	Method of Analysis	Values (mg/24h ± S.E.M.)
242. Dunér, 1961	4	Fl[†]	0.3 - 3.4
268. Evans, 1973	4	GC-FID[†]	14.7 ± 3.4
403. Imamura, 1984	10	REA[†]	1.16± 0.05*
	10	REA	3.30± 0.22* (conj.)
468. Khandelwal, 1985	4	GC-MS[†]	1.01± 0.09 mg/g Cr.
870. Tsuruta, 1987	10	HPLC-Fl[†]	2.04± 0.39

* Originally expressed as nmol/min.

Table 8.   Unconjugated Methylimidazoleacetic Acid in Urine of Normal Subjects

Reference First Author, Year	Number of Subjects	Method of Analysis	Values (mg/24h ± S.E.M.)
859. Tham, 1966	34	GC-FID[†]	2.65 ± 0.19
459. Kelvin, 1970	11	GC-FID	2.45 ± 0.2 (N^τ)
	11	GC-FID	2.53 ± 0.32 (N^π)
871. Turnbull, 1971	21	–	2.72 ± 0.20 (N^τ)
	21	–	2.00 ± 0.27 (N^τ)
463. Keyzer, 1982	20	GC-N[†]	1.85 (N^τ)
467. Khandelwal, 1982	9	GC-MS[†]	2.91 ± 0.18 mg/g Cr. (N^τ)
	9	GC-MS	10.22 ± 5.35 mg/g Cr. (N^π)
870. Tsuruta, 1987	10	HPLC-Fl[†]	2.48 ± 0.35 (N^τ)
	10	HPLC-Fl	2.06 ± 0.51 (N^π)

Table 9. Unconjugated Methylimidazoleacetic and Imidazoleacetic Acid in
Plasma of Normal Subjects

Reference First Author, Year	Number of Subjects	Method of Analysis	Values (ng/mL ± S.E.M.)
467. Khandelwal, 1982	5	GC-MS†	11.84 ± 1.90 (N^τ)
	5	GC-MS	10.30 ± 2.03 (N^π)
841. Swahn, 1983	1	GC-MS†	10.80 (N^τ-Me)
403. Imamura, 1984	10	REA†	277 ± 13 (ImAA)
	10	REA†	25 ± 3 (Conj.ImAA)

Table 10. Unconjugated Methylimidazoleacetic Acid in CSF of Normal

Subjects

Reference First Author, Year	Number of Subjects	Method of Analysis	Values (ng/mL ± S.E.M.)
467. Khandelwal, 1982	10	GC-MS†	3.19 ± 0.29 (N^τ)
	10	GC-MS	11.31 ± 2.65 (N^π)
841. Swahn, 1983	5	GC-MS†	0.14 ± 0.09 (N^τ)
	5	GC-MS	0.82 ± 0.22*

* Schizophrenics.

Section 4

Trace Amines

Tables 11 to 36

Table 11.   Unconjugated Phenylethylamine in Urine of Normal Subjects

Reference First Author, Year	Number of Subjects	Method of Analysis	Values (mg/24h ± S.E.M.)
411. Jepson, 1960	–	Fl	<20
515. Levine, 1964	7	GC	285 ± 14*
279. Fischer, 1968	11	Fl	33.5 mg/L
102. Boulton, 1971	19	Fl[†]	47 ± 10
282. Fischer, 1972	17	Fl[†]	336 ± 45
817. Spatz, 1972	10	Fl[†]	239 ± 26
281. Fischer, 1973	13	GC-FID[†]	400 ±105
371. Heller, 1973	15	Fl	147 ± 9
393. Inwang, 1973	5	Fl	292 ± 45 mg/L
589. Mosnaim, 1973	27	Fl[†]	453 ± 50
764. Schweitzer, 1975	18	GC-ECD[†]	10.3 ± 4.4
693. Reynolds, 1976	12	GC-FID[†]	6.8 ± 0.8
805. Slingsby, 1976	15	MS-SIM[†]	4.9 ± 1.0
15. Anderson, 1977	10 10	GC-MS[†] GC-ECD[†]	8.0 ± 0.3 774 ± 38
838. Suzuki, 1977	9	Fl	15.9 ± 2.1
695. Reynolds, 1978	12	GC-MS	7.4 ± 0.6 mg/g Cr.
92. Blau, 1979	8	GC-ECD[†]	4.1 ± 0.8
396. Huebert, 1979	1 subject (30 times, longitudinal)	MS-SIM[†]	3.2 ± 0.2
449. Karoum, 1979	15	GC-MS	7.1 ± 0.5
674. Potkin, 1979	32	GC-MS	8.0 ± 2.0
744. Sandler, 1979	26 10 (M) 16 (F)	GC-ECD GC-ECD GC-ECD	4.84± 0.57 4.68± 0.70 4.95± 0.82
413. Jeste, 1980	19	GC-MS	4.1 ± 0.5

Table 11. Unconjugated Phenylethylamine in Urine of Normal Subjects
(continued)

Reference First Author, Year	Number of Subjects	Method of Analysis	Values (mg/24h ± S.E.M.)
451. Karoum, 1980	23	GC-MS	5.3 ± 0.5
676. Potkin, 1980	23	GC-MS	5.6
176. Coutts, 1981	12	GC-ECD[†]	22 ± 6
607. Narasimhachari, 1981	4	GC-N[†]	45 – 80
387. Hopkinson, 1982	15	GC-ECD	14.4 mg/g Cr.
441. Karoum, 1982	5	GC-MS[†]	3.0 ± 0.8
837. Suzuki, 1983	19	GC-MS[†]	15.3 ± 1.9
911. Waldmeier, 1983	17	GC-MS[†]	57.1 ± 9.4 mg/g Cr.
511. Lauber, 1984	20	GC-MS[†]	35 ± 5 mg/g Cr.
366. Harris, 1985	10	MS-SIM[†]	13.0 ± 3.3**
49. Baker, 1986	12	GC-ECD[†]	3.40± 0.35 mg/g Cr.
867. Tsuji, 1986	14 (M) 20 (F)	HPLC-Fl[†] HPLC-Fl	7.3 ± 2.9 mg/g Cr. 14.5 ± 3.1 mg/g Cr.
209. Davis, 1987	8	MS-SIM[†]	1.4 ± 0.5
965. Yoshimoto, 1987	24	GC-MS[†]	6.5 ± 3.7
308. Gashkoff, 1988	8	GC-MS[†]	2.85± 0.39 mg/g Cr.

* Originally expressed as mg/8h; ** originally expressed as ng/min.

Table 12. Conjugated Phenylethylamine in Urine of Normal Subjects

Reference First Author, Year	Number of Subjects	Method of Analysis	Values (mg/24h ± S.E.M.)
102. Boulton, 1971	19	Fl[†]	34 - 365
393. Inwang, 1973	5	Fl	276 ± 78 mg/L
589. Mosnaim, 1973	27	Fl[†]	433 ± 47
693. Reynolds, 1976	12	GC-FID[†]	20.9 ± 7.5
695. Reynolds, 1978	12	GC-MS	21.1 ± 6.4 mg/g Cr.
396. Huebert, 1979	1 (longitudinal)	MS-SIM[†]	6.8 ± 0.6
366. Harris, 1985	10	MS-SIM[†]	16.3 ± 5.5*
209. Davis, 1987	8	MS-SIM[†]	24.4 ±10.4

* In original paper expressed as ng/min.

Table 13. Unconjugated Phenylethylamine in Plasma of Normal Subjects

Reference First Author, Year	Number of Subjects	Method of Analysis	Values (pg/mL ± S.E.M.)
449. Karoum, 1979	15	GC-MS	640 ± 50
694. Reynolds, 1980	5	GC-MS	210 ± 18
607. Narasimhachari, 1981	4	GC-N[†]	500 - 2500
867. Tsuji, 1986	8 (M)	HPLC-Fl[†]	4270 ± 430
	11 (F)	HPLC-Fl	5560 ± 750
848. Szymanski, 1987	14	GC-MS	93 ± 30

Table 14. Unconjugated Phenylethylamine in the CSF of Normal Subjects

Reference First Author, Year	Number of Subjects	Method of Analysis	Values (pg/mL ± S.E.M.)
449. Karoum, 1979	15	GC-MS	600 ± 100
607. Narasimhachari, 1981	4	GC-N[†]	300 – 1000
511. Lauber, 1984	15	GC-MS[†]	17300 ± 3300

Table 15. Unconjugated Phenylethylamine in Urine of Depressed Subjects

Reference First Author, Year	Number of Subjects	Method of Analysis	Values (mg/24h ± S.E.M.)
279. Fischer, 1968	12	Fl	n.d.
102. Boulton, 1971	20	Fl[†]	n.d. (<5)
282. Fischer, 1972	14 (endogenous)	Fl[†]	114 ± 13
	4 (manic)	Fl	1047 ± 180
	6 (atypical)	Fl	643 ± 53
281. Fischer, 1973	30 (endogenous)	GC-FID[†]	57 ± 7
	4 (melancholia)	GC-FID	337 ± 132
371. Heller, 1973	15	Fl	18 ± 2
589. Mosnaim, 1973	24 (neurotic)	Fl[†]	352 ± 85
	24	Fl	270 ± 83 (conj.)
744. Sandler, 1979	22 (primary)	GC-ECD	5.42 ± 1.00
	10 (M)	GC-ECD	6.24 ± 1.58
	12 (F)	GC-ECD	4.74 ± 0.94
451. Karoum, 1980	17	GC-MS	7.4 ± 0.8
694. Reynolds, 1980	3	GC-ECD	4.0 ± 1.2 mg/g Cr.
441. Karoum, 1982	6	GC-MS[†]	4.4 ± 1.4
527. Linnoila, 1982	12 (unipolar + bipolar)	GC-MS	8.6 ± 1.7
525. Linnoila, 1982	4 (rapid cyclers)	GC-MS	9.6 ± 3.8
524. Linnoila, 1983	12 (unipolar + bipolar)	GC-MS	13.3 ± 5.6
518. Liebowitz, 1985	8 (atypical)	GC-MS	4 ± 1
612. Nazarali, 1987	13 (dysthymic)	GC-ECD[†]	6.3 ± 2.3 mg/g Cr.

Table 16.   Unconjugated Phenylethylamine in Plasma of Depressed Subjects

Reference First Author, Year	Number of Subjects	Method of Analysis	Values (pg/mL ± S.E.M.)
694. Reynolds, 1980	3	GC-MS	120 ± 60
612. Nazarali, 1987	13 (dysthymic)	GC-ECD[†]	930 ± 220

Table 17.   Unconjugated Phenylethylamine in Urine of Schizophrenic

Subjects

Reference First Author, Year	Number of Subjects	Method of Analysis	Values (mg/24h ± S.E.M.)
279. Fischer, 1968	7	Fl	25 - 800 mg/L
282. Fischer, 1972	4	Fl[†]	1485 ± 410
371. Heller, 1973	3	Fl	650 ± 90
764. Schweitzer, 1975	3	GC-ECD[†]	0 - 2.6
838. Suzuki, 1977	5 (chronic)	Fl	9.3 ± 1.2
674. Potkin, 1979	15 (non-paranoid)	GC-MS	7.0 ± 1.5
	16 (paranoid)	GC-MS	19.0 ± 4.0
413. Jeste, 1980	11 (non-paranoid)	GC-MS	5.0 ± 1.5
	39 (paranoid)	GC-MS	8.3 ± 1.4
451. Karoum, 1980	11 (non-paranoid)	GC-MS	7.9 ± 2.4
	12 (paranoid)	GC-MS	17.4 ± 5.5
676. Potkin, 1980	23 (chronic, all)	GC-MS	13.1
	12 (non-paranoid)	GC-MS	8.6
	11 (paranoid)	GC-MS	18.1
965. Yoshimoto, 1987	25 (non-paranoid)	GC-MS[†]	10.2 ± 2.6
	23 (paranoid)	GC-MS[†]	16.6 ± 3.8

Table 18. Unconjugated Phenylethylamine in Plasma and CSF of

Schizophrenics

Reference First Author, Year	Number of Subjects	Method of Analysis	Values (pg/mL ± S.E.M.)
69. Beckman, 1982	15 (paranoid)	GC–MS	45900 ± 2480 (CSF)
72. Beckman, 1983	9	GC–MS	35500 ± 6700 (CSF)
848. Szymanski, 1987	14 (paranoid)	GC–MS	74 ± 24 (plasma)

Table 19. Unconjugated Phenylethylamine in Urine of Parkinson's

Patients

Reference First Author, Year	Number of Subjects	Method of Analysis	Values (mg/24h ± S.E.M.)
371. Heller, 1973	4	Fl	14 ± 2.2
441. Karoum, 1982	5	GC–MS[†]	3.4 ± 1.0

Table 20. Unconjugated and Conjugated m-Tyramine in Urine of Normal Subjects

Reference First Author, Year	Number of Subjects	Method of Analysis	Values (mg/24h ± S.E.M.)
411. Jepson, 1960	-	Fl	just detectable
647. Perry, 1966	2	Fl	40 ± 8 mg/g Cr.
	2	Fl	680 ±170 mg/g Cr.(conj.)
469. King, 1974	2	GC-MS	20
805. Slingsby, 1976	19	MS-SIM[†]	83 ± 7
396. Huebert, 1979	1 (longitudinal)	MS-SIM[†]	98 ± 2
	1	MS-SIM	106 ± 19 (conjugated)
449. Karoum, 1979	15	GC-MS	86.5 ± 8.4
451. Karoum, 1980	23	GC-MS	54.2 ± 6.3
176. Coutts, 1981	12	GC-ECD[†]	101 ± 12
387. Hopkinson, 1982	15	GC-ECD	76.0 mg/g Cr.
441. Karoum, 1982	5	GC-MS[†]	85 ± 14
366. Harris, 1985	10	MS-SIM[†]	122 ± 18* 57.9 ± 13.0 (conjugated)
209. Davis, 1987	8	MS-SIM[†]	84.4 ± 16.9
	8	MS-SIM	127.9 ± 15.1 (conjugated)

* In original paper expressed as ng/min.

Table 21. Unconjugated m-Tyramine in Urine of Some Mental Disorders

Reference First Author, Year	Number of Subjects	Method of Analysis	Values (mg/24h ± S.E.M.)
103. Boulton, 1967	1 (schizophrenic)	Fl	9.1 mg/g Cr.
	1 (Parkinson's disease)	Fl	25 mg/g Cr.
451. Karoum, 1980	11 (non-paranoid schizophrenics)	GC-MS	49.8 ± 9.6
	12 (paranoid schizophrenics)	GC-MS	37.8 ± 11.6
	17 (depressed)	GC-MS	30.6 ± 4.6
441. Karoum, 1982	5 (Parkinson's disease)	GC-MS[†]	62 ± 16
	6 (depressed)	GC-MS	101 ± 18

Table 22. Unconjugated m-Tyramine in Plasma of Normal Subjects

Reference First Author, Year	Number of Subjects	Method of Analysis	Values (pg/mL ± S.E.M.)
451. Karoum, 1980	10	GC-MS	540 ± 150

Table 23. Unconjugated p-Tyramine in Urine of Normal Subjects

Reference First Author, Year	Number of Subjects	Method of Analysis	Values (mg/24h ± S.E.M.)
796. Sjoerdsma, 1959	4	Fl	316 ± 25
515. Levine, 1964	7	Fl	532 ± 178
647. Perry, 1966	2	Fl	255 ± 110 mg/g Cr.
99. Boulton, 1967	2	Fl	630 ± 75
903. Vogel, 1967	12	Fl	593 ± 55
809. Smith, 1969	15	Fl	554 ± 12
811. Smith, 1971	8	Fl	800 ± 140
967. Youdim, 1971	12	Fl	1128 ± 184*
101. Boulton, 1972	31	Fl	312 ± 29 mg/g Cr.
810. Smith, 1972	9	Fl[†]	1000 ± 171
469. King, 1974	2	GC-MS	1000
806. Slingsby, 1976	21	MS-SIM[†]	489 ± 40
396. Huebert, 1979	1 (longitudinal, 28 days)	MS-SIM[†]	427 ± 12
449. Karoum, 1979	15	GC-MS	608 ± 90
451. Karoum, 1980	23	GC-MS	377 ± 56
176. Coutts, 1981	12	GC-ECD[†]	506 ± 42
387. Hopkinson, 1982	15	GC-ECD	377 mg/g Cr.
441. Karoum, 1982	5	GC-MS[†]	991 ± 204
911. Waldmeier, 1983	5	HPLC-EC[†]	3403 ± 589 mg/g Cr.
366. Harris, 1985	10	MS-SIM[†]	595 ± 74**
722. Roy, 1986	25	GC-MS	425 ± 30
209. Davis, 1987	8	MS-SIM[†]	348 ± 45

* Values expressed in original paper in mg/3h; ** as ng/min.

Table 24.   Conjugated p-Tyramine in Urine of Normal Subjects

Reference First Author, Year	Number of Subjects	Method of Analysis	Values (mg/24h ± S.E.M.)
647. Perry, 1966	2	Fl	4110 ± 280 mg/g Cr.
99. Boulton, 1967	2	Fl	584 ± 362
811. Smith, 1971	8	Fl	2200 ± 670
967. Youdim, 1971	12	Fl	3260 ± 140
810. Smith, 1972	8	Fl[†]	2150 ± 680
396. Huebert, 1979	1 (longitudinal)	MS-SIM[†]	571 ± 142
366. Harris, 1985	10	MS-SIM[†]	343 ± 96*
209. Davis, 1987	8	MS-SIM[†]	557 ± 125

* Values expressed in original paper in mg/3h.

Table 25.   Unconjugated p-Tyramine in Plasma and CSF of Normal Subjects

Reference First Author, Year	Number of Subjects	Method of Analysis	Values (pg/mL ± S.E.M.)
449. Karoum, 1979	15 15	GC-MS GC-MS	680 ± 90 (plasma) 790 ± 250 (CSF)
139. Causon, 1984	3	HPLC-EC[†]	0-3000 (plasma)

Table 26.   p-Tyramine in Urine of Schizophrenic Subjects

Reference First Author, Year	Number of Subjects	Method of Analysis	Values (mg/24h ± S.E.M.)
103. Boulton, 1967	1	Fl	1170 mg/g Cr.
903. Vogel, 1967	28	Fl	496 ± 27
451. Karoum, 1980	11 (non-paranoid)	GC-MS	310 ± 68
	12 (paranoid)	GC-MS	603 ± 287

Table 27.   p-Tyramine in Urine of Depressed Subjects

Reference First Author, Year	Number of Subjects	Method of Analysis	Values (mg/24h ± S.E.M.)
279. Fischer, 1968	4 (endogenous)	Fl	20 - 32 mg/L
451. Karoum, 1980	17	GC-MS	336 ± 30
441. Karoum, 1982	6	GC-MS[†]	686 ± 117
527. Linnoila, 1982	12 (unipolar + bipolar)	GC-MS	969 ± 71
525. Linnoila, 1982	4 (bipolar)	GC-MS	1154 ± 244
724. Roy, 1986	21 (unipolar)	GC-MS	423 ± 39

Table 28. p-Tyramine in Urine of Parkinson's Subjects

Reference First Author, Year	Number of Subjects	Method of Analysis	Values (mg/24h ± S.E.M.)
103. Boulton, 1967	1	Fl	2010 mg/g Cr.
99. Boulton, 1967	1	Fl	452
	1	Fl	1082 (conj.)
809. Smith, 1969	19	Fl	688 ± 10
	8 (severe)	Fl	804 ± 16
	11 (mild)	Fl	604 ± 11
101. Boulton, 1972	28	Fl	500 ± 130 mg/g Cr.

Table 29. Tryptamine in Urine of Normal Subjects

Reference First Author, Year	Number of Subjects	Method of Analysis	Values (mg/24h ± S.E.M.)
709. Rodnight, 1956	6	Fl[†]	61.7 ± 11.1
797. Sjoerdsma, 1959	10	Fl[†]	79
796. Sjoerdsma, 1959	4	Fl	68.3 ± 10.7
710. Rodnight, 1961	19	Fl	61
	13 (M)	Fl	64
	6 (F)	Fl	56
647. Perry, 1966	2	Fl	10.1 ± 5.6
	2	Fl	155 ± 78 (conj.)
33. Arterberry, 1967	23	Fl[†]	169 ± 27*
809. Smith, 1969	15	Fl	83.1 ± 2
101. Boulton, 1972	16	Fl	83 ± 36 mg/g Cr.
679. Prange, 1972	10	Fl	156 ± 28
821. Stachow, 1974	14	Fl	104
805. Slingsby, 1976	18	MS-SIM[†]	100 ± 13
305. Garfinkel, 1977	10	GC-MS	105.0 ± 10.7
304. Garfinkel, 1979	10	GC-MS	103.0 ± 25.7
396. Huebert, 1979	1 (longitudinal)	MS-SIM[†]	79.4 ± 2.8
833. Sullivan, 1980	20	Fl[†]	61.2 ± 3.7
176. Coutts, 1981	12	GC-ECD[†]	96 ± 65
607. Narasimhachari, 1981	4	GC-N[†]	30 - 100
387. Hopkinson, 1982	15	GC-ECD	66.1 mg/g Cr.
366. Harris, 1985	10	MS-SIM[†]	88.8 ± 18.3*
209. Davis, 1987	8	MS-SIM[†]	66.7 ± 11.8

* In original paper expressed as ng/min.

Table 30. Tryptamine in Plasma and CSF of Normal Subjects

Reference First Author, Year	Number of Subjects	Method of Analysis	Values (pg/mL ± S.E.M.)
291. Franzen, 1965	–	–	5000-20000
607. Narasimhachari, 1981	4 4	GC-N[†] GC-N	n.d. (plasma) 1000-6000 (CSF)

Table 31. Tryptamine in Urine of Parkinson's Patients

Reference First Author, Year	Number of Subjects	Method of Analysis	Values (mg/24h ± S.E.M.)
809. Smith, 1969	19	Fl	109 ± 11
123. Brune, 1971	5	Fl	64 ± 17
101. Boulton, 1972	27	Fl	72 ± 8 mg/g Cr.

<u>Table 32.   Tryptamine in Urine of Schizophrenic Subjects</u>

Reference <u>First Author, Year</u>	Number of <u>Subjects</u>	Method of <u>Analysis</u>	<u>Values (mg/24h ± S.E.M.)</u>
710. Rodnight, 1961	17	Fl	62
	9 (M)	Fl	52
	8 (F)	Fl	72
122. Brune, 1962	17 (inactive)	Chemical assay	91.6
	12 (slightly active)	" "	124.9
	7 (moderate)	" "	151.2
	6 (active)	" "	202.8
	2 (markedly active)	" "	382.5
	44 (all)	" "	118
76. Berlet, 1964	–	–	45–182
503. La Brosse, 1964	9	Fl	258.9 ± 22.1
374. Herkert, 1969	10	Fl	113 ± 14
833. Sullivan, 1980	20 (low MAO)	Fl[†]	107.4 ± 1.7
	20 (normal MAO)	Fl	60.1 ± 3.0

Table 33. Tryptamine in Urine of Depressed Subjects

Reference First Author, Year	Number of Subjects	Method of Analysis	Values (mg/24h ± S.E.M.)
710. Rodnight, 1961	18	Fl	34
	8 (M)	Fl	39
	10 (F)	Fl	30
174. Coppen, 1965	13 (depressed)	Fl	39.2 ± 3.5
	13 (recovered)	Fl	66.6 ± 6.3
279. Fischer, 1968	4 (endogenous)	Fl	54–60 mg/L
564. McNamee, 1972	16 (all depressed)	Fl[†]	100.4 ± 11.4
	7 (psychotic)	Fl	102.6 ± 16.3
	9 (neurotic)	Fl	98.9 ± 16.0
	16 (recovered)	Fl	70.5 ± 7.3
679. Prange, 1972	12 (primary)	Fl	140 ± 35
305. Garfinkel, 1977	8 (bipolar)	GC–MS	131.8 ± 42.0
304. Garfinkel, 1979	7 (unipolar)	GC–MS	81.0 ± 28.7
	11 (bipolar)	GC–MS	93.8 ± 8.7

Table 34. p-Octopamine in Urine of Normal Subjects

Reference First Author, Year	Number of Subjects	Method of Analysis	Values (mg/24h ± S.E.M.)
283. Fischer, 1971	11	REA	1.07± 0.27
509. Lam, 1973	23	REA	0.17± 0.01*
552. Manghani, 1975	17	REA[†]	56.4 ± 7.0
51. Baldessarini, 1977	11	–	1.1 ± 0.3
245. Durden, 1978	4	MS-SIM[†]	3.7 ± 0.6**
399. Ibrahim, 1984	10	GC-MS[†]	0.6 ± 0.1 (ortho) mg/g Cr.
	10	GC-MS	2.1 ± 0.3 (meta) mg/g Cr.
	10	GC-MS	25 ± 6 (para) mg/g Cr.

* In original paper expressed as ng/h; ** includes meta isomer.

Table 35. p-Octopamine in Plasma of Normal Subjects

Reference First Author, Year	Number of Subjects	Method of Analysis	Values (pg/mL ± S.E.M.)
509. Lam, 1973	22	REA	18000 ± 200 (serum)
552. Manghani, 1975	17	REA[†]	4600 ± 700 (serum)
717. Rossi-Fanelli, 1976	14	REA	400 ± 60
	5 (arterial)	REA	470 ± 140
	5 (venous)	REA	430 ± 100

Table 36. Synephrine in Urine of Normal Subjects

Reference First Author, Year	Number of Subjects	Method of Analysis	Values (mg/24h ± S.E.M.)
664. Pisano, 1961	12	Fl	650
245. Durden, 1978	4	MS-SIM[†]	6.9 ± 0.7
399. Ibrahim, 1984	10	GC-MS[†]	<0.1 (ortho) mg/g Cr.
	10	GC-MS	1.8 ± 0.2 (meta) mg/g Cr.
	10	GC-MS	16 ± 3 (para) mg/g Cr.

Section 5

Trace Acids and Related Alcohols and Glycols

Tables 37 to 75

<u>Table 37.   Unconjugated Phenylacetic Acid in Urine of Normal Subjects</u>

Reference <u>First Author, Year</u>	Number of <u>Subjects</u>	Method of <u>Analysis</u>	<u>Values (mg/24h ± S.E.M.)</u>
335. Goodwin, 1975	–	GC-FID[†]	0.92 ± 0.49 (S.D.)
558. Martin, 1979	24	GC-MS[†]	8.49 ± 0.99
207. Davis, 1981	1 (longitudinal, 28 days)	GC-MS	0.67
450. Karoum, 1984	31	GC-MS	9.8 ± 1.5
366. Harris, 1985	10	GC-MS[†]	3.3 ± 0.4*
211. Davis, 1986	10	GC-MS[†]	1.7
209. Davis, 1987	8	GC-MS[†]	10.3 ± 6.3

* In original paper expressed as µg/min.

Table 38. Conjugated Phenylacetic Acid in Urine of Normal Subjects

Reference First Author, Year	Number of Subjects	Method of Analysis	Values (mg/24h ± S.E.M.)
766. Seakins, 1971	8	GC-FID[†]	159.3 ± 33.7 (total)
335. Goodwin, 1975	–	GC-FID[†]	118 ± 31
558. Martin, 1979	24	GC-MS[†]	128.8 ± 15.0
744. Sandler, 1979	10 (M) 17 (F) 27	GC-FID GC-FID GC-FID	121.9 ± 18.0 (total) 119.8 ± 20.9 (total) 119.8 ± 15.0 (total)
676. Potkin, 1980	23	GC-MS	156.2 (total)
207. Davis, 1981	1 (longitudinal study)	GC-MS	96.4
441. Karoum, 1982	5	GC-MS[†]	90 ± 9 (total)
733. Sabelli, 1983; 353. Gusovsky, 1984	48	GC-FID	141.1 ± 10.2 (total)
226. De Lisi, 1984	10	GC-MS	166.8 ± 25.6 (total)
450. Karoum, 1984	31	GC-MS	150 ± 19
646. Pennings, 1985	35	HPLC-Fl[†]	168.0 ± 18.8 (total)
207. Davis, 1987	8	GC-MS[†]	106.8 ± 23.2
965. Yoshimoto, 1987	22 15 (F) 32 (M)	GC-MS[†] GC-MS GC-MS	141.0 ± 16.0 (total) 160.9 ± 26.3 (total) 138.1 ± 10.4 (total)
64. Baxter, 1988	21 (M) (F)	GC-FID[†] GC-FID GC-FID	142.0 ± 16.5 (total) 129.0 156.6
333. Gonzalez-Sastre, 1988	32	GC-FID	153 ± 9 (total)
952. Wong, 1988	20	GC-ECD[†]	86.5 ± 14.1 (total)

Table 39.   Unconjugated Phenylacetic Acid in Plasma of Normal Subjects

Reference First Author, Year	Number of Subjects	Method of Analysis	Values (ng/mL ± S.E.M.)
276. Fellows, 1978	21	GC-MS[†]	108 ± 14
741. Sandler, 1978	10 (prisoners)	GC-MS	107.2 ± 10.7
210. Davis, 1982	28 (fasting)	GC-MS[†]	107 ± 12
	14 (not-fasting)	GC-MS	155 ± 22
	12 (M)	GC-MS	79.5 ± 13.5
	7 (F)	GC-MS	119.5 ± 19.1
213. Davis, 1982	14	GC-MS	155.2 ± 21.5
	24 (in institution)	GC-MS	167.7 ± 17.0
743. Sandler, 1982	13 (neurological disorder)	GC-MS	161.8 ± 22.3
100. Boulton, 1983	38 (prisoners)	GC-MS	126.9 ± 9.5
442. Karoum, 1983	10	GC-MS[†]	254 ± 50
972. Yu, 1983	64	GC-MS	132.8 ± 14.3
973. Yu, 1984	10 (prisoners)	GC-MS	124.6
974. Yu, 1985	21 (prisoners)	GC-MS	94.9 ± 9.7
	61 (prisoners)	GC-MS	116.9 ± 13.1
211. Davis, 1986	10	GC-MS[†]	71.4
209. Davis, 1987	14	GC-MS[†]	102.6 ± 13.7

Table 40. Conjugated Phenylacetic Acid in Plasma of Normal Subjects

Reference First Author, Year	Number of Subjects	Method of Analysis	Values (ng/mL ± S.E.M.)
276. Fellows, 1978	21	GC-MS[†]	612 ± 56
741. Sandler, 1978	10 (prisoners)	GC-MS	278.8 ± 40
210. Davis, 1982	28 (fasting)	GC-MS[†]	309 ± 31
	14 (not-fasting)	GC-MS	228 ± 35
	12 (M)	GC-MS	296.4 ± 42.9
	7 (F)	GC-MS	365.6 ± 59.2
213. Davis, 1982	14	GC-MS	228.0 ± 34.1
	24 (in institution)	GC-MS	505.2 ± 43.4
743. Sandler, 1982	13 (neurological disorder)	GC-MS	412.5 ± 68.7
100. Boulton, 1983	38 (prisoners)	GC-MS	361.3 ± 32.4
442. Karoum, 1983	10	GC-MS[†]	205 ± 27
973. Yu, 1984	10 (prisoners)	GC-MS	263.8
974. Yu, 1985	21 (prisoners)	GC-MS	263.5 ± 26.3
	61 (prisoners)	GC-MS	275.5 ± 21.5
209. Davis, 1987	14	GC-MS[†]	132.6 ± 23.7

Table 41. Unconjugated Phenylacetic Acid in the Lumbar CSF of Normal

Subjects

Reference First Author, Year	Number of Subjects	Method of Analysis	Values (ng/mL ± S.E.M.)
276. Fellows, 1978	9 (with lumbar disc lesions)	GC-MS[†]	16.5 ± 2.4
741. Sandler, 1978	14	GC-MS	16.9 ± 2.0
740. Sandler, 1979	30	GC-MS	28.7 ± 2.9
	15 (M)	GC-MS	26.7 ± 2.7
	15 (F)	GC-MS	30.8 ± 5.2
69. Beckman, 1982	15	GC-MS[†]	21.6 ± 3.1
743. Sandler, 1982	13	GC-MS	31.6 ± 6.5
969. Young, 1982	6 (seizures)	GC-MS	7.9 ± 0.7 (lumbar)
	6 (seizures)	GC-MS	10.8 ± 1.6 (cisternal)
442. Karoum, 1983	10	GC-MS[†]	19.7 ± 2.1
309. Gattaz, 1985	16	HPLC-EC	22.2 ± 3.0
457. Kawabata, 1986	18	GC-MS	26.2 ± 3.0

Table 42. Conjugated Phenylacetic Acid in the Lumbar CSF of Normal

Subjects

Reference First Author, Year	Number of Subjects	Method of Analysis	Values (ng/mL ± S.E.M.)
69. Beckman, 1982	15	GC-MS[†]	22.6 ± 5.4
743. Sandler, 1982	13	GC-MS	29.7 ± 4.0
442. Karoum, 1983	10	GC-MS[†]	21.9 ± 2.8
309. Gattaz, 1985	16	HPLC-EC	23.6 ± 5.2

Table 43.   Total Phenylacetic Acid in Urine of Depressed Subjects

Reference First Author, Year	Number of Subjects	Method of Analysis	Values (mg/24h ± S.E.M.)
744. Sandler, 1979	23 (primary)	GC-FID	115.9 ± 12.9
	10 (M)	GC-FID	123.9 ± 9.0
	13 (F)	GC-FID	109.9 ± 19.0
441. Karoum, 1982	6	GC-MS[†]	114 ± 19
733. Sabelli, 1983	18 (unipolar in-patients)	GC-FID	68.6 ± 8.8
	13 (unipolar untreated)	GC-FID	68.8 ± 7.0
	35 (unipolar outpatients, untreated)	GC-FID	86.3 ± 11.8
226. De Lisi, 1984	10 (acute)	GC-MS	84.5 ± 14.6
	21 (chronic)	GC-MS	217.6 ± 37.8
353. Gusovsky, 1984	42	GC-FID[†]	102.8 ± 15.9
450. Karoum, 1984	21 (unipolar)	GC-MS	149.2 ± 17.0
64. Baxter, 1988	33 (unipolar)	GC-FID[†]	144.2 ± 21.5 (total)
	M	GC-FID	164.4
	F	GC-FID	132.0
333. Gonzalez-Sastre, 1988	19 (melancholia)	GC-FID	103 ± 16
	20 (no melancholia)	GC-FID	98 ± 10

Table 44. Unconjugated Phenylacetic Acid in Plasma and CSF of Depressed

Subjects

Reference First Author, Year	Number of Subjects	Method of Analysis	Values (ng/mL ± S.E.M.)
740. Sandler, 1979	24 (primary)	GC-MS	20.8 ± 2.0 (CSF)
	7 (M)	GC-MS	13.8 ± 1.9 (CSF)
	17 (F)	GC-MS	23.6 ± 2.3 (CSF)
972. Yu, 1983	17	GC-MS	82.0 ± 9.7 (plasma)
	29 (agoraphobic)	GC-MS	107.3 ± 2.4 (plasma)
457. Kawabata, 1986	6	GC-MS	14.8 ± 1.9 (CSF)

Table 45. Unconjugated Phenylacetic Acid in Urine of Schizophrenic

Subjects

Reference First Author, Year	Number of Subjects	Method of Analysis	Values (mg/24h ± S.E.M.)
450. Karoum, 1984	23 (chronic)	GC-MS	11.0 ± 2.8
	11 (paranoid)	GC-MS	14 ± 5
	12 (non-paranoid)	GC-MS	8.2 ± 3

Table 46. Conjugated (or Total) Phenylacetic Acid in Urine of

Schizophrenic Subjects

Reference First Author, Year	Number of Subjects	Method of Analysis	Values (mg/24h ± S.E.M.)
676. Potkin, 1980	23 (chronic)	GC-MS	78.6 (T)*
	11 (paranoid)	GC-MS	90.2 (T)
	12 (non-paranoid)	GC-MS	68.9 (T)
450. Karoum, 1984 (chronic)	23	GC-MS	69 ± 8
	11 (paranoid)	GC-MS	83 ± 11
	12 (non-paranoid)	GC-MS	64 ± 18
965. Yoshimoto, 1987	18 (paranoid)	GC-MS[†]	125.1 ± 23.1 (T)
	21 (non-paranoid)	GC-MS	149.7 ± 19.0 (T)

* T = total acid after hydrolysis.

Table 47. Phenylacetic Acid in Plasma of Schizophrenic Subjects

Reference First Author, Year	Number of Subjects	Method of Analysis	Values (ng/mL ± S.E.M.)
213. Davis, 1982	24	GC-MS	174.8 ± 20.2
	18	GC-MS	115.4 ± 12.9
	24	GC-MS	470.6 ± 48.5 (conj.)
	18	GC-MS	360.6 ± 42.5 (conj.)

Table 48. Phenylacetic Acid in CSF of Schizophrenic Subjects

Reference First Author, Year	Number of Subjects	Method of Analysis	Values (ng/mL ± S.E.M.)
742. Sandler, 1978	9	GC-MS	27.2 ± 3.6
69. Beckmann, 1982	13 (paranoid, untreated)	GC-MS[†]	11.6 ± 1.4
	15 (paranoid, treated)	GC-MS	13.5 ± 2.7
	13 (paranoid, untreated)	GC-MS	20.0 ± 5.6 (conj.)
	15 (paranoid, treated)	GC-MS	14.7 ± 2.1 (conj.)
309. Gattaz, 1985	13	HPLC-EC	11.5 ± 1.6
	13	HPLC-EC	20.4 ± 5.5 (conj.)
457. Kawabata, 1986	24	GC-MS	30.1 ± 3.4

Table 49. Phenylacetic Acid in Plasma and CSF of Parkinson's Patients

Reference First Author, Year	Number of Subjects	Method of Analysis	Values (ng/mL ± S.E.M.)
743. Sandler, 1982	6	GC-MS	25.6 ± 6.1 (CSF)
	6	GC-MS	20.2 ± 2.7 (CSF, conj)
	6	GC-MS	105.7 ± 34.5 (plasma)
	6	GC-MS	424.5 ±138.5 (plasma, conj.)

Table 50. Unconjugated Phenylacetic Acid in Plasma of Aggressive Subjects

Reference First Author, Year	Number of Subjects	Method of Analysis	Values (ng/mL ± S.E.M.)
741. Sandler, 1978	10	GC-MS	214.7 ± 40.8
100. Boulton, 1983	35	GC-MS	136.1 ± 18.0
973. Yu, 1984	16	GC-MS	102.6
974. Yu, 1985	82	GC-MS	102.2 ± 10.0
	27	GC-MS	70.6 ± 5.6

Table 51. Conjugated Phenylacetic Acid in Plasma of Aggressive Subjects

Reference First Author, Year	Number of Subjects	Method of Analysis	Values (ng/mL ± S.E.M.)
741. Sandler, 1978	10	GC-MS	446.7 ± 72.3
100. Boulton, 1983	35	GC-MS	270.4 ± 18.3
973. Yu, 1984	16	GC-MS	262.2
974. Yu, 1985	82	GC-MS	246.4 ± 17.5
	27	GC-MS	212.6 ± 19.6

Table 52.   Unconjugated m-Hydroxyphenylacetic Acid in Urine of Normal

Subjects

Reference First Author, Year	Number of Subjects	Method of Analysis	Values (mg/24h ± S.E.M.)
744. Sandler, 1979	27	GC-FID	5.8 ± 0.7
	10 (M)	GC-FID	5.3 ± 1.3
	17 (F)	GC-FID	6.2 ± 0.9
	27	GC-FID	1.0 ± 0.1 (ortho-OH)
	10 (M)	GC-FID	1.3 ± 0.2 (ortho-OH)
	17 (F)	GC-FID	0.8 ± 0.1 (ortho-OH)
451. Karoum, 1980	20	GC-ECD	<1
207. Davis, 1981	1 (longitudinal study)	GC-MS	7.3
366. Harris, 1985	10	GC-MS[†]	10.2 ± 1.6*
211. Davis, 1986	10	GC-MS[†]	5.8
50. Baker, 1987	29	GC-ECD[†]	6.3 ± 0.6
209. Davis, 1987	8	GC-MS[†]	6.2 ± 0.9
	8	GC-MS	1.2 ± 0.7 (conj.)

* In original paper expressed as μg/min.

Table 53. Unconjugated m-Hydroxyphenylacetic Acid in Plasma of Normal

Subjects

Reference First Author, Year	Number of Subjects	Method of Analysis	Values (ng/mL ± S.E.M.)
447. Karoum, 1977	10	GC-MS[†]	1.0 ± 0.3
210. Davis, 1982	28 (fasting)	GC-MS[†]	21.5 ± 3.8
	14 (not-fasting)	GC-MS	17.9 ± 1.4
	12 (M)	GC-MS	16.6 ± 3.7
	7 (F)	GC-MS	22.6 ± 8.3
213. Davis, 1982	14	GC-MS	23.2 ± 5.3
	24 (institutional)	GC-MS	14.8 ± 1.6
100. Boulton, 1983	38 (prisoners)	GC-MS	9.5 ± 1.6
972. Yu, 1983	64	GC-MS	19.2 ± 2.5
973. Yu, 1984	10 (prisoners)	GC-MS	6.7
974. Yu, 1985	21 (prisoners)	GC-MS	7.4 ± 1.2
	61 (prisoners)	GC-MS	6.1 ± 0.6
211. Davis, 1986	10	GC-MS[†]	5.3
209. Davis, 1987	14	GC-MS[†]	11.4 ± 2.7

Table 54. Conjugated m-Hydroxyphenylacetic Acid in Plasma of Normal

Subjects

Reference First Author, Year	Number of Subjects	Method of Analysis	Values (ng/mL ± S.E.M.)
210. Davis, 1982	28 (fasting)	GC–MS[†]	5.4 ± 1.1
	14 (not-fasting)	GC–MS	-1.0 ± 0.7
	12 (M)	GC–MS	10.0 ± 4.3
	7 (F)	GC–MS	5.5 ± 1.8
213. Davis, 1982	14	GC–MS	0.5 ± 0.1
	24 (institutional)	GC–MS	1.5 ± 0.4
100. Boulton, 1983	38 (prisoners)	GC–MS	1.1 ± 0.3
973. Yu, 1984	10 (prisoners)	GC–MS	1.7
974. Yu, 1985	21 (prisoners)	GC–MS	0.9 ± 0.5
	61 (prisoners)	GC–MS	0.9 ± 0.4
209. Davis, 1987	14	GC–MS[†]	0.0 ± 6.0

Table 55. m-Hydroxyphenylacetic Acid in CSF of Non-Psychiatric Patients

Reference First Author, Year	Number of Subjects	Method of Analysis	Values (pg/mL ± S.E.M.)
969. Young, 1982	6 (seizures)	GC-MS	350 ± 120
	6 (seizures)	GC-MS	1350 ± 610 (cisternal)
211. Davis, 1986	10 (neurological)	GC-MS[†]	500

Table 56. m-Hydroxyphenylacetic Acid and o-Hydroxyphenylacetic Acid in

Urine of Depressed Subjects

Reference First Author, Year	Number of Subjects	Method of Analysis	Values (mg/24h ± S.E.M.)
744. Sandler, 1979	23 (primary)	GC-FID	0.8 ± 0.10 (ortho)
	10 (M)	GC-FID	0.89 ± 0.13 (ortho)
	13 (F)	GC-FID	0.75 ± 0.14 (ortho)
	23	GC-FID	4.45 ± 0.63 (meta)
	10 (M)	GC-FID	4.13 ± 0.93 (meta)
	13 (F)	GC-FID	4.70 ± 0.88 (meta)

Table 57. m-Hydroxyphenylacetic Acid in Plasma of Depressed,

Schizophrenic and Aggressive Patients

Reference First Author, Year	Number of Subjects	Method of Analysis	Values (ng/mL ± S.E.M.)
213. Davis, 1982	24 (schizophrenics)	GC-MS	7.8 ± 1.1
	18 (schizophrenics)	GC-MS	7.5 ± 1.3
	24 (schizophrenics)	GC-MS	1.4 ± 0.5 (conjugated)
	18 (schizophrenics)	GC-MS	0.3 ± 0.2 (conjugated)
972. Yu, 1983	17 (depressed)	GC-MS	14.7 ± 3.7
	29 (agoraphobic)	GC-MS	11.9 ± 1.6
100. Boulton, 1983	35 (aggressive)	GC-MS	9.6 ± 1.8
	35 (aggressive)	GC-MS	1.3 ± 0.4 (conjugated)
973. Yu, 1984	16 (violent)	GC-MS	9.6
	16 (violent)	GC-MS	0.9 (conjugated)
974. Yu, 1985	82 (violent)	GC-MS	5.5 ± 0.5
	82 (violent)	GC-MS	0.8 ± 0.3 (conjugated)
	27 (aggressive)	GC-MS	6.2 ± 1.1
	27 (aggressive)	GC-MS	1.0 ± 0.6 (conjugated)

Table 58. Unconjugated p-Hydroxyphenylacetic Acid in Urine of Normal

Subjects

Reference First Author, Year	Number of Subjects	Method of Analysis	Values (mg/24h ± S.E.M.)
943. Williams, 1961	4	GC-FID	19 mg/g Cr.
99. Boulton, 1967	2	Fl	38.8 ± 0.7
	2	Fl	24.9 ± 17.3 (conjugated)
811. Smith, 1971	8	GC-FID	20.9 ± 3.7
	8	GC-FID	6.7 ± 1.6 (conjugated)
967. Youdim, 1971	4	GC-FID	11.0 ± 3.3*
744. Sandler, 1979	27	GC-FID	21.3 ± 2.0
	10 (M)	GC-FID	19.6 ± 3.6
	17 (F)	GC-FID	22.3 ± 2.4
451. Karoum, 1980	20	GC-ECD	13.7 ± 3.5
207. Davis, 1981	1 (longitudinal study)	GC-MS	22.4
441. Karoum, 1982	5	GC-MS[†]	2.3 ± 0.5
218. DeJong, 1983	7	GC-FID[†]	17.5 ± 4.4 mg/g Cr.
366. Harris, 1985	10	GC-MS[†]	25.2 ± 2.7*
211. Davis, 1986	10	GC-MS[†]	25.1
50. Baker, 1987	29	GC-ECD[†]	20.0 ± 1.9
209. Davis, 1987	8	GC-MS[†]	20.2 ± 2.5
	8	GC-MS	0.9 ± 0.3 (conjugated)

* In original paper expressed as µg/min.

Table 59. Unconjugated p-Hydroxyphenylacetic Acid in Plasma of Normal

Subjects

Reference First Author, Year	Number of Subjects	Method of Analysis	Values (ng/mL ± S.E.M.)
447. Karoum, 1977	10	GC-MS[†]	11.3 ± 0.9
210. Davis, 1982	28 (fasting)	GC-MS[†]	54.1 ± 6.4
	14 (not-fasting)	GC-MS	69.0 ± 7.1
	12 (M)	GC-MS	66.6 ± 22.0
	7 (F)	GC-MS	59.6 ± 14.7
213. Davis, 1982	14	GC-MS	69.0 ± 6.9
	24 (institutional)	GC-MS	69.3 ± 5.6
100. Boulton, 1983	38 (prisoners)	GC-MS	99.5 ± 17.9
972. Yu, 1983	64	GC-MS	83.7 ± 6.2
973. Yu, 1984	10 (prisoners)	GC-MS	41.2
974. Yu, 1985	21 (prisoners)	GC-MS	43.7 ± 4.9
	61 (prisoners)	GC-MS	65.6 ± 8.7
211. Davis, 1986	10	GC-MS[†]	68.5
209. Davis, 1987	14	GC-MS[†]	49.4 ± 6.4

Table 60. Conjugated p-Hydroxyphenylacetic Acid in Plasma of Normal

Subjects

Reference First Author, Year	Number of Subjects	Method of Analysis	Values (ng/mL ± S.E.M.)
210. Davis, 1982	28 (fasting)	GC-MS[†]	10.6 ± 3.3
	14 (not-fasting)	GC-MS	1.8 ± 4.4
	12 (M)	GC-MS	17.7 ± 4.1
	7 (F)	GC-MS	13.0 ± 5.9
213. Davis, 1982	14	GC-MS	7.2 ± 3.2
	24 (institutional)	GC-MS	28.6 ± 7.9
100. Boulton, 1983	38 (prisoners)	GC-MS	13.0 ± 4.3
973. Yu, 1984	10 (prisoners)	GC-MS	21.6
974. Yu, 1985	21 (prisoners)	GC-MS	20.0 ± 3.4
	61 (prisoners)	GC-MS	8.9 ± 3.3
209. Davis, 1987	14	GC-MS[†]	9.1 ± 6.1

Table 61. Unconjugated p-Hydroxyphenylacetic Acid in CSF of Normal

Subjects

Reference First Author, Year	Number of Subjects	Method of Analysis	Values (ng/mL ± S.E.M.)
444. Karoum, 1975	5	GC-MS	9.9 ± 3.5 (lumbar)
	8	GC-MS	22.8 ± 3.6 (ventricular)
482. Kobayashi, 1982	11	HPLC-EC[†]	7.8 ± 1.1
	16 (neurological)	HPLC-EC	9.1 ± 1.0
969. Young, 1982	6 (seizures)	GC-MS	6.5 ± 1.0 (lumbar)
	6 (seizures)	GC-MS	8.8 ± 1.0 (cisternal)
211. Davis, 1986	10 (neurological)	GC-MS[†]	6.0

Table 62. Unconjugated p-Hydroxyphenylacetic Acid in Urine of Depressed

Patients

Reference First Author, Year	Number of Subjects	Method of Analysis	Values (mg/24h ± S.E.M.)
744. Sandler, 1979	23 (primary)	GC-FID	13.1 ± 1.3
	10 (M)	GC-FID	12.2 ± 2.2
	13 (F)	GC-FID	13.8 ± 1.5
441. Karoum, 1982	6	GC-MS[†]	1.2 ± 0.1
525. Linnoila, 1982	4 (bipolar)	GC-MS	4.3 ± 0.5

Table 63. m- and p-Hydroxyphenylacetic Acid in Urine of Parkinson's

Patients

Reference First Author, Year	Number of Subjects	Method of Analysis	Values (mg/24h ± S.E.M.)
132. Calne, 1969	14	GC-FID	1.7 ± 0.5 (meta)
	14	GC-FID	7.4 ± 1.5 (para)
451. Karoum, 1980	6	GC-ECD	1.7 ± 0.5 (meta)
	6	GC-ECD	7.4 ± 1.5 (para)

Table 64. p-Hydroxyphenylacetic Acid in Plasma of Depressed,

Schizophrenic and Aggressive Patients

Reference First Author, Year	Number of Subjects	Method of Analysis	Values (ng/mL ± S.E.M.)
213. Davis, 1982	24 (schizophrenics)	GC-MS	52.2 ± 5.7
	18 (schizophrenics)	GC-MS	63.3 ± 8.2
	24 (schizophrenics)	GC-MS	44.3 ± 6.8 (conjugated)
	18 (schizophrenics)	GC-MS	28.6 ± 9.7 (conjugated)
972. Yu, 1983	17 (unipolar + bipolar)	GC-MS	53.8 ± 3.6
	29 (agoraphobic)	GC-MS	62.7 ± 6.0
100. Boulton, 1983	35 (aggressive)	GC-MS	64.5 ± 6.8
	35 (aggressive)	GC-MS	9.8 ± 2.9 (conjugated)
973. Yu, 1984	16 (violent)	GC-MS	56.2
	16 (violent)	GC-MS	19.2 (conjugated)
974. Yu, 1985	82 (violent)	GC-MS	59.8 ± 6.7
	82 (violent)	GC-MS	5.5 ± 1.6 (conjugated)
	27 (aggressive)	GC-MS	44.5 ± 4.1
	27 (aggressive)	GC-MS	5.8 ± 1.8 (conjugated)

Table 65. Unconjugated p-Hydroxyphenylacetic Acid in CSF of Depressed

and Schizophrenic Subjects

Reference First Author, Year	Number of Subjects	Method of Analysis	Values (ng/mL ± S.E.M.)
440. Karoum, 1977	12 (schizophrenics)	GC–MS	6.6 ± 0.8
482. Kobayashi, 1982	10 (schizophrenics)	HPLC–EC[†]	4.8 ± 0.6
	4 (depressed)	HPLC–EC	4.0 ± 0.5
	10 (other psychiatric)	HPLC–EC	8.1 ± 1.2

Table 66. Unconjugated Indoleacetic Acid in Urine of Normal Subjects

Reference First Author, Year	Number of Subjects	Method of Analysis	Values (mg/24h ± S.E.M.)
410. Jepson, 1956	5	–	50 – 200
931. Weissbach, 1959	11	Fl	3.1 – 8.1
	11	Fl	2.1 – 5.7 (conjugated)
943. Williams, 1961	4	GC-FID	1.4 mg/g Cr.
710. Rodnight, 1961	18	Fl	1.25± 0.02 mg/g Cr.
819. Sprince, 1962	11	Fl	2.5 mg/g Cr.
	11	Fl	4.7 mg/g Cr. (conj)
33. Arterberry, 1967	23	Fl[†]	17.6 ± 1.8*
821. Stachow, 1974	14	Fl	6.4
390. Hoskins, 1975	19	GC-MS[†]	2.55± 0.35
237. Domino, 1979	7	GC-MS[†]	14.20± 0.96
387. Hopkinson, 1982	15	HPLC	8.0 mg/g Cr.
366. Harris, 1985	10	GC-MS[†]	5.9 ± 1.6**
211. Davis, 1986	10	GC-MS[†]	10.1
209. Davis, 1987	8	GC-MS[†]	9.14± 2.44

* In original paper, expressed as μg/min; ** as μg/min.

Table 67. Unconjugated Indoleacetic Acid in Plasma of Normal Subjects

Reference First Author, Year	Number of Subjects	Method of Analysis	Values (ng/mL ± S.E.M.)
736. Sakai, 1978	–	GC-MS	350 (serum)
559. Martinez, 1983	15	HPLC-Fl[†]	270 ± 25
298. Friedman, 1984	33	HPLC-EC[†]	208 ± 19 (serum)
836. Suñol, 1984	15	HPLC-Fl	270 ± 27
974. Yu, 1985	21 (prisoners)	GC-MS	201 ± 16
	61 (prisoners)	GC-MS	369 ± 62
211. Davis, 1986	10	GC-MS[†]	292
209. Davis, 1987	14	GC-MS[†]	321 ± 23
749. Sarrias, 1987	6	HPLC-Fl	222

Table 68. Unconjugated Indoleacetic Acid in CSF of Normal Subjects

Reference First Author, Year	Number of Subjects	Method of Analysis	Values (ng/mL ± S.E.M.)
968. Young, 1980*	38	HPLC-Fl	4.56 ± 0.41 (lumbar)
	38	HPLC-Fl	5.39 ± 0.48 (cisternal)
970. Young, 1980*	43 (M)	HPLC-Fl	3.43 ± 0.42 (cisternal)
	36 (F)	HPLC-Fl	4.28 ± 0.56 (cisternal)
	45 (M)	HPLC-Fl	2.84 ± 0.37 (lumbar)
	33 (F)	HPLC-Fl	4.19 ± 0.51 (lumbar)
	21	HPLC-Fl	4.29 ± 0.64 (cisternal)
	21	HPLC-Fl	5.06 ± 0.69 (lumbar)
585. Montplaisir, 1982	11	HPLC-Fl	8.78 ± 2.20
19. Anderson, 1984	36	HPLC-Fl	4.39 ± 0.37
211. Davis, 1986	10	GC-MS[†]	5.1

* Most subjects in these two studies were epileptics.

Table 69. Indoleacetic Acid in Urine of Depressed Subjects

Reference First Author, Year	Number of Subjects	Method of Analysis	Values (mg/24h ± S.E.M.)
710. Rodnight, 1961	15 (depressed)	Fl	2.58 ± 0.49 mg/g Cr.
	3 (hypomania)	Fl	1.51 mg/g Cr.
174. Coppen, 1965	13 (depressed)	Fl	3.4 ± 0.8
	13 (recovered)	Fl	3.2 ± 0.4
564. McNamee, 1972	7 (psychotic)	Fl	4.6 ± 1.2
	9 (neurotic)	Fl	3.1 ± 0.4
	16 (all)	Fl	3.8 ± 0.7
	16 (recovered)	Fl	3.0 ± 0.3

Table 70. Indoleacetic Acid in Urine of Schizophrenic Subjects

Reference First Author, Year	Number of Subjects	Method of Analysis	Values (mg/24h ± S.E.M.)
710. Rodnight, 1961	20	Fl	1.95 ± 0.38 mg/g Cr.
122. Brune, 1962	17 (inactive)	Chemical	16.3
	12 (slightly active)	Chemical	17.3
	7 (moderate)	Chemical	21.2
	6 (active)	Chemical	28.8
	2 (markedly active)	Chemical	43.1
	44 (all)	Chemical	18.1*
819. Sprince, 1962	11 (acute)	Fl	3.2 mg/g Cr.
	11 (acute)	Fl	7.0 mg/g Cr.(conj.)
	11 (chronic)	Fl	6.2 mg/g Cr.
	11 (chronic)	Fl	10.2 mg/g Cr.(conj.)
503. La Brosse, 1964	9	Fl	7.76 ± 0.66
374. Herkert, 1969	10	Fl	7.5 ± 1.0
237. Domino, 1979	7 (chronic)	GC-MS[†]	11.1 ± 0.5

* All values in this paper are for total IAA after hydrolysis.

Table 71. Indoleacetic Acid in CSF (and Plasma) of Depressed,

Schizophrenic and Aggressive Subjects

Reference First Author, Year	Number of Subjects	Method of Analysis	Values (ng/mL ± S.E.M.)
83. Bertilsson, 1972	24 (depressed)	GC-MS[†]	6.1 ± 0.6
37. Åsberg, 1973	36 (depressed)	GC-MS	6.43 ± 0.68
	9 (M)	.GC-MS	6.43 ± 1.41
	27 (F)	GC-MS	6.43 ± 0.79
794. Siwers, 1977	6 (depressed)	GC-MS	5.6 ± 1.1
19. Anderson, 1984	39 (all depressed)	HPLC-Fl	5.23 ± 0.49
	10 (manic depressive)	HPLC-Fl	4.32 ± 0.63
	19 (retarded depressive)	HPLC-Fl	5.90 ± 0.80
	9 (agitated depressive)	HPLC-Fl	4.79 ± 1.12
	17 (schizophrenic)	HPLC-Fl	4.06 ± 0.05
974. Yu, 1985	82 (violent)	GC-MS	332 ± 45 (plasma)
	27 (aggressive)	GC-MS	220 ± 14 (plasma) .
749. Sarrias, 1987	18 (melancholia)	HPLC-Fl	141 (plasma)

Table 72. Alcohol and Glycol Metabolites of the Trace Amines in Urine

of Normal Subjects

Reference First Author, Year	Metabolite	Number of Subjects	Method of Analysis	Values (µg/ 24h/S.E.M.)
253. Edwards, 1979	phenylethyleneglycol	1[†]	GC–MS	22 (total)
	p-hydroxyphenylethanol	1	GC–MS	0
	p-hydroxyphenylethanol	1	GC–MS	11 (conj.)
	p-hydroxyphenylglycol	1	GC–MS	13
	p-hydroxyphenylglycol	1	GC–MS	78 (conj.)

<u>Table 73.   Mandelic Acid, o-, m- and p-Hydroxymandelic Acid in Urine of</u>

<u>Normal and Depressed Subjects</u>

Reference First Author, Year	Number of Subjects	Method of Analysis	Values (µg/24h ± S.E.M.)
573. Midgley, 1979	10	GC-MS[†]	7.3 ± 1.1 µg/g Cr.(ortho)
	10	GC-MS	29.0 ± 6.5 µg/g Cr. (meta)
	10	GC-MS	2200 ± 327 µg/g Cr. (para)
744. Sandler, 1979	10 (M) (normal)	GC-FID	2028 ± 319 (para)
	17 (F) (normal)	GC-FID	1589 ± 220
	27 (combined)	GC-FID	1749 ± 180
	10 (M) (depressed)	GC-FID	1468 ± 309
	13 (F) (depressed)	GC-FID	959 ± 150
	23 (combined)	GC-FID	1179 ± 170
441. Karoum, 1982	5 (normal)	GC-MS[†]	1900 ± 400 (para)
	6 (depressed)	GC-MS	1700 ± 300
208. Davis, 1981	7 (normal)	GC-MS[†]	59.0 ± 13.8 (meta)
366. Harris, 1985	10 (normal)	GC-MS[†]	5200 ± 1300* (para)
211. Davis, 1986	10 (normal)	GC-MS[†]	220 (mandelic acid)
	10	GC-MS	100 (meta)
	10	GC-MS	1910 (para)
209. Davis, 1987	8 (normal)	GC-MS[†]	3580 ± 810 (para)
	8	GC-MS	232 ± 14 (mandelic acid)
	8	GC-MS	118 ± 62 (conj. MA)

* In original paper expressed as µg/min.

<u>Table 74. Mandelic and m- and p-Hydroxymandelic Acids in Plasma of</u>

<u>Normal and Aggressive Subjects</u>

Reference First Author, Year	Number of Subjects	Method of Analysis	Values (ng/mL ± S.E.M.)
447. Karoum, 1977	10 (normals)	GC-MS[†]	16.0 ± 2.5 (para)
538. Luthe, 1983	6 (normals)	GC-MS[†]	41.0 ± 10.5 (MA)
974. Yu, 1985	21 (prisoners)	GC-MS	8.7 ± 0.8 (para)
	61 (prisoners)	GC-MS	8.7 ± 0.4 (para)
	82 (violent)	GC-MS	8.8 ± 0.4 (para)
	27 (aggressive)	GC-MS	9.5 ± 1.2 (para)
211. Davis, 1986	10 (normals)	GC-MS[†]	13.6 (MA)
	10	GC-MS	n.d. (meta)
	10	GC-MS	8.4 (para)
209. Davis, 1987	14 (normals)	GC-MS[†]	11.1 ± 1.7 (para)

Table 75.   p-Hydroxymandelic Acid and p-Hydroxyphenylethanol in CSF

Reference First Author, Year	Number of Subjects	Method of Analysis	Values (ng/mL ± S.E.M.)
444. Karoum, 1975	5 (normals)	GC-MS	1.3 ± 0.4 (lumbar)(pHMA)
	8	GC-MS	7.1 ± 1.0 (ventricular) (pHMA)
	8	GC-MS	12.3 ± 1.7 (pHPE)
440. Karoum, 1977	12 (schizophrenics)	GC-MS	3.0 ± 0.4 (pHMA)

Section 6

Catecholamines and Serotonin

Tables 76 to 135

Table 76. Unconjugated Noradrenaline in Urine of Normal Subjects

Reference First Author, Year	Number of Subjects	Method of Analysis	Values (mg/24h ± S.E.M.)
437. Kärki, 1956	36 (M) 21 (F)	Fl[†] Fl	25.2 ± 1.6 24.9 ± 1.8
921. Watts, 1956	17	Fl,Bio	54.9 ± 6.0*
796. Sjoerdsma, 1959	4	Fl	42.3 ± 18.5
30. Arnett, 1960	7	Fl	14.6 ± 4.3**
60. Barbeau, 1961	24	Fl	42.0 ± 3.2
233. De Quattro, 1964	9	Fl[†]	51.4 ± 7.9**
536. Lovegrove, 1965	30	Fl[†]	40
707. Robinson, 1965	7	Fl[†]	24.9 ± 4.6
368. Hathaway, 1967	9 5 (M) 4 (F)	Fl[†] Fl Fl	27.5 ± 3.1 32.9 ± 5.5 23.6 ± 1.5
561. Mattok, 1967	24	Fl	100.8**
896. Viktora, 1968	9	Fl[†]	15.8 ± 1.6
135. Cardon, 1970	7	Fl	40.3
381. Hoeldtke, 1970	7	Fl[†]	29.3 ± 4.5
278. Fiorica, 1971	12	Fl[†]	45.7 ± 3.3
666. Pollin, 1971	8	GC-ECD	22.9 mg/g Cr.
871. Turnball, 1971	21	–	23.0 ± 1.8
850. Takahashi, 1972	10	Fl[†]	26.2 ± 2.8 mg/g Cr.
654. Peyrin, 1973	25	Fl[†]	90 ± 21
862. Townshend, 1973	30	Fl	29.3 ± 2.6
953. Wong, 1973	8	GC-ECD[†]	52.1 ± 5.3
183. Cuche, 1974	14	Fl	55.9 ± 6.4***
474. Kissinger, 1975	10	HPLC-EC[†]	20 ± 3.2 mg/g Cr.
645. Pedersen, 1975	32	REA	31 mg/g Cr.

Table 76. Unconjugated Noradrenaline in Urine of Normal Subjects (continued)

Reference First Author, Year	Number of Subjects	Method of Analysis	Values (mg/24h ± S.E.M.)
832. Subrahmanyam, 1975	12 12	Fl Fl	40.6 ± 4.2 42.4 ± 5.2
377. Higa, 1977	5	Fl[†]	38.0 ± 5.7
566. Mell, 1977	10 78	HPLC[†] Fl[†]	55 ± 4.4 46 ± 2.4
874. Ueda, 1977	–	Fl[†]	19.4 ± 2.5
923. Weidman, 1977	14	Fl	28.9 ± 4.2 mg/g Cr.
198. Dalmaz, 1978	34	Fl[†]	89 ± 11
234. DeSchaepdryver, 1978	20	Fl[†]	56.9 ± 3.7
401. Imai, 1978	7	HPLC-Fl[†]	35.5 ± 6.3 mg/g Cr.
590. Moyer, 1979	97	Fl[†]	36.2
600. Muskiet, 1979	19	GC-MS[†]	80 ± 5.5 mg/g Cr.
199. Da Prada, 1980	6	REA	40 ± 10
21. Anderson, 1981	44	HPLC-EC[†]	23.6 ± 18.5 mg/L
140. Causon, 1982	10 12	HPLC-EC, Fl[†] HPLC-EC, Fl	43.4 ± 7.0 59.2 ± 14.2
259. Elchisak, 1982	6	HPLC-EC[†]	110.4 ± 15.9
441. Karoum, 1982	5	GC-MS[†]	116 ± 27
460. Kemali, 1982	14	REA[†]	37.2 ± 0.7
625. Oka, 1982	57	Fl[†]	33.6 ± 1.8
933. Westerink, 1982	48	HPLC[†]	41.5 ± 1.6
266. Eriksson, 1983	5	HPLC-EC[†]	30.3 ± 3.1
328. Goldstein, 1983	181	HPLC-EC[†]	37.0 ± 1.9
61. Barbeito, 1984	12	HPLC-EC	27.2 ± 4.0*
195. Dajas, 1984	12	HPLC-EC	44.1 ± 6.3*

Table 76. Unconjugated Noradrenaline in Urine of Normal Subjects (continued)

Reference First Author, Year	Number of Subjects	Method of Analysis	Values (mg/24h ± S.E.M.)
471. Kiriike, 1984	31	Fl	36.7 ± 3.2
196. Dajas, 1986	21	HPLC-EC	17.7 ± 2.0*
290. Frankenhaueser, 1986	19 (M) 30 (F)	GC-MS GC-MS	8.1 ± 0.5* 6.9 ± 0.5*
866. Tsuchiya, 1986	9	HPLC-Fl[†]	16.4 ± 1.6
17. Anderson, 1988	1 –	HPLC-EC[†] HPLC-Fl[†]	15.7 mg/L 17.1 mg/L
431. Julien, 1988	6	HPLC-EC[†]	42 ± 6
537. Lundberg, 1988	30 30	HPLC-EC Fl	37.9 ± 2.4 41.9 ± 2.6

*   In original paper expressed as ng/min.
**   In original paper expressed as mg/h.
*** In original paper expressed as mg/4h.

Table 77. Conjugated Noradrenaline in Urine of Normal Subjects

Reference First Author, Year	Number of Subjects	Method of Analysis	Values (mg/24h ± S.E.M.)
561. Mattok, 1967	24	Fl	43.2**
896. Viktora, 1968	9	Fl[†]	14.9 ± 1.5
381. Hoeldtke, 1970	7	Fl[†]	58.5 ± 8.1
850. Takahashi, 1972	4	Fl[†]	44.2 ± 6.2 mg/g Cr.
474. Kissinger, 1975	6	HPLC-EC[†]	90 ± 12 mg/g Cr.
874. Ueda, 1977	–	Fl[†]	39.8 ± 12.6
199. Da Prada, 1980	6	REA	145 ± 25
259. Elchisak, 1982	6	HPLC-EC[†]	122.9 ± 28.8
25. Arakawa, 1983	11	HPLC[†]	123.8 ± 41.2* (3-sulfate)
	11	HPLC	21.6 ± 6.1* (4-sulfate)
724. Roy, 1986	25	GC-MS	191.0 ± 13.5 (total)
657. Peyrin, 1987	11	Fl mg/g Cr.	732 ± 101 (total)
529. Linnoila, 1988	12	GC-MS	96.3 ± 10.3 (total)

* In original paper expressed as ng/min.
** In original paper expressed as mg/h.

Table 78. <u>Unconjugated Noradrenaline in Plasma of Normal, Supine</u>

<u>Subjects</u>

Reference First Author, Year	Number of Subjects	Method of Analysis	Values (pg/mL ± S.E.M.)
925. Weil-Malherbe, 1953	22 (M) 21 (F)	Fl Fl	5290 ± 230 5160 ± 160
551. Manger, 1954	7	Fl	3960 ± 640
926. Weil-Malherbe, 1954	9 (suspected brain lesions)	Fl	7200 ± 580
31. Aronow, 1956	6	Fl	2100 ± 530 (venous)
168. Cohen, 1957	59	Fl[†]	300 ± 10
680. Price, 1957	12 12	Fl Fl	200 ± 35 (arterial) 340 ± 45 (venous)
689. Reilly, 1957	27	Fl	3000 ± 250
327. Goldfien, 1961	22	Fl[†]	155 ± 13
23. Anton, 1962	5	Fl[†]	970
355. Häggendal, 1963	13	Fl[†]	300 ± 110
563. McCullough, 1968	5	Fl[†]	610
896. Viktora, 1968	9	Fl[†]	290 ± 110 (serum)
265. Engelman, 1970	22	REA[†]	200 ± 17
347. Griffiths, 1970	50	Fl[†]	240 ± 13
624. O'Hanlon, 1970	12	Fl[†]	174 ± 15
692. Renzini, 1970	12	Fl[†]	174 ± 7
791. Siggers, 1970	4	REA[†]	420 ± 110
494. Kotchen, 1971	6	Fl[†]	1500 ± 100
53. Banister, 1972	5	Fl	210 ± 30
32. Aronow, 1973	3 3	REA REA	231 ± 35 (day) 179 ± 62 (night)
159. Christensen, 1973	16	REA	220 ± 22

Table 78. Unconjugated Noradrenaline in Plasma of Normal, Supine

Subjects (continued)

Reference First Author, Year	Number of Subjects	Method of Analysis	Values (pg/mL ± S.E.M.)
312. Geffen, 1973	20	REA	160 ± 40
402. Imai, 1973	6	GC-ECD[†]	1030 ± 270
496. Kozlowski, 1973	102	Fl	950 ± 8
571. Meyer, 1973	5	Fl	390 ± 50
160. Christensen, 1974	9	REA	180 ± 20
182. Cryer, 1974	18	REA[†]	223 ± 92
183. Cuche, 1974	7	Fl	250 ± 60
872. Turton, 1974	12 12	Fl Fl	690 ± 70 (day) 340 ± 40 (night)
157. Chodakowska, 1975	8	Fl	108 ± 9
373. Henry, 1975	7	REA[†]	254 ± 29
645. Pedersen, 1975	26 (M) 6 (F)	REA REA	258 238
914. Wang, 1975	5	GC-ECD[†]	237
181. Cryer, 1976	10	REA	227 ± 23
200. Da Prada, 1976	7	REA[†]	200 ± 23
507. Lake, 1976	74	REA[†]	292 ± 16
572. Michaels, 1976	18	REA	370 ± 40
581. Moerman, 1976	8	REA	160 ± 20 (venous)
929. Weise, 1976	13	REA[†]	208 ± 17
978. Ziegler, 1976	16 (M) 22 (F)	REA REA	270 ± 42 307 ± 31
289. Franco-Morselli, 1977	11	REA	248 ± 56
389. Hörtnagl, 1977	11 (M) 7 (F)	REA REA	444 ± 39 550 ± 33

Table 78. Unconjugated Noradrenaline in Plasma of Normal, Supine

Subjects (continued)

Reference First Author, Year	Number of Subjects	Method of Analysis	Values (pg/mL ± S.E.M.)
475. Klaniecki, 1977	6	REA[†]	182 ± 53
506. Lake, 1977	84	REA	304 ± 20
652. Peuler, 1977	15	REA[†]	279 ± 44
774. Sever, 1977	9	REA	403 ± 61
815. Sole, 1977	3	REA[†]	282 ± 4
946. Winer, 1977	9	REA	162
164. Chryssanthopoulos, 1978	9	Fl	740 ± 160
254. Ehrhardt, 1978	9	GC-ECD[†]	200 ± 40
359. Hallman, 1978	6	HPLC-EC[†]	519 ± 71
423. Jones, 1978	30	REA	560 ± 90
487. Kopin, 1978	15	REA	262 ± 20
704. Robertson, 1978	9	REA	136 ± 12
263. Endert, 1979	20	REA-HPLC[†]	355 ± 28
512. Le Blanc, 1979	12	REA	292 ± 18
706. Robertson, 1979	15	REA[†]	210 ± 11
712. Romoff, 1979	13	REA	116 ± 13
881. Van Loon, 1979	5	REA	274 ± 6
898. Vlachakis, 1979	16	REA[†]	215 ± 28
199. Da Prada, 1980	5	REA	550 ± 50
236. Dimsdale, 1980	9	REA	583 ± 39
421. Johnson, 1980	10	REA	196 ± 17
825. Stene, 1980	4	REA	217 ± 58
920. Watson, 1980	5	REA	429 ± 81

Table 78. Unconjugated Noradrenaline in Plasma of Normal, Supine

Subjects (continued)

Reference First Author, Year	Number of Subjects	Method of Analysis	Values (pg/mL ± S.E.M.)
964. Yoshida, 1980	10	GC-MS[†]	297 ± 30
975. Yui, 1980	10	HPLC-Fl[†]	185 ± 29
141. Causon, 1981	30 (sitting)	HPLC-EC[†]	470 ± 30
247. Demassieux, 1981	4	REA[†]	200 ± 32
330. Goldstein, 1981	7	HPLC-EC	311 ± 20
565. Mefford, 1981	5 (sitting)	HPLC-EC[†]	292 ± 22
687. Raum, 1981	–	RIA[†]	240
860. Thiede, 1981	9	REA[†]	372 ± 39
873. Uchikura, 1981	3	REA[†]	392 ± 82 (serum)
902. Vlachakis, 1981	36	REA	319 ± 46
960. Yamatodani, 1981	10	HPLC[†]	166 ± 14
4. Ackenheil, 1982	200	HPLC-EC	210 ± 14
138. Castellani, 1982	24	REA	201 ± 24
380. Hjemdahl, 1982	13	HPLC-EC	392 ± 46
429. Joyce, 1982	6	REA	252 ± 34
460. Kemali, 1982	45	REA[†]	230 ± 10
504. Lake, 1982	22	REA	280
585. Montplaisir, 1982	11	REA	290 ± 46 (serum)
45. Bagdy, 1983	24 (F) 6 (M)	REA REA	300 ± 30 230 ± 20
166. Claustre, 1983	6	REA	245 ± 51
194. Dajas, 1983	–	HPLC-EC	210 ± 49
244. Dunne, 1983	6	REA	220 ± 40

Table 78. Unconjugated Noradrenaline in Plasma of Normal, Supine

Subjects (continued)

Reference First Author, Year	Number of Subjects	Method of Analysis	Values (pg/mL ± S.E.M.)
916. Wang, 1983	9	REA[†]	190 ± 30
917. Ward, 1983	8	HPLC-EC[†]	347
961. Yoneda, 1983	6	REA	475 ± 55
97. Bondy, 1984	40	HPLC-EC	210 ± 6
331. Goldstein, 1984	9	HPLC-EC[†]	281
559a.Maruta, 1984	–	HPLC-EC[†]	240 ± 7
685. Raskind, 1984	6	REA	253 ± 37
718. Rothschild, 1984	12	HPLC-EC	483 ± 63
789. Siever, 1984	10	REA	232 ± 37
900. Vlachakis, 1984	5	REA[†]	230 ± 54
393. Howes, 1985	6	HPLC-EC[†]	233 ± 24
406. Ishimitsu, 1985	5	HPLC[†]	340 ± 110
408. Izzo, 1985	13	REA	208 ± 24
686. Ratge, 1985	40	REA	288 ± 145
725. Roy, 1985	41	HPLC-EC	147 ± 10
728. Rudorfer, 1985	12	HPLC-EC	264 ± 10
257. Eisenhofer, 1986	62	HPLC-EC	584 ± 47
790. Siever, 1986	21	REA	232 ± 25
74. Benedict, 1987	12	HPLC[†]	208 ± 10
719. Rothschild, 1987	6	HPLC	316 ± 59
720. Roy, 1987	39	HPLC-EC	142 ± 10
872a.Tyce, 1987	6	HPLC-EC	350 ± 40
301. Gaffney, 1988	10	REA	228 ± 22
349. Guillemin, 1988	10	HPLC-EC[†]	232 ± 11

Table 78. Unconjugated Noradrenaline in Plasma of Normal, Supine

Subjects (continued)

Reference First Author, Year	Number of Subjects	Method of Analysis	Values (pg/mL ± S.E.M.)
350a.Gullestad, 1988	8	REA	355 ± 58
358. Halbrügge, 1988	32	HPLC-EC[†]	149 ± 25
400. Imai, 1988	20	HPLC-EC[†]	276 ± 16
775. Sevy, 1989	14	HPLC-EC	87 ± 13

Table 79. Conjugated Noradrenaline in Plasma of Normal, Supine

Subjects

Reference First Author, Year	Number of Subjects	Method of Analysis	Values (pg/mL ± S.E.M.)
402. Imai, 1973	6	GC-ECD[†]	3920 ± 730
914. Wang, 1975	5	GC-ECD[†]	777
199. Da Prada, 1980	5	REA	1260 ± 350
421. Johnson, 1980	10	REA	914 ± 123 (sulfate)
227. Demassieux, 1981	4	REA[†]	345 ± 65
429. Joyce, 1982	6	REA	615 ± 68 (sulfate)
166. Claustre, 1983	6 6	REA REA	139 ± 49 (glucuronide) 723 ± 25 (sulfate)
916. Wang, 1983	9 9	REA[†] REA	trace (glucuronide) 400 ± 40 (sulfate)
961. Yoneda, 1983	6	REA	1259 ± 111
900. Vlachakis, 1984	5	REA[†]	1170 ± 482
184. Cuche, 1985	15	REA	565 ± 31 (sulfate)
406. Ishimitsu, 1985	5	HPLC[†]	1150 ± 130
686. Ratge, 1985	40	REA	748 ± 504
872a.Tyce, 1987	6	HPLC-EC	1150 ± 160 (sulfate)

Table 80. Unconjugated Noradrenaline in CSF of Normal, Supine Subjects

Reference First Author, Year	Number of Subjects	Method of Analysis	Values (pg/mL ± S.E.M.)
926. Weil-Malherbe, 1954	9	Fl	2460 ± 280
230. Dencker, 1966	7	Fl	200 ± 80
571. Meyer, 1973	5	Fl	260 ± 49
653. Peuler, 1977	5	REA[†]	202 ± 27
979. Ziegler, 1977	15	GC-MS	180 ± 35
672. Post, 1978	17	REA	225
162. Christensen, 1980	18	REA	102
332. Gomes, 1980	18	REA	207 ± 11
505. Lake, 1980	29	REA	91 ± 6
827. Sternberg, 1981	40	REA	93 ± 5
901. Vlachakis, 1981	36	REA	156 ± 26
379. Hiramatsu, 1982	75	HPLC-Fl	110 ± 10
460. Kemali, 1982	10	REA[†]	125 ± 6
585. Montplaisir, 1982	11	REA	142 ± 36
45. Bagdy, 1983	24 (F)	REA	160 ± 10
	6 (M)	REA	160 ± 30
310. Gattaz, 1983	15	HPLC-EC	133 ± 10
77. Berrettini, 1984	20	HPLC-EC	54 ± 8
685. Raskind, 1984	6	REA	245 ± 33
773. Seppala, 1984	72	HPLC-EC[†]	88 ± 6
78. Berrettini, 1985	23	HPLC-EC	67 ± 7
309. Gattaz, 1985	16	HPLC-EC	133 ± 9
686. Ratge, 1985	40	REA	128 ± 45
	40	REA	199 ± 137 (conj.)
816. Sparks, 1985	4	HPLC-EC[†]	58 ± 2

Table 80. <u>Unconjugated Noradrenaline in CSF of Normal, Supine Subjects</u>
<u>(continued)</u>

Reference First Author, Year	Number of Subjects	Method of Analysis	Values (pg/mL ± S.E.M.)
735. Saito, 1986	9	HPLC-EC	138 ± 19
723. Roy, 1988	25	HPLC-EC	100 ± 7

<u>Table 81.   Unconjugated Noradrenaline in Urine of Depressed Subjects</u>

Reference First Author, Year	Number of Subjects	Method of Analysis	Values (mg/24h ± S.E.M.)
831. Strom-Olsen, 1958	6 (depressed)	Fl	27.9 ± 3.7
	5 (manic)	Fl	93.9 ± 7.9
536. Lovegrove, 1965	18 (anxiety, psychoneurotic)	Fl[†]	40
	20 (depression, psychoneurotic)	Fl	34
	7 (depressed)	Fl	25 ± 6.9
806. Sloane, 1966	39 (depressed)	Fl	41.1
	7 (manic)	Fl	67.8
126. Bunney, 1967	8 (psychotic (depressive)	Fl	51.2
	8 (neurotic (depressive)	Fl	21.6
849. Takahashi, 1968	1 patient, 4 times (manic depressive)	Fl	33.3 ± 6.8
128. Bunney, 1970	3 (depressed)	Fl	20.7 ± 2.1
	3 (manic)	Fl	56.2 ± 11.6
346. Greenspan, 1970	3 (hypomanic)	Fl	102 ± 15
	2 (normothymic)	Fl	54 ± 2
	3 (agitated depressive)	Fl	53 ± 12
127. Bunney, 1972	6 (depressed)	Fl	36.7 ± 7.1
	6 (manic)	Fl	61.1 ± 13.3
832. Subrahmanyam, 1975	24 (manic depressive psychoses)	Fl	24.6 ± 1.2

Table 81. Unconjugated Noradrenaline in Urine of Depressed Subjects

(continued)

Reference First Author, Year	Number of Subjects	Method of Analysis	Values (mg/24h ± S.E.M.)
592. Murphy, 1977	4 (primary)	Fl	36 ± 6
673. Post, 1977	1 (depressed, 49 days)	Fl	13.6 ± 1.8
	1 (manic, 45 days)	Fl	36.0 ± 3.4
761. Schildkraut, 1978	9 (schizophrenia related)	Fl	33 ± 7
	4 (schizoaffective)	Fl	23 ± 4
	12 (bipolar)	Fl	27 ± 4
	16 (unipolar- endogenous)	Fl	45 ± 4
	13 (unipolar- non-endogenous)	Fl	39 ± 6
	9 (unclassified)	Fl	41 ± 4
441. Karoum, 1982	6	GC-MS[†]	110 ± 11
452. Karoum, 1982	6 (unipolar + bipolar)	GC-MS	232 ± 56
526. Linnoila, 1982 527. Linnoila, 1982	12 (unipolar + bipolar)	GC-MS	201 ± 29 (total)
525. Linnoila, 1982	4 (bipolar)	GC-MS	187 ± 14 (total)
523. Linnoila, 1982	8 (unipolar)	GC-MS	238 ± 36 (total)
	8 (bipolar)	GC-MS	189 ± 40 (total)
524. Linnoila, 1983	12 (unipolar + bipolar)	GC-MS	220 ± 34 (total)

<u>Table 81.   Unconjugated Noradrenaline in Urine of Depressed Subjects</u>

<u>(continued)</u>

Reference First Author, Year	Number of Subjects	Method of Analysis	Values (mg/24h ± S.E.M.)
195. Dajas, 1984	26 (major depressive episode, unipolar)	HPLC-EC	144 ± 18* (total)
	19 (non-psychotic)	HPLC-EC	133 ± 16*
	7 (psychotic)	HPLC-EC	195 ± 58*
	18 (recurrent)	HPLC-EC	159 ± 25*
	8 (first episode)	HPLC-EC	109 ± 16*
548. Maas, 1984	91 (unipolar + bipolar)	Fl	39.7 ± 2.5
196. Dajas, 1986	7 (phobic disorder)	HPLC-EC	29.2 ± 5.6*
	29 (panic disorder)	HPLC-EC	84.5 ± 16.7*
	36 (panic + phobia)	HPLC-EC	55.2 ± 9.9*
724. Roy, 1986	7 (major depression, no melancholia)	GC-MS	211 ± 29 (total)
	5 (history of melancholia)	GC-MS	330 ± 88 (total)
	8 (depression with melancholia)	GC-MS	331 ± 54 (total)
	8 (dysthymic disorder)	GC-MS	235 ± 22 (total)
	7 (M)	GC-MS	360 ± 64 (total)
	21 (F)	GC-MS	240 ± 22 (total)
105. Bowden, 1987	45 (unipolar)	Fl	46.2 ± 3.6
	13 (bipolar)	Fl	23.4 ± 3.1
	58 (combined)	Fl	41.1 ± 3.2
587. Mooney, 1988	9	HPLC-EC	53.4 ± 5.3

* In original paper expressed as ng/min.

Table 82. Unconjugated Noradrenaline in Urine of Schizophrenic Subjects

Reference First Author, Year	Number of Subjects	Method of Analysis	Values (mg/24h ± S.E.M.)
681. Pscheidt, 1964	9	Fl	28 ± 6
536. Lovegrove, 1965	12 (personality disorder)	Fl[†]	35
	10 (acute)	Fl	50 ± 11.6
	5 (chronic)	Fl	43 ± 12.3
806. Sloane, 1966	38	Fl	52.6
561. Mattok, 1967	22 (acute)	Fl	5.1
	22 (acute)	Fl	2.7 (conjugated)
666. Pollin, 1971	30 (15 pairs)	GC-ECD	39.6 mg/g Cr.
832. Subrahmanyam, 1975	30 (acute)	Fl	20.4 ± 1.2
	6 (acute aggressive)	Fl	50.6 ± 3.2
	24 (chronic)	Fl	32.4 ± 2.6
460. Kemali, 1982	16 (all)	REA[†]	35.9 ± 1.2
	12 (paranoid)	REA	35.0 ± 1.2
	4 (hebephrenic)	REA	38.6 ± 4.8
	12 (acute)	REA	35.4 ± 1.4
	4 (chronic)	REA	38.7 ± 3.0
61. Barbeito, 1984	13 (paranoid)	HPLC-EC	151.2 ± 26.6*

* In original paper expressed as ng/min.

Table 83. Unconjugated Noradrenaline in Plasma of Depressed Subjects

Reference First Author, Year	Number of Subjects	Method of Analysis	Values (pg/mL ± S.E.M.)
689. Reilly, 1957	19	Fl	3300 ± 420
175. Corona, 1982	48	Fl	200 ± 140
504. Lake, 1982	6 (depressed)	REA	315 ± 70
	6 (manic)	REA	376 ± 65
	14 (severely depressed)	REA	346 ± 56
	14 (in remission)	REA	322 ± 49
	54 (affective disorder)	REA	450
	15 (unipolar)	REA	550
	30 (bipolar, depressed)	REA	400
	9 (bipolar, manic)	REA	590
725. Roy, 1985	17 (unipolar, melancholia)	HPLC-EC	370 ± 39
	7 (bipolar)	HPLC-EC	122 ± 15
	10 (unipolar, major depressive episode)	HPLC-EC	220 ± 41
	11 (dysthymic disorder)	HPLC-EC	166 ± 18
728. Rudorfer, 1985	12 (bipolar)	HPLC-EC	161 ± 7
	12 (unipolar)	HPLC-EC	233 ± 10
790. Siever, 1986	11 (unipolar)	REA	351 ± 81
	7 (bipolar)	REA	268 ± 30
	18 (combined)	REA	319 ± 52

<u>Table 83.   Unconjugated Noradrenaline in Plasma of Depressed Subjects</u>

<u>(continued)</u>

Reference First Author, Year	Number of Subjects	Method of Analysis	Values (pg/mL ± S.E.M.)
719. Rothschild, 1987	18 (non-psychotic)	HPLC	438 ± 49
	4 (psychotic)	HPLC	366 ± 119
	22 (combined)	HPLC	425 ± 45
720. Roy, 1987	17 (unipolar)	HPLC-EC	318 ± 49
	6 (bipolar)	HPLC-EC	123 ± 17
	30 (all depressed)	HPLC-EC	248 ± 31
301. Gaffney, 1988	10 (panic attacks)	REA	161 ± 14
325. Golden, 1988	8 (unipolar + bipolar)	HPLC-EC	237 ± 51
775. Sevy, 1989	14 (anxiety)	HPLC-EC	199 ± 26
	14 (major depression)	HPLC-EC	103 ± 9

Table 84.   Unconjugated Noradrenaline in Plasma of Schizophrenic Subjects

Reference First Author, Year	Number of Subjects	Method of Analysis	Values (pg/mL ± S.E.M.)
926. Weil-Malherbe, 1954	8	Fl	6070 ± 540
689. Reilly, 1957	21	Fl	3300 ± 390
	4 (paranoid)	Fl	3300 ± 470
602. Naber, 1980	23 (M) (chronic)	REA	770 ± 80
	35 (F) (chronic)	REA	900 ± 80
976. Zander, 1981	13 (chronic)	REA	360 ± 28
138. Castellani, 1982	6 (paranoid)	REA	238 ± 42
	17 (undifferentiated)	REA	197 ± 20
	23 (combined)	REA	208 ± 18
	10 (schizoaffective)	REA	212 ± 50
460. Kemali, 1982	46	REA[†]	262 ± 12
	37 (paranoid)	REA	265 ± 13
	9 (hebephrenic)	REA	249 ± 14
	27 (acute)	REA	265 ± 14
	19 (chronic)	REA	260 ± 18
194. Dajas, 1983	32	HPLC-EC	377 ± 129
61. Barbeito, 1984	13	HPLC-EC	357 ± 32
97. Bondy, 1984	28	HPLC-EC	453 ± 54
	5 (hebephrenic)	HPLC-EC	302 ± 29
	20 (paranoid)	HPLC-EC	426 ± 55
	3 (schizoaffective)	HPLC-EC	913 ± 246

Table 85. Unconjugated Noradrenaline in CSF of Depressed Subjects

Reference First Author, Year	Number of Subjects	Method of Analysis	Values (pg/mL ± S.E.M.)
230. Dencker, 1966	13 (depressed)	Fl	700
	3 (manic)	Fl	500
672. Post, 1978	13 (depressed)	REA	210
	6 (manic)	REA	460
162. Christensen, 1980	15 (unipolar + bipolar)	REA	132
530. Linnoila, 1983	16	HPLC–EC	95 ± 8
77. Berrettini, 1984	10 (bipolar)	HPLC–EC	57 ± 11
789. Siever, 1984	12	REA	319 ± 62
78. Berrettini, 1985	12 (bipolar)	HPLC–EC	76 ± 13
726. Roy, 1985	15 (melancholia)	HPLC–EC	123 ± 15
	8 (major depressive episode)	HPLC–EC	118 ± 18
	5 (dysthymic disorder)	HPLC–EC	71 ± 11
723. Roy, 1988	28	HPLC–EC	131 ± 12

Table 86. Unconjugated Noradrenaline in CSF of Schizophrenic Subjects

Reference First Author, Year	Number of Subjects	Method of Analysis	Values (pg/mL ± S.E.M.)
926. Weil-Malherbe, 1954	8	Fl	3130 ± 190
230. Dencker, 1966	8	Fl	900
332. Gomes, 1980	10 (acute)	REA	216 ± 16
	11 (chronic)	REA	259 ± 14
	14 (psycho-organic)	REA	203 ± 12
	19 (personality disorder)	REA	195 ± 7
505. Lake, 1980	35	REA	125 ± 11
	14 (paranoid)	REA	144 ± 20
	10 (undifferentiated)	REA	101 ± 11
	11 (schizoaffective)	REA	122 ± 21
827. Sternberg, 1981	33	REA	125 ± 11
460. Kemali, 1982	8	REA[†]	151 ± 8
	5 (paranoid)	REA	160 ± 11
	3 (hebephrenic)	REA	138 ± 7
	3 (acute)	REA	159 ± 18
	5 (chronic)	REA	147 ± 9
310. Gattaz, 1983	13	HPLC-EC	163 ± 12
532. Linnoila, 1983	16 (explosive personality)	HPLC-EC	186 ± 25
	7 (antisocial)	HPLC-EC	203 ± 26
	7 (paranoid)	HPLC-EC	254 ± 51
530. Linnoila, 1983	28	HPLC-EC	123 ± 7
	19 (M)	HPLC-EC	123 ± 8
	9 (F)	HPLC-EC	125 ± 16

Table 86.   Unconjugated Noradrenaline in CSF of Schizophrenic Subjects

(continued)

Reference First Author, Year	Number of Subjects	Method of Analysis	Values (pg/mL ± S.E.M.)
755. Scheinin, 1984	46 (chronic)	HPLC-EC[†]	100 ± 5
773. Seppala, 1984	52 (chronic)	HPLC-EC[†]	162 ± 14
46. Bagdy, 1985	15	RIA	170 ± 10
309. Gattaz, 1985	13	HPLC-EC	163 ± 12
735. Saito, 1986	9 (with Parkinson's disease)	HPLC-EC	197 ± 29
	9 (with Tardive dyskinesis)	HPLC-EC	220 ± 36
644. Parnetti, 1987	13	HPLC-EC[†]	338 ± 140

Table 87. Unconjugated Adrenaline in Urine of Normal Subjects

Reference First Author, Year	Number of Subjects	Method of Analysis	Values (mg/24h ± S.E.M.)
437. Kärki, 1956	36 (M) 21 (F)	Fl[†] Fl	6.5 ± 0.7 4.2 ± 0.6
921. Watts, 1956	17	Fl,Bio	11.52 ± 1.87*
89. Bischoff, 1959	7	Fl[†]	8.16 ± 0.96**
796. Sjoerdsma, 1959	3	Fl	12.3 ± 3.8
30. Arnett, 1960	7 7	Bio Fl	6.24 ± 0.48** 5.04 ± 0.96**
60. Barbeau, 1961	24	Fl	17 ± 1.1
233. De Quattro, 1964	9	Fl[†]	12.96 ± 1.68**
536. Lovegrove, 1965	30	Fl[†]	31
648. Persson, 1965	7	Fl	6.7 ± 1.0
368. Hathaway, 1967	9 (M) (F)	Fl[†] Fl Fl	7.5 ± 0.7 8.9 ± 0.8 6.5 ± 0.6
561. Mattok, 1967	24	Fl	<0.48**
896. Viktora, 1968	9	Fl†	1.4 ± 0.17
135. Cardon, 1970	7	Fl	29.4
381. Hoeldtke, 1970	7	Fl[†]	4.66 ± 0.64
278. Fiorica, 1971	12	Fl[†]	9.1 ± 0.5
666. Pollin, 1971	8 (4 pairs of twins)	GC-ECD	5.3 mg/g Cr.
871. Turnbull, 1971	21	–	11 ± 1.3
850. Takahashi, 1972	10	Fl[†]	5.5 ± 0.5 mg/g Cr.
654. Peyrin, 1973	25	Fl[†]	20 ± 4
862. Townshend, 1973	30	Fl	7.1 ± 0.6
953. Wong, 1973	8	GC-ECD[†]	24.2 ± 1.4
183. Cuche, 1974	14	Fl	13.0 ± 1.4***

Table 87. Unconjugated Adrenaline in Urine of Normal Subjects

(continued)

Reference First Author, Year	Number of Subjects	Method of Analysis	Values (mg/24h ± S.E.M.)
474. Kissinger, 1975	10	HPLC-EC[†]	1.2 ± 0.4 mg/g Cr.
645. Pedersen, 1975	32	REA	7 mg/g Cr.
832. Subrahmanyam, 1975	12	Fl	7.9 ± 1.8
	12	Fl	7.2 ± 2.0
377. Higa, 1977	5	Fl[†]	10.6 ± 2.2
874. Ueda, 1977	–	Fl[†]	4.92 ± 0.83
923. Weidmann, 1977	14	Fl	4.38 ± 1.07 mg/g Cr
198. Dalmaz, 1978	34	Fl[†]	19 ± 3
234. DeSchaepdryver, 1978	20	Fl[†]	11.5 ± 0.9
359. Hallman, 1978	6	HPLC-EC[†]	40.3 ±18.3 mg/L
580. Modai, 1979	97	Fl	8.2
600. Muskiet, 1979	18	GC-MS[†]	12 ± 1.4 mg/g Cr.
199. Da Prada, 1980	6	REA	15 ± 4
21. Anderson, 1981	44	HPLC-EC[†]	4.85 ± 0.48 mg/L
140. Causon, 1982	10	HPLC-EC[†]	15.2 ± 3.6
259. Elchisak, 1982	6	HPLC-EC[†]	77.0 ±10.4
460. Kemali, 1982	14	REA[†]	11.2 ± 0.5
625. Oka, 1982	57	Fl[†]	9.3 ± 0.7
933. Westerink, 1982	47	HPLC[†]	12.1 ± 0.7
266. Eriksson, 1983	5	HPLC-EC[†]	8.0 ± 1.5
328. Goldstein, 1983	181	HPLC-EC[†]	7 ± 0.4
61. Barbeito, 1984	12	HPLC-EC	13.5 ± 5.9*
471. Kiriike, 1984	31	Fl	13.1 ± 0.7

Table 87. Unconjugated Adrenaline in Urine of Normal Subjects

(continued)

Reference First Author, Year	Number of Subjects	Method of Analysis	Values (mg/24h ± S.E.M.)
290. Frankenhaueser, 1986	19 (M) 30 (F)	GC-MS GC-MS	3.0 ± 0.3* 2.1 ± 0.2*
866. Tsuchiya, 1986	9	HPLC-Fl[†]	1.3 ± 0.2
17. Anderson, 1988	1 1	HPLC-EC[†] HPLC-Fl[†]	5.8 mg/L 7.0 mg/L
431. Julien, 1988	6	HPLC-EC[†]	6.4 ± 0.6
537. Lundberg, 1988	30 30	HPLC-EC Fl	6.3 ± 1.0* 9.6 ± 1.3*

*   In original paper expressed as ng/min.
**   In original paper expressed as mg/h.
*** In original paper expressed as mg/4h.

Table 88.   Conjugated Adrenaline in Urine of Normal Subjects

Reference First Author, Year	Number of Subjects	Method of Analysis	Values (mg/24h ± S.E.M.)
561. Mattok, 1967	24	Fl	<0.48**
896. Viktora, 1968	9	Fl[†]	0.3 ± 0.05
381. Hoeldtke, 1970	7	Fl[†]	6.06 ± 0.68
850. Takahashi, 1972	4	Fl[†]	16.2 ± 1.4 mg/g Cr
474. Kissinger, 1975	6	HPLC-EC[†]	12.8 ± 4.3 mg/g Cr
874. Ueda, 1977	–	Fl[†]	3.86 ± 0.80
199. Da Prada, 1980	6	REA	35 ± 7
259. Elchisak, 1982	6	HPLC-EC[†]	126.8 ± 44.3
25. Arakawa, 1983	11	HPLC-Fl[†]	18 ± 2.1 (3-sulfate)
	11	HPLC-Fl[†]	3 ± 0.3 (4-sulfate)
657. Peyrin, 1987	11	Fl	94 ± 15 (total) mg/g Cr.
529. Linnoila, 1988	12	GC-MS	9.2 ± 2.1 (total)

** In original paper expressed as mg/h.

Table 89. Unconjugated Adrenaline in Plasma of Normal, Supine Subjects

Reference First Author, Year	Number of Subjects	Method of Analysis	Values (pg/mL ± S.E.M.)
925. Weil-Malherbe, 1953	22 (M) 21 (F)	Fl Fl	1180 ± 40 1460 ± 80
551. Manger, 1954	7	Fl	140 ± 80
926. Weil-Malherbe, 1954	9	Fl	2320 ± 170
31. Aronow, 1956	6	Fl	400 ± 80 (venous)
168. Cohen, 1957	59	Fl[†]	60 ± 7
680. Price, 1957	12 12	Fl Fl	100 ± 3 (arterial) 10 ± 20 (venous)
689. Reilly, 1957	27	Fl	1200 ± 90
327. Goldfien, 1961	22	Fl[†]	48 ± 3
23. Anton, 1962	5	Fl[†]	480
355. Häggendal, 1963	13	Fl[†]	n.d.
563. McCullough, 1968	5	Fl[†]	20
896. Viktora, 1968	9	Fl[†]	n.d. (serum)
265. Engelman, 1970	22	REA[†]	50 ± 6
347. Griffiths, 1970	50	Fl[†]	40 ± 6
624. O'Hanlon, 1970	12	Fl[†]	79 ± 14
692. Renzini, 1970	12	Fl[†]	66 ± 4
791. Siggers, 1970	4	REA[†]	90 ± 50
53. Banister, 1972	5	Fl	90 ± 30
32. Aronow, 1973	3 3	REA REA	37 ± 6 (day) 31 ± 13 (night)
159. Christensen, 1973	16	REA	50 ± 12
402. Imai, 1973	6	GC-ECD[†]	<100
496. Kozlowski, 1973	64	Fl	420 ± 9
571. Meyer, 1973	5	Fl	10 ± 20

Table 89.   Unconjugated Adrenaline in Plasma of Normal, Supine Subjects

(continued)

Reference First Author, Year	Number of Subjects	Method of Analysis	Values (pg/mL ± S.E.M.)
160. Christensen, 1974	9	REA	60 ± 20
182. Cryer, 1974	18	REA[†]	41 ± 23
872. Turton, 1974	12	Fl	360 ± 70 (day)
	12	Fl	150 ± 20 (night)
157. Chodakowska, 1975	8	Fl	329 ± 59
645. Pedersen, 1975	26 (M)	REA	45
	6 (F)	REA	58
914. Wang, 1975	5	GC-MS[†]	800 ± 300
181. Cryer, 1975	10	REA	44 ± 4
200. Da Prada, 1976	7	REA[†]	47 ± 7
572. Michaels, 1976	18	REA	41 ± 5
581. Moerman, 1976	8	REA	160 ± 18 (venous)
929. Weise, 1976	13	REA[†]	67 ± 9
289. Franco-Morselli, 1977	11	REA	41 ± 5
389. Hörtnagl, 1977	11 (M)	REA	124 ± 23
	7 (F)	REA	130 ± 27
475. Klaniecki, 1977	6	REA,HPLC[†]	87 ± 25
653. Peuler, 1977	15	REA[†]	23 ± 5
815. Sole, 1977	3	REA[†]	96 ± 2
164. Chryssanthopoulos, 1978	9	Fl	690 ± 150
254. Ehrhardt, 1978	9	GC-ECD[†]	58 ± 12
704. Robertson, 1978	9	REA	36 ± 5
263. Endert, 1979	20	REA,HPLC[†]	61 ± 6
360. Hamaji, 1979	19	Fl[†]	70 ± 10
512. Le Blanc, 1979	12	REA	67 ± 7

Table 89.   Unconjugated Adrenaline in Plasma of Normal, Supine Subjects

(continued)

Reference First Author, Year	Number of Subjects	Method of Analysis	Values (pg/mL ± S.E.M.)
706. Robertson, 1979	15	REA[†]	29 ± 9
712. Romoff, 1979	13	REA	26 ± 4
881. Van Loon, 1979	5	REA	86 ± 11
898. Vlachakis, 1979	16	REA[†]	83 ± 12
199. Da Prada, 1980	5	REA	50 ± 10
236. Dimsdale, 1980	8	REA	164 ± 13
421. Johnson, 1980	10	REA	36 ± 4
975. Yui, 1980	10	HPLC-Fl[†]	32 ± 8
141. Causon, 1981	30 (sitting)	HPLC-EC[†]	81 ± 7
227. Demassieux, 1981	4	REA[†]	31 ± 8
330. Goldstein, 1981	7	HPLC-EC	53 ± 7
565. Mefford, 1981	5 (sitting)	HPLC-EC[†]	81 ± 16
687. Raum, 1981	–	RIA[†]	22
860. Thiede, 1981	9	REA[†]	39 ± 10
873. Uchikura, 1981	3	REA[†]	165 ± 9 (serum)
901. Vlachakis, 1981	36	REA	84 ± 16
960. Yamatodani, 1981	10	HPLC[†]	59 ± 11
4. Ackenheil, 1982	200	HPLC-EC	60 ± 2
429. Joyce, 1982	6	REA	48 ± 11
460. Kemali, 1982	45	REA[†]	37 ± 2
585. Montplaisir, 1982	11	REA	130 ± 37 (serum)
166. Claustre, 1983	6	REA	41 ± 6
244. Dunne, 1983	6	REA	30 ± 10

Table 89. Unconjugated Adrenaline in Plasma of Normal, Supine Subjects

(continued)

Reference First Author, Year	Number of Subjects	Method of Analysis	Values (pg/mL ± S.E.M.)
916. Wang, 1983	9	REA[†]	20 ± 10
917. Ward, 1983	8	HPLC-EC[†]	57
961. Yoneda, 1983	6	REA	38 ± 5
97. Bondy, 1984	40	HPLC-EC	70 ± 6
331. Goldstein, 1984	9	HPLC-EC[†]	32
559a.Maruta, 1984	–	HPLC-EC[†]	52 ± 2
718. Rothschild, 1984	12	HPLC-EC	216 ± 61
900. Vlachakis, 1984	5	REA[†]	40 ± 20
406. Ishimitsu, 1985	5	HPLC[†]	130 ± 80
686. Ratge, 1985	40	REA	60 ± 39
257. Eisenhofer, 1986	62	HPLC-EC	99 ± 11
74. Benedict, 1987	12	HPLC[†]	42 ± 8
719. Rothschild, 1987	6	HPLC	157 ± 53
872a.Tyce, 1987	6	HPLC-EC	80 ± 8
301. Gaffney, 1988	10	REA	13 ± 3
349. Guillemin, 1988	10	HPLC-EC[†]	57 ± 8
350a.Gullestad, 1988	8	REA	71 ± 17
400. Imai, 1988	6	HPLC-EC	80 ± 8

Table 90. Conjugated Adrenaline in Plasma of Normal, Supine Subjects

Reference First Author, Year	Number of Subjects	Method of Analysis	Values (pg/mL $\pm$ S.E.M.)
402. Imai, 1973	6	GC-ECD[†]	<100
914. Wang, 1975	5	GC-MS[†]	600 ± 200
199. Da Prada, 1980	5	REA	300 ± 75
421. Johnson, 1980	10	REA	286 ± 23 (sulfate)
227. Demassieux, 1981	4	REA[†]	23 ± 6
429. Joyce, 1982	6	REA	525 ± 234 (sulfate)
166. Claustre, 1983	6	REA	22 ± 6 (glucuronide)
	6	REA	82 ± 16 (sulfate)
916. Wang, 1983	9	REA[†]	trace (glucuronide)
	9	REA	100 ± 10 (sulfate)
961. Yoneda, 1983	6	REA	258 ± 20
900. Vlachakis, 1984	5	REA[†]	290 ± 280
184. Cuche, 1985	15	REA	168 ± 11 (sulfate)
406. Ishimitsu, 1985	5	HPLC[†]	640 ± 180
686. Ratge, 1985	40	REA	121 ± 81
872a. Tyce, 1987	6	HPLC-EC	<30 (sulfate)

Table 91. Unconjugated Adrenaline in CSF of Normal Subjects

Reference First Author, Year	Number of Subjects	Method of Analysis	Values (pg/mL ± S.E.M.)
926. Weil-Malherbe, 1954	9	Fl	900 ± 120
571. Meyer, 1973	5	Fl	n.d.
653. Peuler, 1977	5	REA[†]	5 ± 3
162. Christensen, 1980	18	REA	44
901. Vlachakis, 1981	36	REA	34 ± 9
460. Kemali, 1982	10	REA[†]	12.2 ± 0.8
585. Montplaisir, 1982	11	REA	49 ± 19
309. Gattaz, 1985	16	HPLC-EC	159 ± 85
686. Ratge, 1985	40 40	REA REA	27 ± 20 30 ± 34 (conj.)

<u>Table 92.   Unconjugated Adrenaline in Urine of Depressed Subjects</u>

Reference First Author, Year	Number of Subjects	Method of Analysis	Values (mg/24h ± S.E.M.)
831. Strom-Olsen, 1958	6 (depressed)	Fl	9.6 ± 1.1
	5 (manic)	Fl	19.5 ± 1.8
536. Lovegrove, 1965	7	Fl[†]	27 ± 5
806. Sloane, 1966	39 (depressed)	Fl	26.9
	7 (manic)	Fl	35.9
126. Bunney, 1967	8 (psychotic)	Fl	15.7
	8 (neurotic)	Fl	6.6
849. Takahashi, 1968	1 patient, 4 times (manic depressive)	Fl	9.7 ± 0.8
128. Bunney, 1970	3 (depressed)	Fl	5.6 ± 0.8
	3 (manic)	Fl	8.3 ± 1.4
346. Greenspan, 1970	3 (hypomanic)	Fl	20.3 ± 3.5
	2 (normothymic)	Fl	5.5 ± 1.8
	3 (agitated)	Fl	15.6 ± 1.1
127. Bunney, 1972	6 (depressed)	Fl	10.6 ± 1.6
	6 (manic)	Fl	18.6 ± 6.5
592. Murphy, 1977	4 (primary)	Fl	9 ± 2

Table 92. Unconjugated Adrenaline in Urine of Depressed Subjects

(continued)

Reference First Author, Year	Number of Subjects	Method of Analysis	Values (mg/24h ± S.E.M.)
761. Schildkraut, 1978	9 (schizophrenia related)	Fl	5.5 ± 1.0
	4 (schizoaffective)	Fl	10.2 ± 6.8
	12 (bipolar)	Fl	8.2 ± 1.2
	16 (unipolar- endogenous)	Fl	9.8 ± 1.0
	13 (unipolar- non-endogenous)	Fl	10.3 ± 1.4
	9 (unclassified)	Fl	9.5 ± 1.6
548. Maas, 1984	88 (unipolar + bipolar)	Fl	22.2 ± 1.4
105. Bowden, 1987	43 (unipolar)	Fl	25.8 ± 2.1
	17 (bipolar)	Fl	17.7 ± 1.8
	60 (combined)	Fl	23.5 ± 1.7
829. Stokes, 1987	29	GC-MS	26.9 ± 2.7
587. Mooney, 1988	9	HPLC-EC	12.0 ± 1.0

Table 93. Unconjugated Adrenaline in Urine of Schizophrenic Subjects

Reference First Author, Year	Number of Subjects	Method of Analysis	Values (mg/24h ± S.E.M.)
681. Pscheidt, 1964	9	Fl	8 ± 2
536. Lovegrove, 1965	18 (psychoneurotic, anxiety reaction)	Fl[†]	28
	20 (psychoneurotic, depression reaction)	Fl	36
	12 (personality disorder)	Fl	21
	10 (acute)	Fl	31 ± 5.6
	5 (chronic)	Fl	36 ± 10.4
806. Sloane, 1966	38	Fl	34.1
561. Mattok, 1967	22 (acute)	Fl	<0.5
666. Pollin, 1971	30 (15 pairs of twins)	GC-ECD	11.8 mg/g Cr.
832. Subrahmanyam, 1975	30 (acute)	Fl	4.3 ± 0.8
	6 (acute, aggressive)	Fl	10.6 ± 1.2
	24 (chronic)	Fl	6.8 ± 0.6
	24 (manic depressive, psychotic)	Fl	5.2 ± 0.6
460. Kemali, 1982	16	REA[†]	11.8 ± 0.4
	12 (paranoid)	REA	11.9 ± 1.5
	4 (hebephrenic)	REA	12.5 ± 1.7
	12 (acute)	REA	11.7 ± 0.5
	4 (chronic)	REA	12.5 ± 1.0

Table 93.   Unconjugated Adrenaline in Urine of Schizophrenic Subjects

(continued)

Reference First Author, Year	Number of Subjects	Method of Analysis	Values (μg/24h $\pm$ S.E.M.)
61. Barbeito, 1984	13 (paranoid)	HPLC-EC	7.4 $\pm$ 2.3*

* In original paper expressed as ng/min.

Table 94. Unconjugated Adrenaline in Plasma of Schizophrenic Subjects

Reference First Author, Year	Number of Subjects	Method of Analysis	Values (pg/mL ± S.E.M.)
926. Weil-Malherbe, 1954	8	Fl	1610 ± 190
689. Reilly, 1957	21	Fl	1100 ± 170
	4 (paranoid)	Fl	750 ± 220
460. Kemali, 1982	46 (combined)	REA[†]	36.8 ± 1.7
	37 (paranoid)	REA	36.6 ± 1.9
	9 (hebephrenic)	REA	37.7 ± 4.3
	27 (acute)	REA	35.9 ± 1.9
	19 (chronic)	REA	38.1 ± 3.2
97. Bondy, 1984	28 (combined)	HPLC-EC	84 ± 13
	20 (paranoid)	HPLC-EC	90 ± 16
	5 (hebephrenic)	HPLC-EC	59 ± 22
	3 (schizoaffective)	HPLC-EC	99 ± 57

Table 95. Unconjugated Adrenaline in Plasma and CSF of Depressed

Subjects

Reference First Author, Year	Number of Subjects	Method of Analysis	Values (pg/mL ± S.E.M.)
689. Reilly, 1957	19	Fl	1300 ± 160 (plasma)
162. Christensen, 1980	7 (unipolar + bipolar)	REA	16.0 ± 3.4 (CSF)
	7 (recovered)	REA	57.6 ± 13.0 (CSF)
719. Rothschild, 1987	22 (combined)	HPLC	87 ± 9 (plasma)
	18 (non-psychotic)	HPLC	85 ± 10
	4 (psychotic)	HPLC	97 ± 12
301. Gaffney, 1988	10 (panic attacks)	REA	16 ± 3 (plasma)

Table 96. Unconjugated Adrenaline in CSF of Schizophrenic Subjects

Reference First Author, Year	Number of Subjects	Method of Analysis	Values (pg/mL ± S.E.M.)
926. Weil-Malherbe, 1954	8	Fl	930 ± 130
460. Kemali, 1982	8 (combined)	REA[†]	14.2 ± 1.8
	5 (paranoid)	REA	13.3 ± 1.1
	3 (hebephrenic)	REA	15.6 ± 5.0
	3 (acute)	REA	12.1 ± 0.6
	5 (chronic)	REA	15.4 ± 2.8
309. Gattaz, 1985	13	HPLC-EC	225 ± 33

Table 97.   Unconjugated Dopamine in Urine of Normal Subjects

Reference First Author, Year	Number of Subjects	Method of Analysis	Values (mg/24h ± S.E.M.)
796. Sjoerdsma, 1959	3	Fl	245 ± 25
60. Barbeau, 1961	24	Fl	316 ± 15
90. Bischoff, 1962	10	Fl[†]	110 ± 9 mg/g Cr.
165. Clarke, 1967	14	GC-ECD[†]	150 ± 13 mg/g Cr.
561. Mattok, 1967	24	Fl	247**
809. Smith, 1969	15	Fl	176 ± 3
927. Weil-Malherbe, 1969	20 17 (M) 3 (F)	Fl[†] Fl Fl	126 ± 9 161 ± 15 115 ± 14
135. Cardon, 1970	7	Fl	292
381. Hoeldtke, 1970	7	Fl[†]	229 ± 39
569. Messiha, 1970	20	Fl	370 ± 81
256. Eichorn, 1971	28	Fl[†]	267 ± 15 mg/g Cr.
666. Pollin, 1971	8 (4 pairs of twins)	GC-ECD	147 mg/g Cr.
850. Takahashi, 1972	10	Fl[†]	91 ± 8 mg/g Cr.
951. Wong, 1973	8	GC-ECD[†]	402 ± 30
183. Cuche, 1974	14	Fl	588 ± 71***
474. Kissinger, 1975	10	HPLC-EC[†]	213 ± 49 mg/g Cr.
645. Pedersen, 1975	32	REA	222 mg/g Cr.
161. Christensen, 1976	46	REA	248 ± 22
566. Mell, 1977	10 80	HPLC[†] Fl	271 ± 21 235 ± 12
874. Ueda, 1977	–	Fl[†]	320 ± 56
198. Dalmaz, 1978	34	Fl[†]	385 ± 84

Table 97. Unconjugated Dopamine in Urine of Normal Subjects (continued)

Reference First Author, Year	Number of Subjects	Method of Analysis	Values (mg/24h ± S.E.M.)
234. De Schaepdryver, 1978	20	Fl[†]	255 ± 25
401. Imai, 1978	7	HPLC-Fl[†]	182 ± 15 mg/g Cr.
499. Kuchel, 1979	5	REA	547 ± 130*
580. Modai, 1979	97	Fl	204
600. Muskiet, 1979	18	GC-MS[†]	520 ± 53 mg/g Cr.
199. Da Prada, 1980	6	REA	325 ± 40
21. Anderson, 1981	44	HPLC-EC[†]	174 ± 183
259. Elchisak, 1982	6	HPLC-EC[†]	177 ± 31
260. Elchisak, 1982	4	HPLC-EC[†]	230 ± 34
441. Karoum, 1982	5	GC-MS[†]	735 ± 144
460. Kemali, 1982	14	REA[†]	292 ± 11
625. Oka, 1982	57	Fl[†]	120 ± 8
933. Westerink, 1982	48	HPLC[†]	225 ± 9
266. Eriksson, 1983	5	HPLC-EC[†]	208 ± 26
328. Goldstein, 1983	181	HPLC-EC[†]	278 ± 14
61. Barbeito, 1984	12	HPLC-EC	46.4± 7.9*
471. Kiriike, 1984	31	Fl	336 ± 25
866. Tsuchiya, 1986	9	HPLC-Fl[†]	89 ± 14
17. Anderson, 1988	1 1	HPLC-EC[†] HPLC-Fl[†]	90 mg/L 88 mg/L
431. Julien, 1988	6	HPLC-EC[†]	304 ± 18
251. Echizen, 1989	19	HPLC-EC, UV	330 ± 25 mg/g Cr.

*   In original paper expressed as ng/min.
**   In original paper expressed as mg/h.
*** In original paper expressed as mg/4h.

Table 98. Conjugated Dopamine in Urine of Normal Subjects

Reference First Author, Year	Number of Subjects	Method of Analysis	Values (mg/24h ± S.E.M.)
499. Kuchel, 1979	5	REA	2275 ± 300*
199. Da Prada, 1980	6	REA	900 ± 125
259. Elchisak, 1982	6	HPLC-EC[†]	409 ± 98
260. Elchisak, 1982	4	HPLC-EC[†]	415 ± 82
	4	HPLC-EC	329 ± 93 (3-sulfate)
	4	HPLC-EC	n.d. (4-sulfate)
25. Arakawa, 1983	11	HPLC-Fl[†]	420 ± 72 (3-sulfate)
	11	HPLC-Fl[†]	98 ± 17 (4-sulfate)
959. Yamamoto, 1985	5	HPLC-Fl[†]	381 ± 55 (3-sulfate)*
	5	HPLC-Fl	59 ± 4 (4-sulfate)*
724. Roy, 1986	25	GC-MS	642 ± 79 (total)
844. Swann, 1986	6	HPLC-EC[†]	861 ± 483 (3-sulfate)
	6	HPLC-EC	558 ± 337 (4-sulfate)
657. Peyrin, 1987	11	Fl	737 ± 86 (total) mg/g Cr.
529. Linnoila, 1988	12	GC-MS	688 ± 118 (total)

* In original paper expressed as ng/min.

Table 99. Unconjugated Dopamine in Plasma of Normal Subjects

Reference First Author, Year	Number of Subjects	Method of Analysis	Values (pg/mL ± S.E.M.)
158. Christensen, 1973	6	REA[†]	200 ± 25
402. Imai, 1973	6	GC-ECD[†]	700 ± 360
914. Wang, 1975	5	GC-MS[†]	2000 ± 900
161. Christensen, 1976	46	REA	330 ± 60
200. Da Prada, 1976	7	REA[†]	127 ± 20
131. Buu, 1977	17	REA[†]	n.d.
289. Franco-Morselli, 1977	11	REA	46 ± 6
475. Klaniecki, 1977	6	REA, HPLC[†]	33 ± 28
653. Peuler, 1977	15	REA[†]	34 ± 8
815. Sole, 1977	3	REA[†]	53 ± 1
254. Ehrhardt, 1978	9	GC-ECD[†]	48 ± 10
359. Hallman, 1978	6	HPLC-EC[†]	<8
360. Hamaji, 1979	26	Fl[†]	220 ± 30
499. Kuchel, 1979	5	REA	n.d.
706. Robertson, 1979	15	REA[†]	55 ± 16
712. Romoff, 1979	13	REA	108 ± 9
771. Seki, 1979	26	Fl[†]	230 ± 33
881. Van Loon, 1979	5	REA	55 ± 9
199. Da Prada, 1980	5	REA	50 ± 10
421. Johnson, 1980	10	REA	62 ± 5
141. Causon, 1981	30	HPLC-EC[†]	n.d.
237. Demassieux, 1981	4	REA[†]	19 ± 12
565. Mefford, 1981	5	HPLC-EC[†]	29 ± 3
860. Thiede, 1981	9	REA	63 ± 25

Table 99. Unconjugated Dopamine in Plasma of Normal Subjects (continued)

Reference First Author, Year	Number of Subjects	Method of Analysis	Values (pg/mL ± S.E.M.)
873. Uchikura, 1981	3	REA[t]	186 ± 30 (serum)
941. Wilkes, 1981	6	REA	42 ± 9
4. Ackenheil, 1982	200	HPLC-EC	<30
460. Kemali, 1982	45	REA[t]	55 ± 4
585. Montplaisir, 1982	11	REA	90 ± 23 (serum)
166. Claustre, 1983	6	REA	285 ± 30
244. Dunne, 1983	6	REA	n.d.
916. Wang, 1983	9	REA[t]	50 ± 10
961. Yoneda, 1983	6	REA	10 ± 6
97. Bondy, 1984	40	HPLC-EC	18 ± 1.4
331. Goldstein, 1984	9	HPLC-EC[t]	66
559a.Maruta, 1984	–	HPLC-EC[t]	26 ± 1
718. Rothschild, 1984	12	HPLC-EC	50 ± 5
900. Vlachakis, 1984	5	REA[t]	80 ± 22
406. Ishimitsu, 1985	5	HPLC[t]	290 ± 80
686. Ratge, 1985	40	REA	47 ± 22
257. Eisenhofer, 1986	62	HPLC-EC	63 ± 4
74. Benedict, 1987	12	HPLC[t]	39 ± 6
719. Rothschild, 1987	6	HPLC	43 ± 4
872a.Tyce, 1987	6	HPLC-EC	<30
349. Guillemin, 1988	10	HPLC-EC[t]	40 ± 4
350a.Gullestad, 1988	8	REA	72 ± 20
400. Imai, 1988	20	HPLC-EC[t]	14 ± 1

Table 100. Conjugated Dopamine in Plasma of Normal Subjects

Reference First Author, Year	Number of Subjects	Method of Analysis	Values (pg/mL ± S.E.M.)
402. Imai, 1973	6	GC-ECD[†]	3570 ± 1110
914. Wang, 1975	5	GC-MS[†]	14000 ± 900
131. Buu, 1977	17	REA[†]	740 ± 170
499. Kuchel, 1979	5	REA	980 ± 100
199. Da Prada, 1980	5	REA	2800 ± 200
421. Johnson, 1980	10	REA	6288 ± 773 (sulfate)
227. Demassieux, 1981	4	REA[†]	1060 ± 160
166. Claustre, 1983	6	REA	924 ± 121 (glucuronide)
	6	REA	3426 ± 356 (sulfate)
916. Wang, 1983	9	REA[†]	trace (glucuronide)
	9	REA	2490 ± 300 (sulfate)
961. Yoneda, 1983	6	REA	4066 ± 529
900. Vlachakis, 1984	5	REA[†]	8500 ± 4240
184. Cuche, 1985	15	REA	3115 ± 174 (sulfate)
406. Ishimitsu, 1985	5	HPLC[†]	1700 ± 260
500. Kuchel, 1985	34	REA	1714 ± 122 (sulfate)
686. Ratge, 1985	40	REA	2783 ± 1461
959. Yamamoto, 1985	10	HPLC-Fl[†]	4054 ± 537 (3-sulfate)
	10	HPLC-Fl	410 ± 16 (4-sulfate)
861. Toth, 1986;	6	HPLC-EC[†]	3718 ± 780 (3-sulfate)
765. Scott, 1987	6	HPLC-EC[†]	1377 ± 230 (4-sulfate)
872a. Tyce, 1987	6	HPLC-EC	4070 ± 780 (sulfate)

Table 101. Unconjugated (and Conjugated) Dopamine in CSF of Normal

Subjects

Reference First Author, Year	Number of Subjects		Method of Analysis	Values (pg/mL ± S.E.M.)
653. Peuler, 1977	5		REA[†]	3600 ± 1000
162. Christensen, 1980	18		REA	n.d.
379. Hiramatsu, 1982	75		HPLC-Fl	1400 ± 67
	55	(M)	HPLC-Fl	1440 ± 85
	20	(F)	HPLC-Fl	1180 ± 96
460. Kemali, 1982	10		REA[†]	53 ± 2
585. Montplaisir, 1982	11		REA	158 ± 28
45. Bagdy, 1983	21	(F)	REA	2810 ± 230
	6	(M)	REA	2920 ± 390
310. Gattaz, 1983	15		HPLC-EC	207 ± 68
755. Scheinin, 1984	54		HPLC-EC[†]	719 ± 46 (conj.)
773. Seppala, 1984	25		HPLC-EC[†]	37 ± 8*
78. Berrettini, 1985	23		HPLC-EC	522 ± 62 (sulfate)
309. Gattaz, 1985	16		HPLC-EC	207 ± 66
686. Ratge, 1985	40		REA	41 ± 19
	40		REA	610 ± 218 (conj.)

* 72 samples measured; in 47 no dopamine was detected; this value is the mean for the 25 samples in which dopamine was detected.

Table 102.   Unconjugated (and Conjugated) Dopamine in Urine of Depressed

Subjects

Reference First Author, Year	Number of Subjects	Method of Analysis	Values (mg/24h ± S.E.M.)
831. Strom-Olsen, 1958	6 (depressed)	Fl	324 ± 88
	5 (manic)	Fl	423 ± 46
806. Sloane, 1966	39 (depressed)	Fl	185.0
	7 (manic)	Fl	344.0
126. Bunney, 1967	8 (psychotic)	Fl	280
	8 (neurotic)	Fl	212
849. Takahashi, 1968	1 patient, 3 times (manic-depressive)	Fl	430 ± 30
128. Bunney, 1970	3 (depressed)	Fl	153 ± 31
	3 (manic)	Fl	276 ± 81
569. Messiha, 1970	6 (depressed)	Fl	520
	7 (manic)	Fl	710
	6 (depressed)	Fl	180 (conjugated)
	7 (manic)	Fl	410 (conjugated)
127. Bunney, 1972	6 (depressed)	Fl	193.0 ± 20.0
	6 (manic)	Fl	218.0 ± 19.0
593. Murphy, 1973	6 (bipolar)	Fl	170 ± 40
	6 (unipolar)	Fl	210 ± 30
441. Karoum, 1982	6	GC-MS[†]	604 ±160
451. Karoum, 1982	6 (unipolar + bipolar)	GC-MS	483 ± 69

Table 102. Unconjugated (and Conjugated) Dopamine in Urine of Depressed

Subjects (continued)

Reference First Author, Year	Number of Subjects	Method of Analysis	Values (mg/24h ± S.E.M.)
525. Linnoila, 1982	4 (bipolar)	GC-MS	636 ± 134 (total)
528. Linnoila, 1983	7 (unipolar + bipolar)	GC-MS	762 ± 111 (total)
524. Linnoila, 1983	12 (unipolar + bipolar)	GC-MS	964 ± 199 (total)
724. Roy, 1986	7 (no melancholia)	GC-MS	716 ± 136 (total)
	5 (melancholia history)	GC-MS	571 ± 113 (total)
	8 (with melancholia)	GC-MS	662 ± 118 (total)
	8 (dysthymic disorder)	GC-MS	794 ± 175 (total)

Table 103. Unconjugated Dopamine in Urine of Schizophrenic Patients

Reference First Author, Year	Number of Subjects	Method of Analysis	Values (mg/24h ± S.E.M.)
681. Pscheidt, 1964	9	Fl	155 ± 30
806. Sloane, 1966	38	Fl	199
561. Mattok, 1967	22 (acute)	Fl	127*
	22 (acute)	Fl	446* (conjugated)
666. Pollin, 1971	30 (15 pairs of twins)	GC-ECD	196 mg/g Cr.
460. Kemali, 1982	16	REA[†]	291 ± 21
	12 (paranoid)	REA	283 ± 10
	4 (hebephrenic)	REA	318 ± 25
	12 (acute)	REA	293 ± 7
	4 (chronic)	REA	320 ± 16
61. Barbeito, 1984	13 (paranoid)	HPLC-EC	115.5 ± 5.2**

*   In original paper expressed as mg/h.
** In original paper expressed as ng/min.

Table 104. Unconjugated Dopamine in Plasma of

Schizophrenic Patients

Reference First Author, Year	Number of Subjects	Method of Analysis	Values (pg/mL ± S.E.M.)
460. Kemali, 1982	46 (combined)	REA[†]	54.0 ± 3.2
	37 (paranoid)	REA	53.5 ± 3.6
	9 (hebephrenic)	REA	54.2 ± 6.9
	27 (acute)	REA	50.2 ± 3.3
	19 (chronic)	REA	59.3 ± 6.1
97. Bondy, 1984	28 (combined)	HPLC-EC	42 ± 7.2
	20 (paranoid)	HPLC-EC	42 ± 9.8
	5 (hebephrenic)	HPLC-EC	24 ± 6.7
	3 (schizoaffective)	HPLC-EC	59 ± 12

Table 105. Unconjugated (and Conjugated) Dopamine in CSF of

Schizophrenic Patients

Reference First Author, Year	Number of Subjects	Method of Analysis	Values (pg/mL ± S.E.M.)
460. Kemali, 1982	8	REA[†]	54.9 ± 1.4
	5 (paranoid)	REA	55.7 ± 1.9
	3 (hebephrenic)	REA	53.5 ± 2.4
	3 (acute)	REA	55.9 ± 2.6
	5 (chronic)	REA	54.3 ± 1.8
310. Gattaz, 1983; 309. Gattaz, 1985	13	HPLC-EC	200 ± 35
755. Scheinin, 1984	46 (chronic)	HPLC-EC[†]	673 ± 47 (conjugated)
	46 (chronic)	HPLC-EC	566 ± 36 (sulfate)
46. Bagdy, 1985	15 (chronic)	REA	3090 ± 830
644. Parnetti, 1987	13	HPLC-Fl[†]	3060 ± 1100

Table 106. Unconjugated (and Conjugated) Dopamine in Plasma and CSF of

Depressed Subjects

Reference First Author, Year	Number of Subjects	Method of Analysis	Values (pg/mL ± S.E.M.)
162. Christensen, 1980	7	REA	12 (CSF)
755. Scheinin, 1984	161 (primary affective disorder)	HPLC-EC[†]	765 ± 30 (conj.) (CSF)
77. Berrettini, 1984; 78. Berrettini, 1985	7 (euthymic, bipolar)	HPLC-EC	771 ± 118 (sulfate) (CSF)
726. Roy, 1985	15 (melancholic)	HPLC-EC	679 ± 98 (sulfate) (CSF)
	8 (major episode)	HPLC-EC	642 ± 65 (sulfate) (CSF)
	5 (dysthymic disorder)	HPLC-EC	845 ± 320 (sulfate) (CSF)
719. Rothschild, 1987	22 (all depressed)	HPLC	93 ± 20 (plasma)
	18 (non-psychotic)	HPLC	51 ± 4 (plasma)
	4 (psychotic)	HPLC	282 ± 12 (plasma)

Table 107.   Catecholamines in Urine of Subjects with Parkinson's Disease

Reference First Author, Year	Number of Subjects	Method of Analysis	Values (mg/24h ± S.E.M.)
60. Barbeau, 1961	16	Fl	40 ± 5 (NA)
	16	Fl	15 ± 0.4 (A)
	16	Fl	241 ± 21.5 (DA)
90. Bischoff, 1962	7	Fl[†]	168 ± 24 (DA)*
632. O'Reilly, 1965	6	Fl	330 ± 78 (DA) mg/g Cr.
809. Smith, 1969	19	Fl	204 ± 11 (DA)
927. Weil-Malherbe, 1969	34	Fl[†]	67.5 ± 3.2 (DA)
	20 (M)	Fl	97.8 ± 7.0 (DA)
	14 (F)	Fl	73.3 ± 5.5 (DA)
	34	Fl	230 ± 11.9 (conj.)
	20 (M)	Fl	281 ± 20.1 (conj.)
	14 (F)	Fl	299 ± 38 (conj.)

* In original paper expressed as mg/h.

Table 108. Catecholamines in CSF of Subjects with Alzheimer's Disease

Reference First Author, Year	Number of Subjects	Method of Analysis	Values (pg/mL ± S.E.M.)
685. Raskind, 1984	7 (advanced Alzheimer's disease)	REA	411 ± 25 (NA)
	7 (moderate Alzheimer's disease)	REA	250 ± 27 (NA)
816. Sparks, 1985	4 (Alzheimer's disease)	HPLC-EC†	34 ± 9 (NA)
644. Parnetti, 1987	12 (Alzheimer's disease)	HPLC†	338 ± 147 (NA)
	12 (Alzheimer's disease)	HPLC†	2142 ± 884 (DA)

Table 109. Unconjugated 5-Hydroxytryptamine in Urine of Normal Subjects

Reference First Author, Year	Number of Subjects	Method of Analysis	Values (mg/24h ± S.E.M.)
709. Rodnight, 1956	11	Fl[†]	90 ± 7
710. Rodnight, 1961	26	Fl	68
	20 (M)	Fl	72
	6 (F)	Fl	55
216. Davis, 1965	21	Fl[†]	131
33. Arterberry, 1967	23	Fl[†]	127 ± 10*
890. Van Praag, 1968	4	Fl	149 ± 18
491. Korf, 1970	5	Fl	79.6 ± 17.7
176. Coutts, 1981	12	GC-ECD[†]	139 ± 65

* In original paper expressed as mg/h.

Table 110. Conjugated 5-Hydroxytryptamine in Urine of Normal Subjects

Reference First Author, Year	Number of Subjects	Method of Analysis	Values (mg/24h ± S.E.M.)
216. Davis, 1965	21	Fl[†]	93 (glucuronide)
	21	Fl	59 (sulfate)
491. Korf, 1970	5	Fl	34 ± 9.3 (glucuronide)
	5	Fl	52 ± 13.2 (sulfate)

<u>Table 111.   5-Hydroxytryptamine in Plasma of Normal Subjects</u>

Reference First Author, Year	Number of Subjects	Method of Analysis	Values (ng/mL ± S.E.M.)
215. Davis, 1959	50	Fl[†]	210 (serum)
274. Feldstein, 1959	15 (M)	Fl	190 ± 20
	2 (F)	Fl	150 ± 10
641. Pare, 1960	7	Fl	130 ± 16 (serum)
178. Crawford, 1963	18	Fl	20.9 ± 2.5
179. Crawford, 1965	27	Fl	13 ± 1.2
348. Guilbaut, 1974	25	Fl[†]	98 ± 1.6 (serum)
227a.Demet, 1978	6	Fl[†]	0.0
750. Sasa, 1978	23	HPLC-EC[†]	146 ± 46 (serum)
293. Frattini, 1979	10	Fl[†]	122 ± 13.5 (platelet-rich)
	10	Fl	7.1 ± 0.75 (platelet-poor)
483. Koch, 1979	7	HPLC-EC[†]	13.3 ± 3.0 (plasma)
	7	HPLC-EC	39.5 ± 15.5 (serum)
484. Koch, 1980	1	HPLC-EC[†]	3.31 (plasma)
	1	HPLC-EC[†]	72.1 (serum)
782. Shen, 1979	68	Bio	68 ± 4
398. Hussain, 1981	–	REA[†]	3.98 (platelet-poor)
	–	REA	256.6 (platelet-rich)
264. Engbaek, 1982	14	RIA[†]	1.58± 0.14 (plasma)
	10 (M)	RIA	91.5 ± 5.2 (serum)
	10 (F)	RIA	122.3 ± 6.1 (serum)
44. Baba, 1984	5	GC-MS[†]	295.0 ± 9.2
378. Hindberg, 1984	39	REA[†]	1.44 (platelet-poor)
35. Artigas, 1985	15	HPLC[†]	2.60 ± 0.23
658. Picard, 1985	10 (M)	HPLC-EC[†]	2.71 ± 0.20
	10 (F)	HPLC-EC	1.83 ± 0.28

Table 111. 5-Hydroxytryptamine in Plasma of Normal Subjects (continued)

Reference First Author, Year	Number of Subjects	Method of Analysis	Values (ng/mL ± S.E.M.)
34. Artigas, 1986	58	HPLC-Fl	0.88 ± 0.08
18. Anderson, 1987	7	HPLC-Fl[†]	0.587± 0.105 (platelet-poor)
	7	HPLC-Fl	0.387± 0.084 (ultrafiltrate)
397a.Hussain, 1987	22	REA	1.04 ± 0.06
636. Palmerini, 1987	15	HPLC-Fl[†]	2.1 ± 0.21 (platelet-poor)
749. Sarrias, 1987	20	HPLC-EC,Fl	2.57
400. Imai, 1988	20	HPLC-EC[†]	2.4 ± 0.3

Table 112.   Unconjugated 5-Hydroxytryptamine in CSF of Normal Subjects

Reference First Author, Year	Number of Subjects	Method of Analysis	Values (ng/mL ± S.E.M.)
461. Kemerer, 1979	–	Fl	0 – 13
584. Montplaisir, 1982	11	REA	1.965 ± 0.333
378. Hindberg, 1984	9	REA[†]	0.026 – 3.52
35. Artigas, 1985	8	HPLC[†]	0.302 ± 0.099
906. Volicer, 1985	17	HPLC-EC	12.7 ± 2.6
907. Volicer, 1985	9	HPLC-EC[†]	0.40 ± 0.14 (caudal)
522. Linnoila, 1986	20	HPLC-EC[†]	1.03 ± 0.07
495. Koyama, 1988	5	HPLC-EC[†]	0.37 ± 0.10

Table 113.   Unconjugated 5-Hydroxytryptamine in Urine of

Schizophrenic and Depressed Subjects

Reference First Author, Year	Number of Subjects	Method of Analysis	Values (mg/24h ± S.E.M.)
710. Rodnight, 1961	22 (schizophrenics)	Fl	51
	12 (M)	Fl	54
	10 (F)	Fl	47
	18 (depressed)	Fl	47
	8 (M)	Fl	40
	10 (F)	Fl	54
890. Van Praag, 1968	20 (depressed)	Fl	183 ± 18
524. Linnoila, 1983	12 (unipolar + bipolar)	HPLC	143 ± 61

Table 114. Unconjugated 5-Hydroxytryptamine in Plasma and CSF of

Depressed and Schizophrenic Subjects

Reference First Author, Year	Number of Subjects	Method of Analysis	Values (ng/mL ± S.E.M.)
274. Feldstein, 1959	22 (chronic)	Fl	170 ± 10
	13 (M) (acute)	Fl	130 ± 20
	2 (F) (acute)	Fl	70 ± 20
641. Pare, 1960	3	Fl	89 ± 3 (serum)
782. Shen, 1979	100	Bio	50 ± 3
	60 (other psychoses)	Bio	66 ± 3
644. Parnetti, 1987	13	HPLC-EC[†]	0.53 ± 0.44 (CSF)
749. Sarrias, 1987	18 (melancholic, depressed)	HPLC-EC,Fl	0.85

Table 115. Unconjugated 5-Hydroxytryptamine in CSF of

Alzheimer's Disease Subjects

Reference First Author, Year	Number of Subjects	Method of Analysis	Values (ng/mL ± S.E.M.)
906. Volicer, 1985	9 (Alzheimer's)	HPLC-EC	12.1 ± 3.9
	2 (pre-senile)	HPLC-EC	14.3 ± 5.1
	7 (senile)	HPLC-EC	11.5 ± 5.0
	10 (Parkinson's)	HPLC-EC	7.8 ± 2.3
907. Volicer, 1985	10 (caudal Alzheimer's)	HPLC-EC[†]	0.11± 0.01
	14 (rostral Alzheimer's)	HPLC-EC	0.30± 0.13
644. Parnetti, 1987	12	HPLC-EC[†]	n.d.
495. Koyama, 1988	6	HPLC-EC[†]	0.47± 0.09

Table 116. Unconjugated Normetanephrine in Urine of Normal Subjects

Reference First Author, Year	Number of Subjects	Method of Analysis	Values (mg/24h ± S.E.M.)
663. Pisano, 1960	30	Fl[†]	600 ± 55 (incl. MN)
664. Pisano, 1961	12	Fl	400 (incl. MN)
966. Yoshinaga, 1961	8	Fl[†]	176 ± 20
855. Taniguchi, 1964	6	Fl[†]	21.2 ± 2.4
433. Kahane, 1967	15	Fl[†]	196 ± 23
561. Mattok, 1967	24	Fl	216*
86. Bigelow, 1968	16	Fl[†]	130 ± 16
936. Wilk, 1968	45	Fl	78 mg/g Cr.
79. Bertani, 1970	16	GC-ECD[†]	116 ± 7 mg/g Cr.
135. Cardon, 1970	7	Fl	366
666. Pollin, 1971	8 (4 pairs of twins)	GC-ECD	141 mg/g Cr.
879. Van de Calseyde, 1971	18	GC-FID[†]	670 ± 50 (incl. MN)
679. Prange, 1972	10	Fl	250 ± 33
223. De Leon-Jones, 1973	12	Fl	191
224. De Leon-Jones, 1975	21	Fl	207 ± 27
541. Maas, 1975	19 (M) 21 (F)	– –	196 ± 17 223 ± 33
786. Shoup, 1977	–	HPLC-EC[†]	238 ± 80 (S.D.)
234. De Schaepdryver, 1977	20	Fl[†]	136 ± 14
704. Robertson, 1978	9	GC-MS	469 ± 22*
705. Robertson, 1978	7	GC-MS[†]	379 ± 13
899. Vlachakis, 1978	22	REA[†]	24 ± 2.6 mg/g Cr.

Table 116. Unconjugated Normetanephrine in Urine of Normal Subjects

(continued)

Reference First Author, Year	Number of Subjects	Method of Analysis	Values (mg/24h ± S.E.M.)
600. Muskiet, 1979	13	GC-MS[†]	212 ± 25 mg/g Cr.
614. Nelson, 1979	12	GC-ECD[†]	167 ± 27
81. Bertani-Dziedzic, 1981	7	HPLC-EC[†]	140 ± 8
176. Coutts, 1981	12	GC-ECD[†]	28 ± 5
441. Karoum, 1982	5	GC-MS[†]	275 ± 41
430. Jouve, 1983	30	HPLC-EC[†]	138 ± 12 mg/g Cr.
489. Kopin, 1983	12	REA[†]	274 ± 20
493. Koslow, 1983	77	Fl	192 ± 8
	41 (F)	Fl	189 ± 12
	36 (M)	Fl	195 ± 11
471. Kiriike, 1984	31	Fl	118 ± 8
790. Siever, 1986	18	GC-MS	293 ± 24
287. Foti, 1987	6	HPLC-EC	424*
	6	Fl	445*
431. Julien, 1988	6	HPLC-EC[†]	18.7 ± 3.4

* In original paper expressed in mg/h.

Table 117. Conjugated Normetanephrine in Urine of Normal Subjects

Reference First Author, Year	Number of Subjects	Method of Analysis	Values (mg/24h ± S.E.M.)
807. Smith, 1962	19	Fl[†]	159 ± 18 (total)
233. De Quattro, 1964	9	Fl[†]	235 ± 26 (total)*
855. Taniguchi, 1964	6	Fl[†]	223 ± 28
730. Ruthven, 1965	18	Fl[†]	500 ± 33 (total) (incl. MN)
177. Coward, 1966	17	Fl[†]	130 ± 10 mg/g Cr. (total)
561. Mattok, 1967	24	Fl	139*
544. Maas, 1968	11	Fl	117 ± 21 mg/g Cr.
352. Gupta, 1973	100	Fl[†]	500 mg/g Cr. (total) (incl. MN)
526. Linnoila, 1982	12	GC-MS	258 ± 56 (total)
911. Waldmeier, 1983	5	HPLC-EC[†]	232 ± 22 mg/g Cr. (total)
724. Roy, 1986	25	GC-MS	137 ± 9 (total)
657. Peyrin, 1987	11	Fl	762 ±124 mg/g Cr. (total)
529. Linnoila, 1988	12	GC-MS	322 ± 34 (total)

* In original paper expressed in mg/h.

Table 118. Unconjugated Normetanephrine in Urine of Depressed Subjects

Reference First Author, Year	Number of Subjects	Method of Analysis	Values (mg/24h ± S.E.M.)
807. Smith, 1962	10 (anxiety)	Fl[†]	173 ± 46 (total)
613. Nelson, 1966	6 (includes schizophrenics)	Fl	190 ± 9 mg/g Cr.
757. Schildkraut, 1966	3 (depressed)	Fl	308 ± 16
	3 (depressed)	Fl	508 ± 39
126. Bunney, 1967	8 (psychotic)	Fl	49.6
	8 (neurotic)	Fl	40.5
544. Maas, 1968	16 (severe)	Fl	112 ± 20 mg/g Cr.
346. Greenspan, 1970	3 (hypomanic)	Fl	512 ± 45
	2 (normothymic)	Fl	388 ± 72
	3 (agitated)	Fl	509 ±162
679. Prange, 1972	12 (primary)	Fl	316 ± 70
223. De Leon-Jones, 1973	1 (depressed)	Fl	99
	1 (manic)	Fl	206
224. De Leon-Jones, 1975	5 (bipolar)	Fl	187 ± 30
	14 (single episode, (unipolar)	Fl	207 ± 25
	13 (recurrent unipolar)	Fl	182 ± 27
541. Maas, 1975;	20 (M)	–	172 ± 17
542. Mass, 1978	48 (F)	–	214 ± 17
592. Murphy, 1977	4 (primary)	Fl	320 ± 30

<u>Table 118.   Unconjugated Normetanephrine in Urine of Depressed Subjects</u>

<u>(continued)</u>

Reference First Author, Year	Number of Subjects	Method of Analysis	Values (mg/24h ± S.E.M.)
761. Schildkraut, 1978	9 (schizophrenia (related)	Fl	214 ± 44
	4 (schizoaffective)	Fl	285 ± 34
	12 (bipolar)	Fl	225 ± 26
	16 (unipolar endogenous)	Fl	323 ± 43
	13 (unipolar (non-endogenous)	Fl	247 ± 27
	9 (unclassified)	Fl	209 ± 12
441. Karoum, 1982	6	GC-MS[†]	273 ± 35
452. Karoum, 1982	6 (unipolar + bipolar)	GC-MS	505 ±146
527. Linnoila, 1982	12 (unipolar + bipolar)	GC-MS	379 ± 83
525. Linnoila, 1982	4 (bipolar)	GC-MS	303 ± 70
526. Linnoila, 1982	12 (unipolar + bipolar)	GC-MS	258 ± 56
523. Linnoila, 1982	8 (unipolar)	GC-MS	324 ± 74
	8 (bipolar)	GC-MS	260 ± 74
493. Koslow, 1983; 548. Maas, 1984	117 (depressed)	Fl	279 ± 16
	63 (M)	Fl	280 ± 23
	54 (F)	Fl	278 ± 22
	17 (manic)	Fl	299 ± 35
	11 (M)	Fl	329 ± 49
	6 (F)	Fl	246 ± 34
524. Linnoila, 1983	12 (unipolar + (bipolar)	GC-MS	421 ± 95

Table 118. Unconjugated Normetanephrine in Urine of Depressed Subjects

(continued)

Reference First Author, Year	Number of Subjects	Method of Analysis	Values (mg/24h ± S.E.M.)
724. Roy, 1986	7 (without melancholia)	GC-MS	145 ± 24 (total)
	5 (melancholia history)	GC-MS	245 ± 39 (total)
	8 (with melancholia)	GC-MS	227 ± 21 (total)
	8 (dysthymic disorder)	GC-MS	174 ± 16 (total)
790. Siever, 1986	14	GC-MS	293 ± 24
	10 (unipolar)	GC-MS	293 ± 23
	4 (bipolar)	GC-MS	275 ± 46
105. Bowden, 1987	91	Fl	283 ± 18
	62 (unipolar)	Fl	310 ± 22
	29 (bipolar)	Fl	227 ± 31
587. Mooney, 1988	9	HPLC-EC	264 ± 7

Table 119. Normetanephrine and Metanephrine in Urine of Schizophrenic

Subjects

Reference First Author, Year	Number of Subjects	Method of Analysis	Values (mg/24h ± S.E.M.)
561. Mattok, 1967	22 (acute)	Fl	242 (NMN)*
	22 (acute)	Fl	154 (conjugated NMN)*
	22 (acute)	Fl	9.6 (MN)*
	22 (acute)	Fl	55.2 (conjugated MN)*
666. Pollin, 1971	30 (15 pair of twins)	GC-ECD	193 mg/g Cr. (NMN)
	30 (15 pair of twins)	GC-ECD	91 mg/g Cr. (MN)

* In original paper expressed as mg/h.

Table 120. Normetanephrine and Metanephrine in Plasma of Normal

Subjects

Reference First Author, Year	Number of Subjects	Method of Analysis	Values (pg/mL ± S.E.M.)
915. Wang, 1975	3	GC-MS[†]	274 ± 37 (NMN)
	3	GC-MS	494 ± 37 (conj. NMN)
	3	GC-MS	118 ± 92 (MN)
	3	GC-MS	335 ± 63 (conj. MN)
902. Vlachakis, 1979	10	REA[†]	1200 ± 100 (total NMN)
481. Kobayashi, 1980	9	REA[†]	64 ± 10 (NMN)
901. Vlachakis, 1981	36	REA	2071 ± 220 (total NMN)

Table 121. Normetanephrine and Metanephrine in CSF of Normal and Other

Subjects

Reference First Author, Year	Number of Subjects	Method of Analysis	Values (pg/mL ± S.E.M.)
901. Vlachakis, 1981	36	REA	1601 ± 143 (total NMN)
557. Martin, 1982	13	GC-MS[†]	2200 ± 500 (NMN)
67. Beck, 1985	6	GC-MS[†]	950 ± 250 (NMN)
	6	GC-MS	80 ± 20 (MN)
644. Parnetti, 1987	12 (Alzheimer's)	HPLC-Fl[†]	n.d. (NMN)
	13 (schizophrenic)	HPLC-Fl	360 ± 200 (NMN)

Table 122.   Unconjugated Metanephrine in Urine of Normal Subjects

Reference First Author, Year	Number of Subjects	Method of Analysis	Values (mg/24h ± S.E.M.)
966. Yoshinaga, 1961	8	Fl[†]	205 ± 22
855. Taniguchi, 1964	6	Fl[†]	29.5 ± 2.3
433. Kahane, 1967	15	Fl[†]	130 ± 13
561. Mattok, 1967	24	Fl	315*
86. Bigelow, 1968	16	Fl[†]	70 ± 9
79. Bertani, 1970	16	GC-ECD[†]	93 ± 7 mg/g Cr.
135. Cardon, 1970	7	Fl	176
666. Pollin, 1971	8 (4 pairs of twins)	GC-ECD	55 mg/g Cr.
679. Prange, 1972	10	Fl	135 ± 20
224. De Leon-Jones, 1975	21	Fl	75 ± 6
541. Maas, 1975	19 (M) 21 (F)	– –	86 ± 9 83 ± 9
510. Lam, 1977	15	RIA[†]	3.5 ± 0.3
786. Shoup, 1977	–	HPLC-EC[†]	174 ± 79 (S.D.)
234. De Schaepdryver, 1977	20	Fl[†]	48.6 ± 3.5
704. Robertson, 1978	9	GC-MS	142 ± 10**
705. Robertson, 1978	7	GC-MS[†]	157 ± 16
600. Muskiet, 1979	13	GC-MS[†]	71 ± 5 mg/g Cr.
614. Nelson, 1979	12	GC-ECD[†]	116 ± 21
81. Bertani-Dziedzic,	7	HPLC-EC[†]	40 ± 4 mg/g Cr.
430. Jouve, 1983	30	HPLC-EC[†]	128 ± 6 mg/g Cr.
493. Koslow, 1983	37 (M) 40 (F)	Fl Fl	107 ± 7 88 ± 5
911. Waldmeier, 1983	5	HPLC-EC[†]	104 ± 11 mg/g Cr.

Table 122.   Unconjugated Metanephrine in Urine of Normal Subjects (continued)

Reference First Author, Year	Number of Subjects	Method of Analysis	Values (mg/24h ± S.E.M.)
471. Kiriike, 1984	31	Fl	107 ± 7
790. Siever, 1986	18	GC-MS	130 ± 15
431. Julien, 1988	6	HPLC-EC[†]	16.0 ± 3.4

*   In original paper expressed in mg/h.
** In original paper expressed in mg/3h.

Table 123.   Conjugated Metanephrine in Urine of Normal Subjects

Reference First Author, Year	Number of Subjects	Method of Analysis	Values (mg/24h ± S.E.M.)
807. Smith, 1962	19	Fl[†]	72 ± 6 (total)
233. De Quattro, 1964	9	Fl[†]	127 ± 17 (total)*
855. Taniguchi, 1964	6	Fl[†]	134 ± 10.5
177. Coward, 1966	10	Fl[†]	98 ± 10 mg/g Cr. (total)
561. Mattok, 1967	24	Fl	177*
544. Maas, 1968	11	Fl	53 ± 12 mg/g Cr. (total)
510. Lam, 1977	15	RIA[†]	13.4 ± 2.7
657. Peyrin, 1987	11	Fl	579 ± 76 mg/g Cr. (total)
529. Linnoila, 1988	12	GC-MS	156 ± 19 (total)

* In original paper expressed in mg/h.

Table 124. Unconjugated Metanephrine in Urine of Depressed Patients

Reference First Author, Year	Number of Subjects	Method of Analysis	Values (mg/24h ± S.E.M.)
807. Smith, 1962	10 (anxiety)	Fl[†]	91 ± 17 (total)
613. Nelson, 1966	6 (includes schizophrenics)	Fl	133 ± 30 mg/g Cr.
126. Bunney, 1967	8 (psychotic)	Fl	43.2
	8 (neurotic)	Fl	24.5
544. Maas, 1968	16 (severe)	Fl	68 ± 7 mg/g Cr.
346. Greenspan, 1970	3 (hypomanic)	Fl	142 ± 30
	2 (normothymic)	Fl	149 ± 62
	3 (agitated)	Fl	206 ± 13
679. Prange, 1972	12 (primary)	Fl	148 ± 27
224. De Leon-Jones, 1975	5 (bipolar)	Fl	85 ± 16
	14 (single episode (unipolar)	Fl	92 ± 7
	13 (recurrent unipolar)	Fl	90 ± 9
541. Maas, 1975;	20 (M)	–	114 ± 22
542. Maas, 1978	48 (F)	–	97 ± 6
592. Murphy, 1977	4 (primary)	Fl	125 ± 20

Table 124. Unconjugated Metanephrine in Urine of Depressed Patients

(continued)

Reference First Author, Year	Number of Subjects	Method of Analysis	Values (mg/24h ± S.E.M.)
761. Schildkraut, 1978	9 (schizophrenia (related)	Fl	72 ± 14
	4 (schizoaffective)	Fl	224 ± 15
	12 (bipolar)	Fl	161 ± 19
	16 (unipolar endogenous)	Fl	144 ± 11
	13 (unipolar (non-endogenous)	Fl	168 ± 16
	9 (unclassified)	Fl	137 ± 74
493. Koslow, 1983; 548. Maas, 1984	64 (M) (depressed)	Fl	149 ± 8
	55 (F) (depressed)	Fl	122 ± 7
	11 (M) (manic)	Fl	157 ± 23
	6 (F) (manic)	Fl	91 ± 11
790. Siever, 1986	14	GC–MS	132 ± 11
	10 (unipolar)	GC–MS	138 ± 19
	4 (bipolar)	GC–MS	138 ± 49
105. Bowden, 1987	93	Fl	138 ± 6
	63 (unipolar)	Fl	141 ± 7
	30 (bipolar)	Fl	133 ± 10
587. Mooney, 1988	9	HPLC-EC	138 ± 12

Table 125. 3-Methoxytyramine in Urine of Normal and Depressed Patients

Reference First Author, Year	Number of Subjects	Method of Analysis	Values (mg/24h ± S.E.M.)
456. Käser, 1970	14	Fl[†]	88.4 ± 14.4
197. Dalmaz, 1976	43	Fl[†]	98.4 ± 8.3 (total)
786. Shoup, 1977	–	HPLC-EC[†]	137 ± 60 (S.D.)
600. Muskiet, 1979	13	GC-MS[†]	106 ± 13 mg/g Cr.
614. Nelson, 1979	12	GC-ECD[†]	82 ± 20
176. Coutts, 1981	12	GC-ECD[†]	48 ± 9
441. Karoum, 1982	5	GC-MS[†]	14.6 ± 7.4
	6 (depressed)	GC-MS	7 ± 1.5
525. Linnoila, 1982	4 (bipolar)	GC-MS	21.7 ± 7.4
430. Jouve, 1983	30	HPLC-EC[†]	87 ± 4 mg/g Cr.
911. Waldmeier, 1983	5	Fl[†]	74 ± 5 mg/g Cr.
431. Julien, 1988	6	HPLC-EC[†]	37 ± 3

Table 126. 3-Methoxytyramine in Plasma and CSF of Normal and Other Subjects

Reference First Author, Year	Number of Subjects	Method of Analysis	Values (pg/mL ± S.E.M.)
915. Wang, 1975	3	GC-MS[†]	418 ± 84 (plasma)
	3	GC-MS	668 ± 217 (conjugated)
67. Beck, 1985	6	GC-MS[†]	635 ± 184 (CSF)
644. Parnetti, 1987	12 (Alzheimer's)	HPLC-Fl[†]	n.d. (CSF)
	13 (schizophrenic)	HPLC-Fl	n.d. (CSF)

Table 127. 3,4-Dimethoxyphenylethylamine in Urine of Normal and

Schizophrenic Subjects

Reference First Author, Year	Number of Subjects	Method of Analysis	Values (mg/24h ± S.E.M.)
271. Faurbye, 1964	10 (normal)	Fl[†]	n.d.
	15 (chronic schizophrenic)	Fl	n.d.
647. Perry, 1966	– (psychotics)	Fl	n.d.
180. Creveling, 1967	2 (schizophrenic)	MS	trace
697. Rinne, 1967	9 (neurological)	Fl	6.8 ± 1.2
	20 (Parkinson's disease)	Fl	4.4 ± 0.3
904. Vogel, 1967	8 (normal)	Fl[†]	trace
	9 (schizophrenic)	Fl	trace
424. Jones, 1969	– (normal)	GC-MS,GC-ECD[†]	n.d.
	– (schizophrenic)	GC-MS,GC-ECD	n.d.
820. Stabenau, 1970	– (normal)	MS	trace
787. Siegel, 1971	– (normal)	MS[†]	trace
	– (schizophrenic)	MS	trace
477. Knoll, 1976	80 (normal)	RIA[†]	0.077
297. Friedhoff, 1977	16 (normal)	TLC-radioactivity	1.71± 0.41
	15 (schizophrenic)	TLC-radioactivity	4.3 ± 0.98

Table 127.   3,4-Dimethoxyphenylethylamine in Urine of Normal and

Schizophrenic Subjects (continued)

Reference First Author, Year	Number of Subjects	Method of Analysis	Values (mg/24h ± S.E.M.)
372. Hempel, 1982	– (normal)	Fl[†]	n.d.
	– (schizophrenic)	Fl	n.d.

Table 128. N,N-Dimethyltryptamine in Urine of Normal, Depressed and

Schizophrenic Subjects

Reference First Author, Year	Number of Subjects	Method of Analysis	Values (mg/24h ± S.E.M.)
291. Franzen, 1965	37 (normal)	–	43.0 ± 8.6
609. Narasimhachari, 1973	– (schizophrenic)	Fl[†]	≈1
	– (normal)	Fl	n.d.
606. Narasimhachari, 1974	– (schizophrenic)	GC-MS	<1
631. Oon, 1977	– (schizophrenic)	GC-ECD[†]	1.1
	– (manic)	GC-ECD	1.0
	– (psychotic depressed)	GC-ECD	0.5
	– (neurotic depressed)	GC-ECD	0.45
	– (normal)	GC-ECD	0.35
630. Oon, 1977	19 (normal)	GC-N	0.38± 0.12
594. Murray, 1979	26 (schizophrenic)	GC-N	1.22
	10 (manic psychotic)	GC-N	1.02
	4 (depressed psychotic)	GC-N	0.32
684. Räisänen, 1979	26	GC-MS[†]	0.096 mg/g Cr.

Table 129. N-Methyltryptamine in Urine of Normal, Schizophrenic and

Depressive Subjects

Reference First Author, Year	Number of Subjects	Method of Analysis	Values (ng/24h ± S.E.M.)
630. Oon, 1977	19 (normal)	GC-N	856 ± 224
594. Murray, 1979	26 (schizophrenic)	GC-N	678
	10 (manic (psychotic)	GC-N	897
	4 (depressive psychotic)	GC-N	501

Table 130. Bufotenin (N,N-Dimethyl-5-tryptamine) in Urine of Normal and

Schizophrenic Subjects

Reference First Author, Year	Number of Subjects	Method of Analysis	Values (mg/24h ± S.E.M.)
647. Perry, 1964	– (psychotic)	Fl	n.d.
291. Franzen, 1965	46 57	– –	62.8 ± 7.2 36.6 ± 5.2 (methylether)
280. Fischer, 1967	– (schizophrenic)	Fl[†]	trace
792. Sireix, 1969	20 (normal) 20 (schizophrenic)	Fl Fl	21 ± 2.2 mg/L 155 ±19.7 mg/L
608. Narasimhachari, 1972	– (normal) – (schizophrenic)	GC,Fl GC,Fl	n.d. trace
609. Narasimhachari, 1973	– (normal) – (schizophrenic)	Fl[†] Fl	n.d. ≈3
606. Narasimhachari, 1974	– (schizophrenic)	GC-MS	3
136. Carpenter, 1975	10 (normal) 26 (schizophrenic)	GC-MS GC-MS	1.71 1.14
684. Räisänen, 1979	26 (normal)	GC-MS[†]	0.95 mg/g Cr.
683. Räisänen, 1984	10 (normal) 10	GC-MS[†] GC-MS[†]	1.10 ± 0.54 mg/g Cr. (unconj.) 2.18 ± 1.35 mg/g Cr. (conj.)
438. Kärkkäinen, 1988	51 (normal) 75 (psychotic)	GC-MS[†] GC-MS[†]	0.37 mg/g Cr. 1.88 mg/g Cr.

Table 131. Melatonin in Urine of Normal and Depressed Subjects

Reference First Author, Year	Number of Subjects	Method of Analysis	Values (mg/24h ± S.E.M.)
417. Jimerson, 1977	5 (normal)	Bio-Assay	9.6 ± 1.2
	5 (normal)	Bio-Assay	2.0 ± 0.1 (day, mg/12h)
	5 (normal)	Bio-Assay	6.5 ± 1.3 (night, mg/12h)
	5 (depressed)	Bio-Assay	11.6 ± 1.1
	5 (depressed)	Bio-Assay	2.0 ± 0.1 (day, mg/12h)
	5 (depressed)	Bio-Assay	8.0 ± 0.9 (night, mg/12h)
540. Lynch, 1978	4	RIA	1.3 ± 0.1 ng/4h (day)
	4	RIA	4.3 ± 0.4 ng/4h (night)

<u>Table 132. Unconjugated (and Conjugated) 6-Hydroxymelatonin in Urine of</u>

<u>Normal and Depressed Subjects</u>

Reference First Author, Year	Number of Subjects	Method of Analysis	Values (mg/24h ± S.E.M.)
793. Sisak, 1979	1	GC-MS[†]	20 mg/L
275. Fellenberg, 1980	10 (M) 10 (F)	GC-MS[†] GC-MS	21.0 (sulfate) 16.0 (sulfate)
858. Tetsuo, 1980	7	GC-MS	15.5 ± 0.9
857. Tetsuo, 1981	10 (M) 4 (F)	GC-MS[†] GC-MS	12.4 (total) 11.9 (total)
376. Higa, 1985	23	GC-MS[†]	14.4 ± 2.0
93. Bojkowski, 1987	9 (M)	RIA[†]	1.69± 0.17 (day,mg/12h) (sulfate)
	9 (M)	RIA	7.42± 0.68 (night,mg/12h) (sulfate)
	9 (M)	RIA	9.14± 0.78 (sulfate)
	9 (F)	RIA	1.72± 0.37 (day,mg/12h) (sulfate)
	9 (F)	RIA	8.47± 2.32 (night,mg/12h) (sulfate)
	9 (F)	RIA	10.18± 2.67 (sulfate)
324. Golden, 1988	27 (depressed)	NCI-MS	7.2 ± 1.2

Table 133. N,N-Dimethyltryptamine in Plasma of Normal, Schizophrenic

and Depressed Subjects

Reference First Author, Year	Number of Subjects	Method of Analysis	Values (ng/mL ± S.E.M.)
291. Franzen, 1965	37 (normal)	–	8–55
	46	–	1–40 (5-hydroxy)
	57	–	2–80 (5-methoxy)
912. Walker, 1973	39 (normal)	GC-MS[†]	<0.5
955. Wyatt, 1973	5 (normal)	GC-MS	0.9
	– (schizophrenic)	GC-MS	n.d.
	– (depressed)	GC-MS	n.d.
913. Walker, 1979	4 (normal)	GC-MS[†]	n.d.
	9 (schizophrenic)	GC-MS[†]	26.9 ± 12.1 (arterial)
	9 (schizophrenic)	GC-MS[†]	28.0 ± 12.3 (venous)
944. Wilson, 1979	3	GC-MS	0.005–0.025 (5-methoxy)

Table 134. Melatonin in Plasma of Normal, Depressed and Schizophrenic

Subjects

Reference First Author, Year	Number of Subjects	Method of Analysis	Values (pg/mL ± S.E.M.)
28. Arendt, 1975	5	RIA[†]	132 ± 10 (noon)
	5	RIA	188 ± 15 (midnight)
29. Arendt, 1977	3 (F)	RIA	45 ± 5 (serum, day)
	3 (F)	RIA	130 ± 7 (serum, night)
	3 (M)	RIA	70 ± 5 (serum, day)
	3 (M)	RIA	140 ± 11 (serum, night)
812. Smith, 1977	5	RIA	20 ± 3 (2 p.m.)
	5	RIA	78 ± 13 (2 a.m.)
945. Wilson, 1977	5	GC-MS[†]	28.2 ± 8.1
516. Lewy, 1978	4	GC-MS[†]	1.5 (day)
	4	GC-MS	42.6 (night)
540. Lynch, 1978	2	RIA	23 ± 7 (day)
	2	RIA	97 ± 33 (night)
934. Wetterberg, 1978	1	RIA[†]	107 (midnight, plasma)
	1	RIA	111 (midnight, serum)
116. Branchey, 1982	4 (unipolar + bipolar)	RIA	188 ± 38 (day-night mean)
	4 (depressed)	RIA	166 ± 23 (day)
	4 (depressed)	RIA	224 ± 66 (night)
292. Fraser, 1983	13	RIA[†]	50.1 ± 8.0
27. Arendt, 1985	9	RIA[†]	10 ± 0.5 (day, 6 p.m.)
	9	RIA	29 ± 6 (night, 2 a.m.)
	9	RIA	<13 (day, 6 p.m.) (6-hydroxy, sulfate)
	9	RIA	52 ± 11 (night, 2 a.m.) (6-hydroxy, sulfate)
229. Demisch, 1987	10	RIA	4.2 ± 1.0 (day)
	10	RIA	37 ± 3.8 (night)
788. Sieghart, 1987	15 (psychiatric)	RIA[†]	13.5 ± 1.0 (day)
	15 (psychiatric)	RIA	86 ± 11.6 (night)

Table 134. Melatonin in Plasma of Normal, Depressed and Schizophrenic

Subjects (continued)

Reference First Author, Year	Number of Subjects	Method of Analysis	Values (pg/mL ± S.E.M.)
269. Fanget, 1989	26 (normal)	RIA	75.5 ± 3.7 (night)
	23 (schizophrenic)	RIA	52.3 ± 8.7 (night)
777. Sharma, 1989	– (young)	RIA	119 ± 13 (peak)
	– (middle age)	RIA	72 ± 18 (peak)
	– (old age)	RIA	59 ± 13 (peak)
828. Stewart, 1989	113 (depressed)	RIA	64 ± 4

Table 135. Methylated Tryptamines in CSF of Normal and Schizophrenic

Subjects

Reference First Author, Year	Number of Subjects	Method of Analysis	Values (pg/mL ± S.E.M.)
163. Christian, 1975	– (normal)	GC-ECD[†]	traces of DMT and 5-MeO-DMT
29. Arendt, 1977	8 (M)	RIA	59 ± 33 (melatonin)
	7 (F)	RIA	57 ± 28 (melatonin)
945. Wilson, 1977	2	GC-MS[†]	68 ± 9 (melatonin)
813. Smythies, 1979	6 (normal)	GC-MS[†]	1500 ± 1100 (DMT)
	3 (schizophrenic)	GC-MS	2000 ± 1000 (DMT)

Section 7

Catecholic Acids, 5-Hydroxyindoleacetic Acid, and Related Alcohols and Glycols

Tables 136 to 207

Table 136. Unconjugated 5-Hydroxyindoleacetic Acid in Urine of Normal

Subjects

Reference First Author, Year	Number of Subjects	Method of Analysis	Values (mg/24h ± S.E.M.)
369. Haverback, 1956	9	Fl	4.1 ± 0.32
273. Feldstein, 1958	29	Fl	5.2 ± 0.3
274. Feldstein, 1959	36 (M)	Fl	4.87 ± 0.31*
	8 (F)	Fl	5.14 ± 1.37*
486. Kopin, 1959	6	Fl	5.50 ± 1.63*
641. Pare, 1960	18	Fl	3.9 ± 0.40 mg/g Cr.
73. Benassi, 1961	5	Fl	4.09 ± 0.12
943. Williams, 1961	4	GC-FID	1.1 mg/g Cr.
891. Van Praag, 1963	15	Fl	5.7 ± 0.1
185. Curran, 1965	10	Fl	5.61 ± 0.66
216. Davis, 1965	21	Fl†	3.04
632. O'Reilly, 1965	4	Fl	6.59 ± 1.00 mg/g Cr.
143. Cazzullo, 1966	6	Fl	2.70 ± 0.48*
189. Curzon, 1966	4	Fl	2.65 ± 0.22 mg/g Cr.
33. Arterberry, 1967	23	Fl†	4.84 ± 0.10*
491. Korf, 1970	5	Fl	3.64 ± 0.53
119. Brown, 1971	30	HPLC†	3.5 ± 1.1
871. Turnball, 1971	21	-	6.7 ± 0.4
679. Prange, 1972	10	Fl	5.2 ± 0.6
326. Goldenberg, 1973	50	Fl†	3.9 ± 0.1
390. Hoskins, 1975	19	GC-MS†	3.36 ± 0.18
832. Subrahmanyam, 1975	12	Fl	4.36 ± 0.9
	12	Fl	4.00 ± 0.4
839. Swahn, 1976	5	GC-MS†	6.88 mg/L
	5	GC-MS	0.38 mg/L (conj.)

<u>Table 136.   Unconjugated 5-Hydroxyindoleacetic Acid in Urine of Normal</u>

<u>Subjects (continued)</u>

Reference First Author, Year	Number of Subjects	Method of Analysis	Values (mg/24h ± S.E.M.)
305. Garfinkel, 1977	10	Fl	3.83 ± 0.25
962. Yoshida, 1977	7	HPLC	3.7 ± 0.4
284. Fornstedt, 1978	10	HPLC[†]	6.0 ± 1.2
958. Yamaguchi, 1978	38	Fl	8.3 ± 0.62
237. Domino, 1979	7	GC-MS[†]	9.82 ± 0.64 or 4.87 ± 0.32 mg/g Cr.
782. Shen, 1979	68	Bio-Assay	7.0 ± 0.5
285. Fornstedt, 1980	12	HPLC[†]	4.5 ± 0.2
306. Garnier, 1981	112	HPLC-Fl[†]	4.78 ± 0.36
863. Tracy, 1981	40	HPLC[†]	3.8 ± 0.44
387. Hopkinson, 1982	15	HPLC	10.4 mg/g Cr.
715. Rosano, 1982	27	HPLC-Fl[†]	3.9
933. Westerink, 1982	6	HPLC[†]	3.4 ± 0.4
935. Wiesel, 1982	33 (M) 33 (F)	GC-MS GC-MS	5.21 ± 0.32* 4.35 ± 0.26*
218. De Jong, 1983	7	GC-FID[†]	5.58 ± 0.68 mg/g Cr.
804. Skrinska, 1984	47	HPLC[†]	3.2 ± 0.25 mg/g Cr.
20. Anderson, 1985	11	HPLC-EC[†]	5.0 ± 0.8
211. Davis, 1986	10	GC-MS[†]	4.78
290. Frankenhaueser, 1986	19 (M) 30 (F)	GC-MS GC-MS	5.31 ± 0.69** 3.11 ± 0.36**
50. Baker, 1987	29	GC-ECD[†]	5.2 ± 0.6
445. Karoum, 1987	–	GC-MS[†]	8.8 ± 1.0
201. Davidson, 1988	47	HPLC-EC[†]	3.40 ± 0.22
319. Gironi, 1988	120	HPLC-Fl[†]	3.78 ± 0.17

Table 136.   Unconjugated 5-Hydroxyindoleacetic Acid in Urine of Normal

Subjects (continued)

Reference First Author, Year	Number of Subjects	Method of Analysis	Values (mg/24h ± S.E.M.)
623. Odink, 1988	6 (M)	HPLC-EC[†]	4.41
	6 (F)	HPLC-EC[†]	4.34

*   In original paper expressed as μg/h.
** In original paper expressed as nmol/min.

Table 137.   5-Hydroxyindoleacetic Acid in Plasma of Normal and Depressed

Subjects

Reference First Author, Year	Number of Subjects	Method of Analysis	Values (ng/mL ± S.E.M.)
227a.Demet, 1978	6	Fl[†]	78.3 ± 5.3
483. Koch, 1979	7	HPLC-EC[†]	16.5 ± 2.8 (plasma)
	7	HPLC-EC	10.2 ± 1.3 (serum)
547. Maas, 1980	6	GC-MS	7.1 ± 0.7
559. Martinez, 1983	16	HPLC-Fl[†]	9.9 ± 1.0
529. Linnoila, 1984	8 (euthymic, depressed)	HPLC-EC	9.6 ± 2.6
575. Minegishi, 1984	6	HPLC-EC[†]	9.22 ± 1.24
836. Suñol, 1984	16	HPLC-Fl	9.9 ± 1.0
211. Davis, 1986	10	GC-MS[†]	34
749. Sarrias, 1987	19 18 (melancholia)	HPLC-Fl HPLC-Fl	7.4 6.1
9. Alfredsson, 1988	10	GC-MS	9.9 ± 0.4 (serum)

Table 138. Unconjugated 5-Hydroxyindoleacetic Acid in CSF of Normal

Subjects

Reference First Author, Year	Number of Subjects	Method of Analysis	Values (ng/mL ± S.E.M.)
42. Ashcroft, 1960	10	Fl	32.2 ± 2.8
648. Persson, 1965	34	Fl	29
41. Ashcroft, 1966	28	Fl	33.3 ± 2.1 (air-encephal)
	7	Fl	17.4 ± 2.0 (lumbar puncture)
	6	Fl	88.1 ± 9.2 (ventricular)
231. Dencker, 1966	34	Fl	20 – 60
314. Gerbode, 1968	11	Fl	153 ± 21 (ventricular)
	51	Fl	34 ± 2 (lumbar)
627. Olsson, 1968	7	Fl	40 ± 1.5
110. Bowers, 1969	18	Fl	43.5 ± 4.0
342. Gottfries, 1969	25	Fl	40 ± 2
492. Korf, 1969	5	Fl[†]	5 – 30
152. Chase, 1970	10	–	30 ± 3.2
425. Jonsson, 1970	7	Fl[†]	32 ± 1
582. Moir, 1970	20	Fl	105 ± 11 (ventricular)
	1	Fl	85 (cisternal)
	21	Fl	19 ± 0.9 (lumbar)
682. Pullar, 1970	21	Fl	19 ± 0.9
186. Curzon, 1971	11	Fl	23 ± 2.7
323. Godwin-Austen, 1971	9	Fl	27 ± 3.3
338. Gordon, 1971	4	GC-ECD[†]	91 (ventricular)
	40	GC-ECD	29 (lumbar)
341. Gottfries, 1971	35	Fl	28.3 ± 1.4 µg/mL
637. Papeschi, 1971	10	Fl	28 ± 3
642. Parkes, 1971	11	Fl	23 ± 2.7
696. Rimon, 1971	17	Fl	29.7 ± 3.3

Table 138. Unconjugated 5-Hydroxyindoleacetic Acid in CSF of Normal

Subjects (continued)

Reference First Author, Year	Number of Subjects	Method of Analysis	Values (ng/mL ± S.E.M.)	
885. Van Praag, 1971	15	Fl	40 ± 4.6	
884. Van Praag, 1971	11	Fl	40 ± 7.2	
108. Bowers, 1972	15	Fl	57.1 ± 3.9	
155. Chase, 1972	8	Fl	28 ± 3.1	
172. Coppen, 1972	20	Fl	42.3 ± 3.2	
	15 (M)	Fl	42.7 ± 3.8	
	5 (F)	Fl	41.0 ± 6.4	
435. Kangasniemi, 1972	6	Fl[†]	26.1 ± 3.0	
638. Papeschi, 1972	18	Fl	31 ± 3	
699. Rinne, 1972	22	Fl	36.7 ± 3.8	
888. Van Praag, 1972	10	Fl	31.1 ± 4.5	
154. Chase, 1973	11	Fl	102 ± 14	(ventricular)
	7	Fl	28 ± 1.3	(lumbar)
303. Garelis, 1973	17	Fl	29.2 ± 2.4	
336. Goodwin, 1973	29	Fl	27.3 ± 2.2	
339. Gordon, 1973	5	Fl	29.4 ± 7.7	
344. Gottfries, 1973	25	Fl	40 ± 2.4	
669. Post, 1973	29	Fl	27.3 ± 1.6	
700. Rinne, 1973	31	Fl	33.9 ± 3.3	
887. Van Praag, 1973	12	Fl	29 ± 3	
643. Parkes, 1974	11	Fl	26 ± 2	
420. Johansson, 1975	8	Fl	83	(cisternal)
667. Post, 1975	10	Fl	27	
803. Sjöström, 1975	11	GS-MS	33.4 ± 2.9	(first fraction)
832. Subrahmanyam, 1975	12	Fl	40.6 ± 4.2	

Table 138. Unconjugated 5-Hydroxyindoleacetic Acid in CSF of Normal

Subjects (continued)

Reference First Author, Year	Number of Subjects	Method of Analysis	Values (ng/mL ± S.E.M.)
971. Young, 1975	20	Fl	31.7 ± 4.1
117. Bridges, 1976	5	Fl	87 ± 10 (ventricular)
839. Swahn, 1976	5	GC-MS[†]	32.3 ± 0.8
	5	GC-MS	25.8 (total)
54. Banki, 1977	32	Fl	27.5 ± 1.2
202. Davidson, 1977	7	Fl	21 ± 4
88. Bioulac, 1978	6	Fl	21 ± 3
800. Sjöquist, 1978	7	GC-MS	30.8 ± 2.0
894. Vestergaard, 1978	22	Fl	28 ± 6
270. Faull, 1979	23	GC-MS[†]	29.4 ± 2.6
550. Major, 1979	7	GC-MS	18.8 ± 2.2
	7	Fl	22.6 ± 3.0
75. Berger, 1980	23	GC-MS	27.7 ± 2.4
188. Curzon, 1980	23	Fl	22 ± 2.1 (lumbar)
	5	Fl	87 ± 10.3 (ventricular)
332. Gomes, 1980	19	Fl	35.5 ± 2.1
768. Sedvall, 1980	32 (no family history)	GC-MS	19.5 ± 0.7
	28 (family history of psychiatric morbidity)	GC-MS	20.4 ± 1.5
968. Young, 1980	29 (epileptic)	HPLC-Fl	22.0 ± 12.4 (lumbar)
	29 (epileptic)	HPLC-Fl	27.7 ± 13.1 (cisternal)

Table 138.   Unconjugated 5-Hydroxyindoleacetic Acid in CSF of Normal

Subjects (continued)

Reference First Author, Year	Number of Subjects	Method of Analysis	Values (ng/mL ± S.E.M.)	
970. Young, 1980	43 (M) (epileptic)	HPLC-Fl	27.5 ±	1.5 (cisternal)
	29 (F)	HPLC-Fl	32.4 ±	2.4 (cisternal)
	44 (M)	HPLC-Fl	19.2 ±	1.2 (lumbar)
	28 (F)	HPLC-Fl	25.3 ±	2.3 (lumbar)
	17	HPLC-Fl	33.0 ±	3.0 (cisternal)
	15	HPLC-Fl	27.1 ±	3.6 (lumbar)
16. Anderson, 1981	5	GC-MS[†]	18.5 ±	1.7
57. Banki, 1981	4	Fl	53.0 ±	6.1 (cisternal)
	32	Fl	27.0 ±	1.8 (lumbar)
616. Nicoletti, 1981	5	Fl	14.2 ±	0.9 (6 a.m.)
	5	Fl	19.8 ±	0.9 (noon)
	5	Fl	21.4 ±	2.1 (6 p.m.)
	5	Fl	28.7 ±	2.6 (midnight)
633. Oreland, 1981	28 (M)	GC-MS	17.0 ±	1.1
	14 (F)	GC-MS	23.1 ±	1.9
814. Soininen, 1981	13	Fl	42 ±	3
865. Träskman, 1981	45	GC-MS	19.8 ±	1.1
629. Bareggi, 1982	8	Fl	32.5 ±	2.0
311. Gattaz, 1982	16	HPLC-EC[†]	15.3 ±	4.4
585. Montplaisir, 1982	11	HPLC-Fl	19.6 ±	3.3
605. Nair, 1982	16	Fl	14.8 ±	0.8
954. Wood, 1982	32	GC-MS	22.9 ±	2.3
55. Banki, 1983	32	Fl	27.0 ±	1.8
620. Nybäck, 1983	43	GC-MS	19.1 ±	1.0
843. Swann, 1983	29 (M)	GC-MS	20.6 ±	0.8
	29 (F)	GC-MS	21.8 ±	1.3
	58	GC-MS	21.2 ±	0.8
878. Van Bockstaele, 1983	11	HPLC-EC[†]	19.8 ±	1.5
36. Åsberg, 1984	66	GC-MS	19.9 ±	0.9

Table 138. Unconjugated 5-Hydroxyindoleacetic Acid in CSF of Normal

Subjects (continued)

Reference First Author, Year	Number of Subjects	Method of Analysis	Values (ng/mL ± S.E.M.)
77. Berrettini, 1984	20	HPLC-EC	14.3 ± 0.9
98. Bottiglieri, 1984	9	HPLC-EC[†]	16.7 ± 4.1
316. Gerner, 1984	37	HPLC-EC	22.2 ± 1.8
386. Honegger, 1984	8	HPLC[†]	23.2 ± 2.2
409. Javors, 1984	7	HPLC-EC[†]	22.4 ± 3.7
458. Kay, 1984	12	HPLC[†]	10.8 ± 0.4
635. Palmer, 1984	23	HPLC-EC[†]	21.4 ± 1.8
690. Reimherr, 1984	7 (M)	GC-MS	15.7 ± 3.4
	6 (F)	GC-MS	33.8 ± 5.3
	13	GC-MS	24.0 ± 3.9
35. Artigas, 1985	8	HPLC[†]	24.8 ± 3.9
78. Berrettini, 1985	25	HPLC-EC	13.8 ± 0.8
309. Gattaz, 1985	16	HPLC-EC	15.3 ± 1.1
517. Lidberg, 1985	39	GC-MS	17.4 ± 0.9
520. Lindstrom, 1985	21	GC-MS	20.6 ± 1.0
535. Lopez-Ibor, 1985	16	Fl	16.8 ± 1.7
816. Sparks, 1985	4	HPLC-EC[†]	23 ± 3
822. Stahl, 1985	36	GC-MS	26.1 ± 1.9
824. Stanley, 1985	48	HPLC	34.4
906. Volicer, 1985	17	HPLC-EC	25.5 ± 2.4
907. Volicer, 1985	8	HPLC-EC[†]	20.2 ± 1.8 (caudal)
211. Davis, 1986	10	GC-MS[†]	18.6
354. Guthrie, 1986	24	HPLC-EC	10.9 ± 0.9

Table 138. Unconjugated 5-Hydroxyindoleacetic Acid in CSF of Normal

Subjects (continued)

Reference First Author, Year	Number of Subjects	Method of Analysis	Values (ng/mL ± S.E.M.)
634. Oxenstierna, 1986	30 (monozygotic twins)	GC-MS	18.0 ± 1.0
	30 (dizygotic twins)	GC-MS	14.2 ± 0.8
	30 (brothers)	GC-MS	13.6 ± 1.2
	30 (unrelated men)	GC-MS	13.4 ± 1.0
735. Saito, 1986	9	HPLC-EC	21.2 ± 2.9
11. Almay, 1987	35	HPLC-EC	21.2 ± 0.8
	16 (M)	HPLC-EC	19.3 ± 1.2
	19 (F)	HPLC-EC	22.8 ± 1.0
262. Emanuelsson, 1987	11	GC-MS	18.0 ± 1.5
322. Gjerris, 1987	15	GC-MS	24.4
621. Nybäck, 1987	18	GC-MS	22.0 ± 2.8
834. Sunderland, 1987	7	HPLC-EC	20.8 ± 2.1
9. Alfredsson, 1988	10	GC-MS	10.7 ± 1.3
495. Koyama, 1988	5	HPLC-EC[†]	14.3 ± 1.3
723. Roy, 1988	39	HPLC-EC	14.7 ± 0.9
932. Westenberg, 1988	48	HPLC-EC[†]	23.7 ± 0.1
	27 (F)	HPLC-EC[†]	25.0 ± 0.2
	21 (M)	HPLC-EC[†]	22.0 ± 2.8

Table 139. Unconjugated 5-Hydroxyindoleacetic Acid in Urine of

Depressed Subjects

Reference First Author, Year	Number of Subjects	Method of Analysis	Values (mg/24h ± S.E.M.)
640. Pare, 1959	9	Fl	3.7 ± 0.7 mg/g Cr.
891. Van Praag, 1963	7	Fl	2.7 ± 0.3
	6	Fl	5.7 ± 0.8
143. Cazzullo, 1966	12 (depressed)	Fl	4.07 ± 1.56*
	6 (manic)	Fl	2.91 ± 0.42*
849. Takahashi, 1968	1 patient, 8 times (manic- depressive)	Fl	11.8 ± 1.4
890. Van Praag, 1968	20	Fl	4.40 ± 0.59
127. Bunney, 1972	6 (depressed)	Fl	4.40 ± 0.80
	6 (manic)	Fl	7.60 ± 1.3
564. McNamee, 1972	7 (psychotic)	Fl	6.0 ± 1.2
	9 (neurotic)	Fl	6.0 ± 0.9
	16 (combined)	Fl	6.0 ± 0.8
	16 (recovered)	Fl	3.85 ± 0.2
679. Prange, 1972	12 (primary)	Fl	10.3 ± 1.3
832. Subrahmanyam, 1975	24	Fl	3.2 ± 0.6
305. Garfinkel, 1977	8 (bipolar)	Fl	4.13 ± 0.51
525. Linnoila, 1982	4 (rapid cyclers)	HPLC-EC	4.43 ± 1.12
524. Linnoila, 1983	12 (unipolar + bipolar)	HPLC-EC	2.35 ± 0.35

Table 139.   Unconjugated 5-Hydroxyindoleacetic Acid in Urine of

Depressed Subjects (continued)

Reference First Author, Year	Number of Subjects	Method of Analysis	Values (mg/24h ± S.E.M.)
539. Lykouras, 1988	18 (delusional)	GC-ECD	3.04 ± 0.26 mg/g Cr.
	22 (non-delusional)	GC-ECD	3.30 ± 0.23 mg/g Cr.

Table 140.   Unconjugated 5-Hydroxyindoleacetic Acid in CSF of

Depressed Subjects

Reference First Author, Year	Number of Subjects	Method of Analysis	Values (ng/mL ± S.E.M.)
42. Ashcroft, 1960	9 (depressive psychosis)	Fl	13.2 ± 2.5
286. Fotherby, 1963	11	Fl	12.2 ± 2.5
	11	Fl	114 ± 24 (plasma)
41. Ashcroft, 1966	24	Fl	11.1 ± 0.8
	4 (hypomanic)	Fl	18.7 ± 2.7
231. Dencker, 1966	17 (depressed)	Fl	<10-30
	8 (manic)	Fl	<10-30
314. Gerbode, 1968	33	Fl	30 ± 2
110. Bowers, 1969	18 (psychiatric)	Fl	28.8 ± 2.8
	8 (depressed)	Fl	34.0 ± 4.1
	8 (manic)	Fl	32.0 ± 3.6
854. Tamarkin, 1970	9	Fl	25 ± 1.5
619. Nordin, 1971	20 (endogenous)	Fl	31.1 ± 2.8

Table 140.   Unconjugated 5-Hydroxyindoleacetic Acid in CSF of

Depressed Subjects (continued)

Reference First Author, Year	Number of Subjects	Method of Analysis	Values (ng/mL ± S.E.M.)
637. Papeschi, 1971	12 (endogenous)	Fl	22 ± 2
885. Van Praag, 1971	15 (endogenous)	Fl	23 ± 4.4
884. Van Praag, 1971	14 (vital)	Fl	17 ± 4.5
109. Bowers, 1972	11 (unipolar)	Fl	62 ± 6
108. Bowers, 1972	44	Fl	58.5 ± 4.3
172. Coppen, 1972	31 (depressed)	Fl	19.8 ± 1.5
	14 (M)	Fl	21.4 ± 2.0
	17 (F)	Fl	18.5 ± 2.3
	18 (manic)	Fl	19.7 ± 1.6
	11 (M)	Fl	20.3 ± 2.3
	7 (F)	Fl	18.7 ± 2.3
	8 (recovered)	Fl	19.9 ± 2.5
502. Kupfer, 1972	9	Fl	69.2 ±15.6
567. Mendels, 1972	6 (depressed)	Fl	15.8 ± 2.7
	3 (manic)	Fl	8.8 ± 1.8
	6 (unipolar)	Fl	10.1 ± 2.0
	7 (psychotic)	Fl	12.8 ± 5.0
	8 (neurotic)	Fl	15.9 ± 2.0
888. Van Praag, 1972	10 (endogenous)	Fl	21.7 ± 2.4
37. Åsberg, 1973	43	GC-MS	19.7 ± 1.2
	11 (M)	GC-MS	15.8 ± 2.1
	32 (F)	GC-MS	21.0 ± 1.4

Table 140. Unconjugated 5-Hydroxyindoleacetic Acid in CSF of

Depressed Subjects (continued)

Reference First Author, Year	Number of Subjects	Method of Analysis	Values (ng/mL ± S.E.M.)
40. Ashcroft, 1973	11 (unipolar)	Fl	10 ± 2
	9 (bipolar depressed)	Fl	18 ± 3
	11 (bipolar manic)	Fl	15 ± 2
336. Goodwin, 1973	58 (depressed)	Fl	25.6 ± 1.3
	17 (hypomanic)	Fl	29.2 ± 2.4
339. Gordon, 1973	41	Fl	28.3 ± 2.2
671. Post, 1973	10 (hypomanic)	Fl	24.6 ± 1.8
	55 (depressed)	Fl	25.5 ± 1.3
	9 (depressed)	Fl	29.2 ± 3.7
	9 (simulated mania)	Fl	42.4 ± 4.4
887. Van Praag, 1973	28 (endogenous)	Fl	27 ± 2.0
	10 (neurotic)	Fl	23 ± 2.4
668. Post, 1974	46 (unipolar + bipolar)	Fl	25.4 ± 1.4
299. Fyrö, 1975	13 (manic)	GC-MS	20.1 ± 1.9
	5 (M)	GC-MS	19.7 ± 2.1
	8 (F)	GC-MS	20.2 ± 2.9
426. Jori, 1975	26 (psychotic)	Fl	22 ± 1
667. Post, 1975	21 (manic)	Fl	28
	77 (depressed)	Fl	25

Table 140.   Unconjugated 5-Hydroxyindoleacetic Acid in CSF of

Depressed Subjects (continued)

Reference First Author, Year	Number of Subjects	Method of Analysis	Values (ng/mL ± S.E.M.)
832. Subrahmanyam, 1975	24 (manic-depressive psychosis)	Fl	26.2 ± 4.2
3. Abrams, 1976	6 (endogenous)	Fl	32.8 ± 8.6
39. Åsberg, 1976	9 (endogenous)	GC-MS	19.6 ± 3.4
	6 (reactive)	GC-MS	17.0 ± 1.8
117. Bridges, 1976	10 (severe)	Fl	56 ± 5.4
	11 (less severe)	Fl	75 ± 7.8
	21 (combined)	Fl	66 ± 5.2
187. Curzon, 1976	37 (includes schizophrenia)	Fl	73 ± 4.3 (ventricular)
473. Kirstein, 1976	10 (unipolar + bipolar)	Fl[†]	88.2 ± 9.4
38. Åsberg, 1977	14 (endogenous, neurotic)	GC-MS	21.6 ± 1.9
54. Banki, 1977	55 (unipolar)	Fl	16.4 ± 0.9
	16 (bipolar depressed)	Fl	14.6 ± 1.7
	10 (bipolar-manic)	Fl	13.9 ± 2.9
794. Siwers, 1977	6	GC-MS	18.1 ± 3.1

<u>Table 140. Unconjugated 5-Hydroxyindoleacetic Acid in CSF of</u>

<u>Depressed Subjects (continued)</u>

Reference First Author, Year	Number of Subjects	Method of Analysis	Values (ng/mL ± S.E.M.)
894. Vestergaard, 1978	28 (before recovery)	Fl	29 ± 2.3
	14 (unipolar)	Fl	32 ± 3.2
	6 (bipolar)	Fl	23 ± 2.9
	15 (after recovery)	Fl	24 ± 3.9
	8 (unipolar)	Fl	21 ± 4.6
	4 (bipolar)	Fl	20 ± 3.5
	4 (manic)	Fl	40 ± 8
52. Ballenger, 1979	28 (personality disorder)	Fl	31.7 ± 2.0
	31 (alcoholic)	Fl	21.8 ± 1.9
864. Träskman, 1979	28 (endogenous)	GC-MS	17.4 ± 1.2
5. Ågren, 1980	21 (unipolar)	GC-MS	21.0 ± 1.8
	12 (bipolar)	GC-MS	17.8 ±10.5
75. Berger, 1980	13 (M) (primary)	GC-MS	36.2 ± 7.2
188. Curzon, 1980	6 (at worst)	Fl	9 ± 0.8 (lumbar)
	6 (not at worst)	Fl	21 ± 3.3 (lumbar)
	2 (agitated)	Fl	26 ± 4.2 (lumbar)
	20 (at worst)	Fl	71 ± 4.5 (ventricular)
	20 (not at worst)	Fl	80 ± 5.3 (ventricular)
	4 (agitated)	Fl	91 ± 9.5 (ventricular)
2. Åberg-Wistedt, 1981	25 (endogenous)	GC-MS	23.7 ± 2.3

Table 140. Unconjugated 5-Hydroxyindoleacetic Acid in CSF of

Depressed Subjects (continued)

Reference First Author, Year	Number of Subjects	Method of Analysis	Values (ng/mL ± S.E.M.)
57. Banki, 1981; 59. Banki, 1981	33 11 (severe)	Fl Fl	25.4 ± 2.2 (lumbar) 49.8 ± 5.3 (cisternal)
106. Bowden, 1981	17 (M) (unipolar) 26 (F) (unipolar)	GC-MS GC-MS	18.7 ± 0.7 24.1 ± 1.0
214. Davis, 1981	14 (unipolar + bipolar)	GC-MS	28.4
568. Mendlewicz, 1981	7 (unipolar)	-	51.8 ± 5.8
633. Oreland, 1981	6 (M) (depressed) 14 (F) (depressed) 5 (M) (recovered) 6 (F) (recovered)	GC-MS GC-MS GC-MS GC-MS	16.9 ± 1.8 20.0 ± 1.9 19.7 ± 2.3 23.9 ± 3.4
192. Dahl, 1982	25 (endogenous, combined) 9 (M) 16 (F)	GC-MS GC-MS GC-MS	17.6 ± 1.4 18.7 ± 2.7 16.8 ± 1.6
546. Maas, 1982	40 (F) 43 (M) (unipolar + bipolar)	- -	25.3 ± 1.3 19.3 ± 1.0
605. Nair, 1982	16 (unipolar + bipolar)	Fl	10.0 ± 0.2
732. Rydin, 1982	14 (endogenous, depressed) 14 (endogenous, depressed)	GC-MS GC-MS	22.1 ± 1.8 10.5 ± 1.1
7. Ågren, 1983	100	GC-MS	18.0 ± 1.0

Table 140. Unconjugated 5-Hydroxyindoleacetic Acid in CSF of

Depressed Subjects (continued)

Reference First Author, Year	Number of Subjects	Method of Analysis	Values (ng/mL ± S.E.M.)
55. Banki, 1983	43 (includes schizophrenics)	Fl	25.9 ± 2.0
56. Banki, 1983	32 (combined)	Fl	26.4 ± 2.0
	17 (unipolar)	Fl	29.4 ± 2.2
	9 (bipolar)	Fl	22.0 ± 3.4
493. Koslow, 1983; 548. Maas, 1984	26 (M) (unipolar)	GC-MS	19.7 ± 0.9
	31 (F) (unipolar)	GC-MS	25.4 ± 1.2
	23 (M) (bipolar)	GC-MS	20.4 ± 1.4
	12 (F) (bipolar)	GC-MS	23.3 ± 1.7
	9 (M) (manic)	GC-MS	22.5 ± 2.8
	5 (F) (manic)	GC-MS	30.8 ± 3.5
	49 (M) (depressed)	GC-MS	20.1 ± 0.8
	43 (F) (depressed)	GC-MS	24.8 ± 1.0
843. Swann, 1983	14 (manic)	GC-MS	25.6 ± 2.3
36. Åsberg, 1984	83 (melancholia)	GC-MS	17.8 ± 0.8
77. Berrettini, 1984	10 (bipolar)	HPLC-EC	17.6 ± 2.5
98. Bottiglieri, 1984	18 (primary)	HPLC-EC[†]	16.3 ± 1.6
316. Gerner, 1984	38 (depressed)	HPLC-EC	22.7 ± 1.5
	13 (manic)	HPLC-EC	22.8 ± 2.9
78. Berrettini, 1985	10 (bipolar)	HPLC-EC	17.6 ± 2.5

Table 140.   Unconjugated 5-Hydroxyindoleacetic Acid in CSF of

Depressed Subjects (continued)

Reference First Author, Year	Number of Subjects	Method of Analysis	Values (ng/mL ± S.E.M.)
104. Bowden, 1985	33 (M) 27 (F) (unipolar + bipolar)	GC-MS GC-MS	19.7 ± 1.0 25.2 ± 1.4
382. Hoffman, 1985	8 (unipolar + bipolar)	HPLC	17.6 ± 3.1
517. Lidberg, 1985	22 (suicide attempters)	GC-MS	13.7 ± 1.1
535. Lopez-Ibor, 1985	21 (melancholia)	Fl	15.0 ± 1.7
679. Potter, 1985	11 (unipolar + bipolar)	HPLC-EC[†]	22.2 ± 2.3
726. Roy, 1985	15 (melancholia) 8 (major depressive episode) 5 (dysthymic disorder)	HPLC-EC HPLC-EC HPLC-EC	16.6 ± 1.5 19.3 ± 2.6 17.7 ± 1.7
8. Ågren, 1986	52 27 (M) 25 (F)	GC-MS GC-MS GC-MS	16.4 ± 0.9 16.0 ± 1.3 17.0 ± 1.1
688. Redmond, 1986	164 (includes controls) 92 (depressed) 14 (manic)	GC-MS GC-MS GC-MS	22.1 ± 0.5 22.2 ± 0.7 25.2 ± 2.4
823. Standish-Barry, 1986	15 (severe, endogenous)	Fl	70 ± 8

Table 140. Unconjugated 5-Hydroxyindoleacetic Acid in CSF of

Depressed Subjects (continued)

Reference First Author, Year	Number of Subjects	Method of Analysis	Values (ng/mL ± S.E.M.)
625. Gjerris, 1987	33 (endogenous)	GC-MS[†]	25.8
	7 (non-endogenous)	GC-MS	22.3
394. Hsiao, 1987	40 (unipolar + bipolar)	HPLC-EC	18.9 ± 0.9
829. Stokes, 1987	23	GC-MS	18.9 ± 1.3
325. Golden, 1988	6 (unipolar + bipolar)	HPLC-EC	15.2 ± 1.8
723. Roy, 1988	27	HPLC-EC	17.3 ± 1.3
932. Westenberg, 1988	38	HPLC-EC[†]	21.6 ± 0.2
	21 (F)	HPLC-EC[†]	23.5 ± 0.4
	17 (M)	HPLC-EC[†]	19.3 ± 0.5

Table 141. 5-Hydroxyindoleacetic Acid in Urine of Schizophrenic

Subjects

Reference First Author, Year	Number of Subjects	Method of Analysis	Values (mg/24h ± S.E.M.)
273. Feldstein, 1958	30 (chronic)	Fl	5.3 ± 0.4
	7 (paranoid)	Fl	4.3
	3 (catatonic)	Fl	5.5
	5 (hebephrenic)	Fl	6.2
	3 (simple)	Fl	6.2
	12 (undifferentiated)	Fl	5.4
	23 (acute)	Fl	5.5 ± 0.9
274. Feldstein, 1959	32 (chronic)	Fl	5.4 ± 0.4*
	23 (M) (acute)	Fl	8.0 ± 2.1*
	12 (F) (acute)	Fl	6.6 ± 3.4*
486. Kopin, 1959	16	Fl	4.6 ± 2.2*
73. Benassi, 1961	8	Fl	2.82 ± 0.06
124. Brune, 1961	14 (inactive)	Chem	5.9
	10 (slightly active)	Chem	6.2
	6 (moderately)	Chem	9.8
	6 (active)	Chem	8.8
	2 (markedly active)	Chem	17.8
10. Allegranza, 1965	9	Fl	5.16 ± 0.30
	9	Fl	4.94 ± 0.26
115. Bozzi, 1965	11	Fl	5.34 ± 0.31
374. Herkert, 1969	10	Fl	5.8 ± 0.6

Table 141.   5-Hydroxyindoleacetic Acid in Urine of Schizophrenic
Subjects (continued)

Reference First Author, Year	Number of Subjects	Method of Analysis	Values (mg/24h ± S.E.M.)
832. Subrahmanyam, 1975	30 (acute)	Fl	2.6 ± 0.4
	6 (acute, aggressive)	Fl	6.4 ± 1.0
	24 (chronic)	Fl	3.8 ± 0.4
237. Domino, 1979	7 (chronic)	GC-MS[†]	6.62 ± 0.38
782. Shen, 1979	100 (combined)	Bio-Assay	5.9 ± 0.4
	60 (various psychoses)	Bio-Assay	6.8 ± 0.6
	22 (acute)	Bio-Assay	4.7 ± 0.4
	16 (not acute)	Bio-Assay	7.5 ± 0.5

* In original paper expressed as μg/h.

<u>Table 142.   5-Hydroxyindoleacetic Acid in CSF of Schizophrenic Subjects</u>

Reference First Author, Year	Number of Subjects	Method of Analysis	Values (ng/mL ± S.E.M.)
286. Fotherby, 1963	11	Fl	11.5 ± 1.2
	11	Fl	82 ± 17 (plasma)
648. Persson, 1965	40	Fl	26
41. Ashcroft, 1966	7 (acute)	Fl	10.9 ± 0.9
	7 (chronic)	Fl	16.4 ± 1.1
649. Persson, 1968	4	Fl	35 ± 5
110. Bowers, 1969	7	Fl	26.8 ± 3.9
662. Pind, 1970	8 (with tardive dyskinesia)	Fl	30 ± 7
341. Gottfries, 1971	40	Fl	31.4 ± 1.4 (µg/mL)
696. Rimon, 1971	9 (paranoid)	Fl	32.7 ± 3.8
	8 (other paranoid)	Fl	31.6 ± 5.9
	17 (all paranoid)	Fl	32.2 ± 3.3
	13 (non-paranoid)	Fl	27.7 ± 3.1
	9 (other non- paranoid)	Fl	31.5 ± 3.6
	22 (all non- paranoid)	Fl	29.3 ± 3.0
883. Van Praag, 1973	12	Fl	28 ± 5
295. Fri, 1974	5	GC-MS[†]	19.5 ± 3.2
426. Jori, 1975	7	Fl	20 ± 1
667. Post, 1975	18	Fl	26
832. Subrahmanyam, 1975	30 (acute)	Fl	20.6 ± 2.8
	6 (acute, aggressive)	Fl	43.4 ± 4.2
	24 (chronic)	Fl	28.4 ± 2.2

Table 142. 5-Hydroxyindoleacetic Acid in CSF of Schizophrenic Subjects

(continued)

Reference First Author, Year	Number of Subjects	Method of Analysis	Values (ng/mL ± S.E.M.)
473. Kirstein, 1976	10	Fl[†]	99.2 ± 12.5
91. Bjerkenstedt, 1977	34	GC-MS	26.0 ± 11.1
	29	GC-MS	24.3 ± 1.3
363. Härnryd, 1979	12	GC-MS	21.2 ± 2.5
604. Nagao, 1979	15	Fl	22.5 ± 1.4
	12 (with tardive dyskinesia)	Fl	22.5 ± 1.4
75. Berger, 1980	9	GC-MS	34.3 ± 3.5
332. Gomes, 1980	10 (acute)	Fl	31.4 ± 1.6
	10 (chronic)	Fl	34.8 ± 3.1
	15 (pseudo-organic)	Fl	32.4 ± 2.0
	19 (personality disorder)	Fl	32.3 ± 1.3
770. Sedvall, 1980	11 (with family history)	GC-MS	26.5 ± 3.2
	25 (no family history)	GC-MS	20.6 ± 1.3
311. Gattaz, 1982	15 (on neuroleptics)	HPLC-EC[†]	9.9 ± 3.7
	13 (off drugs)	HPLC-EC	11.8 ± 4.6
	28 (combined)	HPLC-EC	10.8 ± 4.2
650. Petrucelli, 1982	20	HPLC-EC[†]	24.3 ± 2.4
954. Wood, 1982	9	GC-MS	26.0 ± 4.8

Table 142.   5-Hydroxyindoleacetic Acid in CSF of Schizophrenic Subjects

(continued)

Reference First Author, Year	Number of Subjects	Method of Analysis	Values (ng/mL ± S.E.M.)
56. Banki, 1983	32 (combined)	Fl	21.4 ± 1.2
	10 (acute)	Fl	17.6 ± 1.2
	6 (catatonic)	Fl	22.7 ± 3.8
	4 (disorganized)	Fl	17.0 ± 3.3
	12 (paranoid)	Fl	24.1 ± 2.5
72. Beckmann, 1983	9	HPLC	9.3 ± 1.3
530. Linnoila, 1983	28	HPLC-EC	24.4 ± 1.7
	19 (M)	HPLC-EC	23.9 ± 2.1
	9 (F)	HPLC-EC	25.4 ± 3.1
620. Nybäck, 1983	26	GC-MS	19.1 ± 1.7
675. Potkin, 1983	15	HPLC-EC	8.5
316. Gerner, 1984	20	HPLC-EC	26.9 ± 5.4
617. Ninan, 1984	8 (non-suicidal)	HPLC-EC	28.3
	8 (suicidal)	HPLC-EC	18.0
755. Scheinin, 1984	46 (chronic)	HPLC-EC[†]	15.5 ± 0.6
46. Bagdy, 1985	15 (chronic)	Fl	29.2 ± 2.9
309. Gattaz, 1985	13	HPLC-EC	11.8 ± 1.3
520. Lindstrom, 1985	40	GC-MS	21.2 ± 1.2
735. Saito, 1986	9 (with Parkinson's disease)	HPLC-EC	21.3 ± 3.3
	9 (with Tardive dyskinesis)	HPLC-EC	20.3 ± 2.2

Table 143.   5-Hydroxyindoleacetic Acid in Urine of Parkinson's Disease

Patients

Reference First Author, Year	Number of Subjects	Method of Analysis	Values (± S.E.M.)
632. O'Reilly, 1965	6	Fl	8.73 ± 1.68 mg/g Cr.
123. Brune, 1971	8	Fl	6.4 ± 0.7 mg/24 h.

Table 144.   5-Hydroxyindoleacetic Acid in CSF of Parkinson's Disease

Patients

Reference First Author, Year	Number of Subjects	Method of Analysis	Values (ng/mL ± S.E.M.)
627. Olsson, 1968	8	Fl	20 ± 12.4
342. Gottfries, 1969	24	Fl	20 ± 2.0
152. Chase, 1970	10	Fl	29 ± 2.9
682. Pullar, 1970	26	Fl	13 ± 1.0
892. Van Woert, 1970	10	Fl	20 ± 2
186. Curzon, 1971	18	Fl	21 ± 2.6
642. Parkes, 1971	12	Fl	17 ± 3.5
153. Chase, 1972	6	Fl	27 ± 4.2
154. Chase, 1972	15	Fl	24 ± 3.1
508. Lakke, 1972	27	Fl	20.4 ± 2.3
638. Papeschi, 1972	17	Fl	46 ± 7 (ventricular)
	4	Fl	24 ± 9 (lumbar)
699. Rinne, 1972	80	Fl	26.3 ± 1.5
	28 (M)	Fl	25.3 ± 2.6
	52 (F)	Fl	26.8 ± 1.9
700. Rinne, 1973	116	Fl	24.0 ± 1.3

Table 144.   5-Hydroxyindoleacetic Acid in CSF of Parkinson's Disease

Patients (continued)

Reference First Author, Year	Number of Subjects	Method of Analysis	Values (ng/mL ± S.E.M.)
643. Parkes, 1974	5 (old)	Fl	12 ± 4
	16 (young)	Fl	17 ± 2
202. Davidson, 1977	74	Fl	14 ± 1
568. Mendlewicz, 1981	–	–	52.8 ± 9.8
317. Gibson, 1985	4 (mild)	HPLC-EC[†]	15.2 ± 1.5
	8 (moderate)	HPLC-EC	18.5 ± 3.6
	9 (severe)	HPLC-EC	19.7 ± 3.1
	21 (combined)	HPLC-EC	18.3 ± 1.8
822. Stahl, 1985	6 (tardive dyskinesis)	GC-MS	27.8 ± 5.6
	9 (dystonia)	GC-MS	23.4 ± 2.9
906. Volicer, 1985	10	HPLC-EC	21.6 ± 3.6

Table 145. 5-Hydroxyindoleacetic Acid in CSF of Alzheimer's Disease

Patients

Reference First Author, Year	Number of Subjects	Method of Analysis	Values (ng/mL ± S.E.M.)
342. Gottfries, 1969	18 (senile)	Fl	30 ± 2.4
	10 (presenile)	Fl	20 ± 3.2
344. Gottfries, 1973	15	Fl	35 ± 3.4
643. Parkes, 1974	8 (senile)	Fl	31 ± 3
568. Mendlewicz, 1981	7 (senile)	–	62.5 ± 7.5
814. Soininen, 1981	28	Fl	35 ± 2
	9 (less severe)	Fl	38 ± 5
	9 (severe)	Fl	37 ± 5
	10 (very severe)	Fl	31 ± 3
62. Bareggi, 1982	16	Fl[†]	29.5 ± 4.5
	8 (mild)	Fl	35.6 ± 6.8
	8 (severe)	Fl	23.5 ± 4.2
954. Wood, 1982	11	GC-MS	22.5 ± 2.7
458. Kay, 1984	28	HPLC[†]	14.4 ± 0.2
635. Palmer, 1984	16 (presenile)	HPLC-EC[†]	16.0 ± 1.5
	4 (senile)	HPLC-EC	13.7 ± 2.9
317. Gibson, 1985	32	HPLC-EC[†]	19.4 ± 3.5
	17 (mild)	HPLC-EC	19.1 ± 3.2
	10 (moderate)	HPLC-EC	21.5 ± 3.0
	5 (severe)	HPLC-EC	16.1 ± 1.3
816. Sparks, 1985	4	HPLC-EC[†]	17 ± 1

Table 145.   5-Hydroxyindoleacetic Acid in CSF of Alzheimer's Disease

Patients (continued)

Reference First Author, Year	Number of Subjects	Method of Analysis	Values (ng/mL ± S.E.M.)
906. Volicer, 1985	9	HPLC-EC	27.9 ± 2.9
	2 (presenile)	HPLC-EC	26.2 ±15.8
	7 (senile)	HPLC-EC	28.4 ± 1.5
907. Volicer, 1985	10 (caudal)	HPLC-EC[†]	12.9 ± 1.3
	14 (rostral)	HPLC-EC	18.0 ± 1.4
621. Nybäck, 1987	15	GC-MS	24.1 ± 1.9
701. Risby, 1987	12	HPLC-EC	19.7 ± 2.1
834. Sunderland, 1987	13	HPLC-EC	20.6 ± 1.9
495. Koyama, 1988	6	HPLC-EC[†]	8.1 ± 1.9

Table 146. 5-Hydroxyindoleacetic Acid in CSF of Aggressive and Suicidal

Subjects

Reference First Author, Year	Number of Subjects	Method of Analysis	Values (ng/mL ± S.E.M.)
88. Bioulac, 1978	5 (aggressive)	Fl	21.6 ± 1.9
118. Brown, 1979	3 (antisocial)	Fl	23.5 ± 5.8
	4 (explosive)	Fl	17.6 ± 4.4
	5 (immature)	Fl	23.3 ± 3.5
	3 (passive-aggressive)	Fl	41.3 ± 7.6
	3 (passive-depressed)	Fl	35.5 ± 0.8
	3 (schizoid)	Fl	41.0 ± 7.9
	2 (obsessional- compulsive)	Fl	40.8 ± 9.2
	24 (more impulsive)	Fl	21.5 ± 2.4
	24 (less impulsive)	Fl	40.0 ± 2.7
	24 (history of (suicide)	Fl	22.2 ± 3.1
	24 (no history of suicide)	Fl	35.8 ± 3.1
633. Oreland, 1981	5 (M) (suicidal, not depressed)	GC-MS	10.1 ± 1.8
	10 (F) (suicidal, not depressed)	GC-MS	15.4 ± 1.3
865. Träskman, 1981	30 (suicide attempters)	GC-MS	16.3 ± 0.9
	8 (depressed)	GC-MS	14.2 ± 1.3
	22 (not depressed)	GC-MS	17.0 ± 1.1

Table 146.   5-Hydroxyindoleacetic Acid in CSF of Aggressive and Suicidal

Subjects (continued)

Reference First Author, Year	Number of Subjects	Method of Analysis	Values (ng/mL ± S.E.M.)
55. Banki, 1983	6 (violent suicide)	Fl	16.3 ± 1.8
	13 (non-violent)	Fl	25.6 ± 3.2
532. Linnoila, 1983	21 (murderers)	HPLC	15.6 ± 0.9
	15 (attempted murder)	HPLC	13.9 ± 1.2
	17 (more than one violent crime)	HPLC	13.0 ± 0.6
	– (only one violent crime)	HPLC	16.6 ± 4.5 (S.D.)
	– (violent, suicide attempt)	HPLC	12.9 ± 3.7 (S.D.)
	– (violent, no suicide attempt)	HPLC	17.4 ± 4.2 (S.D.)
517. Lidberg, 1985	15 (homicidal)	GC-MS	17.4 ± 1.4
535. Lopez-Ibor, 1985	– (self-aggressive)	Fl	9.1 ± 2.8 (S.D.)
	– (not self-aggressive)	Fl	16.8 ± 8.1 (S.D.)
	– (suicidal)	Fl	12.4 ± 7.0 (S.D.)
	– (non-suicidal)	Fl	17.2 ± 8.3 (S.D.)
897. Virkkunen, 1987	20 (violent)	HPLC-EC	13.0 ± 0.7

Table 147. Unconjugated Homovanillic Acid in Urine of Normal Subjects

Reference First Author, Year	Number of Subjects	Method of Analysis	Values (mg/24h ± S.E.M.)
942. Williams, 1960	5	Fl[†]	9.6 ± 0.8
943. Williams, 1961	4	GC-FID	3.6 mg/g Cr.
729. Ruthven, 1962	14	Fl[†]	6.0 ± 0.3
745. Sankoff, 1963	18	Fl[†]	8.23 ± 0.70
751. Sato, 1965	5	Fl[†]	5.4 ± 0.6
731. Ruthven, 1966	15	Fl[†]	5.4 ± 0.3
241. Duke, 1968	12	Fl[†]	5.2 ± 0.4
313. Geissbühler, 1969	46	Fl[†]	5.4 ± 0.5
439. Karoum, 1969	20	GC-FID	4.2 ± 0.3
927. Weil-Malherbe, 1969	20	Fl[†]	2.17 ± 0.17
	17 (M)	Fl	3.53 ± 0.28
	3 (F)	Fl	1.36 ± 0.23
169. Comoy, 1971	10	Fl[†]	5.4
	10	Fl	0.05 (iso-HVA)
256. Eichorn, 1971	14	Fl[†]	6.89 ± 0.76 mg/g Cr.
434. Kahane, 1971	7	Fl	4.25 ± 0.87
808. Smith, 1971	8	Fl	4.45 ± 0.62
	8	Fl	-0.60 (conjugated)
247. Dziedzic, 1972	30	GC-ECD[†]	3.30 ± 0.20 mg/g Cr.
	19 (M)	GC-ECD	3.26 ± 0.23 mg/g Cr.
	11 (F)	GC-ECD	3.33 ± 0.39 mg/g Cr.
850. Takahashi, 1972	10	Fl[†]	1.61 ± 0.15 mg/g Cr.
895. Vidi, 1972	10	Fl[†]	1.71
193. Dailey, 1973	10	GC-FlD[†]	3.42 ± 0.54 mg/g Cr.
248. Dziedzic, 1973	20	GC-ECD[†]	3.72 mg/g Cr.
	20	GC-ECD	0.28 mg/g Cr. (iso-HVA)
570. Messiha, 1973	12	Fl[†]	9.41 ± 0.71
611. Narasimhachari, 1974	6	GC-MS[†]	3.4

Table 147. Unconjugated Homovanillic Acid in Urine of Normal Subjects

(continued)

Reference First Author, Year	Number of Subjects	Method of Analysis	Values (mg/24h ± S.E.M.)
711. Roginsky, 1974	25	GC-FID[†]	4.1 ± 0.36
830. Stott, 1975	123	Fl[†]	4.9 ± 0.1
	80 (M)	Fl	4.9 ± 0.1
	43 (F)	Fl	4.9 ± 0.1
839. Swahn, 1976	5	GC-MS[†]	27.7 mg/L
	5	GC-MS	5.8 mg/L (conj.)
910. Wadman, 1976	9	GC-FID[†]	7.6 ± 0.4
963. Yoshida, 1976	14	HPLC	4.0 ± 0.3
234. De Schaepdryver, 1978	20	Fl[†]	6.9 ± 0.7
598. Muskiet, 1978	25	GC-MS[†]	4.0 ± 0.3 mg/g Cr.
237. Domino, 1979	7	GC-MS[†]	11.3 ± 1.1
744. Sandler, 1979	27	GC-FID	4.06 ± 0.18
	10 (M)	GC-FID	4.59 ± 0.40
	17 (F)	GC-FID	3.75 ± 0.25
156. Chauhan, 1980	5	GC-ECD[†]	6.7 ± 1.0
	5	GC-ECD	0.48 ± 0.10 (iso-HVA)
714. Rosano, 1981	31	Fl[†]	3.6
	26	Fl	2.7 mg/g Cr.
441. Karoum, 1982	5	GC-MS[†]	2.9 ± 0.2
933. Westerink, 1982	6	HPLC[†]	3.9 ± 0.3
935. Wiesel, 1982	33 (M)	GC-MS	5.01 ± 0.19*
	33 (F)	GC-MS	4.58 ± 0.35*
218. De Jong, 1983	7	GC-FID[†]	4.03 ± 0.48 mg/g Cr.
87. Binder, 1984	110	HPLC-EC[†]	3.14 ± 0.15
471. Kiriike, 1984	31	Fl	5.4 ± 0.5
560. Mathieu, 1984	62	GC-ECD[†]	4.60 ± 0.26
211. Davis, 1986	10	GC-MS[†]	5.37

Table 147. Unconjugated Homovanillic Acid in Urine of Normal Subjects

(continued)

Reference First Author, Year	Number of Subjects	Method of Analysis	Values (mg/24h ± S.E.M.)
290. Frankenhaueser, 1986	19 (M) 30 (F)	GC-MS GC-MS	5.53 ± 0.55* 3.51 ± 0.24*
485. Kodama, 1986	18	HPLC[†]	6.2 ± 0.45 mg/g Cr.
724. Roy, 1986	25	GC-MS	4.40 ± 0.19 (total)
50. Baker, 1987	29	GC-ECD[†]	6.4 ± 1.2
209. Davis, 1987	8	GC-MS[†]	3.94 ± 0.33
628. Ong, 1987	200	HPLC-EC[†]	3.3 ± 0.8
319. Gironi, 1988	120	HPLC-EC[†]	3.79 ± 0.13
431. Julien, 1988	6	HPLC-EC[†]	5.2 ± 0.7
488. Kopin, 1988	18	GC-MS	5.19 ± 0.35
529. Linnoila, 1988	12	GC-MS	5.18 ± 0.62 (total)
623. Odink, 1988	6 (M) 6 (F)	HPLC-EC[†] HPLC-EC[†]	5.19 3.73

* In original paper expressed as nmol/min.

Table 148. Unconjugated Homovanillic Acid in Plasma of Normal Subjects

Reference First Author, Year	Number of Subjects	Method of Analysis	Values (ng/mL ± S.E.M.)
313. Geissbühler, 1969	5	Fl[†]	160 (serum)
22. Ånggard, 1973	11	GC-MS[†]	18.2 ± 1.8 (serum)
801. Sjöquist, 1973	1	GC-MS[†]	8.7
610. Narasimhachari, 1975	17	GC-MS[†]	44 ± 6.8 (serum)
447. Karoum, 1977	10	GC-MS[†]	11.7 ± 1.9
853. Takahashi, 1978	5	GC-MS[†]	10.2 ± 2.5
547. Maas, 1980	6	GC-MS	13.3 ± 1.9
599. Muskiet, 1980	23	GC-MS[†]	11.3 ± 0.9 (serum)
842. Swan, 1980	–	GC-MS	10.5 ± 1.3 (S.D.)
603. Naber, 1981	14	GC-MS	5.9 ± 0.5
113. Bowers, 1983	22 14 (F) 8 (M)	GC-MS GC-MS GC-MS	12.9 ± 0.8 13.2 ± 0.8 12.5 ± 1.7
397. Hunneman, 1983	16	GC-MS[†]	12.0 ± 1.0
588. Moore, 1983	25 12 (M) 13 (F)	GC-MS GC-MS GC-MS	13.3 12.5 14.1
364. Harris, 1984	22	HPLC-EC[†]	9.8 ± 0.5
660. Pickar, 1984	8	HPLC	9.8 ± 1.3
235. Devanand, 1985	7 (M) 11 (F)	GC-MS GC-MS	13.1 ± 1.1 12.3 ± 0.7
950. Wolkowitz, 1985	12	HPLC-EC	9.1 ± 0.8
974. Yu, 1985	21 (prisoners) 61 (prisoners)	GC-MS GC-MS	7.9 ± 0.6 8.5 ± 0.4
217. De Jong, 1986	10	GC-MS[†]	12.1 ± 2.1
315. Gerhardt, 1986	6	HPLC-EC[†]	12.8 ± 2.0

Table 148. Unconjugated Homovanillic Acid in Plasma of Normal Subjects

(continued)

Reference First Author, Year	Number of Subjects	Method of Analysis	Values (ng/mL ± S.E.M.)
112. Bowers, 1987	65 (M) 112 (F)	GC–MS GC–MS	13.3 ± 0.6 14.0 ± 0.5
209. Davis, 1987	14	GC–MS[†]	8.2 ± 2.8
949. Wolkowitz, 1987	35	HPLC–EC	10.0 ± 0.9
9. Alfredsson, 1988	10	GC–MS	14.9 ± 2.9 (serum)
203. Davidson, 1988	14	GC–MS	9.5 ± 0.7
772. Semba, 1988	13	HPLC–EC[†]	10.8 ± 0.9

Table 149. Unconjugated Homovanillic Acid in CSF of Normal Subjects

Reference First Author, Year	Number of Subjects	Method of Analysis	Values (ng/mL ± S.E.M.)
13. Andén, 1963	–	Fl[†]	75, 100
648. Persson, 1965	29	Fl	36
177. Coward, 1966	–	Fl[†]	20-50
314. Gerbode, 1968	18	Fl	40 ± 7 (total)
627. Olsson, 1968	7	Fl	50 ± 5
698. Rinne, 1968	15	Fl	85.9 ± 7.7
313. Geissbühler, 1969	5	Fl[†]	160
342. Gottfries, 1969	15	Fl	60 ± 8
152. Chase, 1970	10	Fl	31 ± 5.1
582. Moir, 1970	18	Fl	466 ± 38 (ventricular)
	1	Fl	185 (cisternal)
	11	Fl	53 ± 11 (lumbar)
186. Curzon, 1971	11	Fl	39 ± 4
323. Godwin-Austen, 1971	9	Fl	45 ± 3
338. Gordon, 1971	4	GC-ECD[†]	370 (ventricular)
	40	GC-ECD	37 (lumbar)
341. Gottfries, 1971	20 (old)	Fl	60.4 ± 7.2
	24 (young)	Fl	30.8 ± 2.6
637. Papeschi, 1971	18	Fl	50 ± 6
642. Parkes, 1971	11	Fl	39 ± 4
696. Rimon, 1971	27	Fl	24.6 ± 2.8
886. Van Praag, 1971	12	Fl	42 ± 4.6
108. Bowers, 1972	15	Fl	92.9 ± 7
155. Chase, 1972	8	Fl	28 ± 6.8
412. Jequier, 1972	20	Fl	87.2 ± 9.2
435. Kangasniemi, 1972	6	Fl[†]	26.0 ± 6.0
638. Papeschi, 1972	25	Fl	53 ± 1

Table 149. Unconjugated Homovanillic Acid in CSF of Normal Subjects

(continued)

Reference First Author, Year	Number of Subjects	Method of Analysis	Values (ng/mL ± S.E.M.)
699. Rinne, 1972	63	Fl	34.6 ± 1.9
154. Chase, 1973	11	Fl	352 ± 54 (ventricular)
	7	Fl	30 ± 2.8 (lumbar)
303. Garelis, 1973	19	Fl	49.1 ± 3.4
336. Goodwin, 1973	28	Fl	22.4 ± 2
339. Gordon, 1973	5	Fl	23.6 ± 8.2
344. Gottfries, 1973	20	Fl	60 ± 7
671. Post, 1973	29	Fl	22.4 ± 2.4
700. Rinne, 1973	64	Fl	34.4 ± 1.9
801. Sjöquist, 1973	1	GC-MS[†]	76.4
887. Van Praag, 1973	12	Fl	35 ± 3.9
249. Dziedzic, 1974	–	GC-ECD[†]	40
643. Parkes, 1974	16	Fl	40 ± 6
691. Renaud, 1974	5	Fl	47 ± 8
340. Gordon, 1975	13	GC-MS	23.7 ± 3.5
420. Johansson, 1975	7	Fl	143 (cisternal)
444. Karoum, 1975	5	GC-MS	51 ± 8 (lumbar)
	8	GC-MS	154 ± 14.4 (cisternal)
610. Narasimhachari, 1975	19	GC-MS[†]	22 ± 19
667. Post, 1975	10	Fl	22
803. Sjöström, 1975	11	GC-MS	46.4 ± 8.6
832. Subrahmanyam, 1975	12	Fl	40.2 ± 4
	12	Fl	42.4 ± 3.8
889. Van Praag, 1975	12	–	42 ± 16
919. Watson, 1975	22	GC-ECD[†]	23
117. Bridges, 1976	4	Fl	165 ± 28 (ventricular)

Table 149. Unconjugated Homovanillic Acid in CSF of Normal Subjects

(continued)

Reference First Author, Year	Number of Subjects	Method of Analysis	Values (ng/mL ± S.E.M.)
839. Swahn, 1976	5 5	GC-MS[†] GC-MS	61.9 ± 1.8 60.1 (total)
54. Banki, 1977	32	Fl	33.4 ± 1.0
202. Davidson, 1977	5	Fl	31 ± 5.8
88. Bioulac, 1978	6	Fl	47 ± 8
800. Sjöquist, 1978	7	GC-MS	60.2 ± 5.3
894. Vestergaard, 1978	23	GC-ECD	45 ± 5.4
270. Faull, 1979	23 23	GC-MS[†] GC-MS	43.6 ± 3.7 0.25± 0.58 (conj.)
550. Major, 1979	7	GC-MS	26.9 ± 2.6
188. Curzon, 1980	5	Fl	165 ± 25 (ventricular)
332. Gomes, 1980	20	Fl	33.1 ± 2.3
768. Sedvall, 1980	32 (no family history) 28 (family history of psychiatric morbidity)	GC-MS GC-MS	34.4 ± 1.4 34.4 ± 2.8
905. Vogt, 1980	10	GC-MS[†]	30.9
16. Andersen, 1981	5	GC-MS[†]	39.7 ± 3.1
59. Banki, 1981	32	Fl	27.7 ± 2.2
107. Bowen, 1981	12	–	33 ± 4.6
633. Oreland, 1981	28 (M) 14 (F)	GC-MS GC-MS	39.1 ± 3.8 47.8 ± 3.5
814. Soininen, 1981	13	Fl	78 ± 7
865. Träskman, 1981	45	GC-MS	44.4 ± 3.3
62. Bareggi, 1982	8	Fl	67.5 ± 3.7
311. Gattaz, 1982	16	HPLC-EC[†]	33.9 ± 18.1

Table 149. Unconjugated Homovanillic Acid in CSF of Normal Subjects

(continued)

Reference First Author, Year	Number of Subjects	Method of Analysis	Values (ng/mL ± S.E.M.)
455. Kasa, 1982	16	Fl[†]	41.8 ± 4.2
585. Montplaisir, 1982	11	Fl	40.7 ± 5.4
954. Wood, 1982	32	GC-MS	52.1 ± 4.7
45. Bagdy, 1983	21 (F)	Fl	19.9 ± 1.3
	6 (M)	Fl	22.9 ± 4.1
493. Koslow, 1983	32 (F)	GC-MS	43.7 ± 2.6
	30 (M)	GC-MS	40.0 ± 2.3
620. Nybäck, 1983	43	GC-MS	32.6 ± 1.8
843. Swann, 1983	62	GC-MS	41.9 ± 1.8
878. Van Bockstaele, 1983	11	HPLC-EC[†]	40.7 ± 6.0
36. Åsberg, 1984	66	GC-MS	44.8 ± 2.6
77. Berrettini, 1984	20	HPLC-EC	32.8 ± 2.2
98. Bottiglieri, 1984	9	HPLC-EC[†]	53.3 ± 10.7
316. Gerner, 1984	37	HPLC-EC	28.6 ± 2.5
386. Honegger, 1984	8	HPLC[†]	31.8 ± 2.6
409. Javors, 1984	7	HPLC-EC[†]	39.9 ± 8.1
458. Kay, 1984	12	HPLC[†]	26.3 ± 0.7
635. Palmer, 1984	25	HPLC-EC[†]	42.3 ± 3.4
690. Reimherr, 1984	13	GC-MS	37.1 ± 3.3
78. Berrettini, 1985	28	HPLC-EC	32.0 ± 2.0
309. Gattaz, 1985	16	HPLC-EC	33.9 ± 4.5
517. Lidberg, 1985	39	GC-MS	40.0 ± 3.0
520. Lindstrom, 1985	21	GC-MS	48.0 ± 3.8
816. Sparks, 1985	4	HPLC-EC[†]	35 ± 21
822. Stahl, 1985	36	GC-MS	45.6 ± 3.3

Table 149. Unconjugated Homovanillic Acid in CSF of Normal Subjects

(continued)

Reference First Author, Year	Number of Subjects	Method of Analysis	Values (ng/mL ± S.E.M.)
824. Stanley, 1985	48	HPLC	71.6
211. Davis, 1986	10	GC-MS[†]	20.1
217. De Jong, 1986	14	GC-MS[†]	34.1 ± 5.6
354. Guthrie, 1986	27	HPLC-EC	27.7 ± 11.1
634. Oxenstierna, 1986	30 (monozygotic twins)	GC-MS	34.6 ± 2.3
	30 (dizygotic twins)	GC-MS	27.5 ± 1.9
	30 (brothers)	GC-MS	25.1 ± 2.8
	30 (unrelated men)	GC-MS	25.3 ± 2.2
735. Saito, 1986	9	HPLC-EC	45.0 ± 4.6
11. Almay, 1987	35	HPLC-EC	37.8 ± 2.0
	16 (M)	HPLC-EC	35.3 ± 2.5
	19 (F)	HPLC-EC	39.8 ± 2.9
262. Emanuelsson, 1987	11	GC-MS	35.7 ± 4.1
322. Gjerris, 1987	15	GC-MS	42.0
621. Nybäck, 1987	18	GC-MS	39.1 ± 5.2
834. Sunderland, 1987	7	HPLC-EC	41.5 ± 3.8
9. Alfredsson, 1988	10	GC-MS	22.4 ± 0.3
495. Koyama, 1988	5	HPLC-EC[†]	42.2 ± 4.5
723. Roy, 1988	38	HPLC-EC	27.6 ± 1.9
932. Westenberg, 1988	48	HPLC-EC[†]	37.2 ± 0.3
	27 (F)	HPLC-EC[†]	39.6 ± 0.7
	21 (M)	HPLC-EC[†]	34.1 ± 0.6

Table 150. Unconjugated Homovanillic Acid in Urine of Depressed

Subjects

Reference First Author, Year	Number of Subjects	Method of Analysis	Values (mg/24h ± S.E.M.)
849. Takahashi, 1968	1 patient, 4 times (manic-depressive)	Fl	4.9 ± 0.4
593. Murphy, 1973	6 (bipolar)	Fl	4.97 ± 0.67
	6 (unipolar)	Fl	5.82 ± 0.71
744. Sandler, 1979	23	GC-FID	3.55 ± 0.24
	10 (M)	GC-FID	3.93 ± 0.47
	13 (F)	GC-FID	3.28 ± 0.18
441. Karoum, 1982	6	GC-MS[†]	4.3 ± 0.6
452. Karoum, 1982	6 (unipolar + bipolar)	GC-MS	3.14 ± 0.51
525. Linnoila, 1982	4 (F) (rapid cyclers)	GC-MS	4.9 ± 1.0
528. Linnoila, 1983	7 (unipolar + bipolar)	GC-MS	4.64 ± 0.61
524. Linnoila, 1983	12 (unipolar + bipolar)	GC-MS	3.33 ± 0.31
724. Roy, 1986	7 (no melancholia)	GC-MS	5.41 ± 0.65 (total)
	5 (history of melancholia)	GC-MS	4.30 ± 0.66 (total)
	8 (with melancholia)	GC-MS	3.89 ± 0.37 (total)
	8 (dysthymic disorder)	GC-MS	4.99 ± 0.34 (total)
539. Lykouras, 1988	18 (delusional)	GC-ECD	3.33 ± 0.25 mg/g Cr.
	22 (non-delusional)	GC-ECD	2.97 ± 0.31 mg/g Cr.

<u>Table 151.   Unconjugated Homovanillic Acid in Plasma of Depressed</u>

<u>Subjects</u>

Reference First Author, Year	Number of Subjects	Method of Analysis	Values (ng/mL ± S.E.M.)
364. Harris, 1984	25 (psychiatric)	HPLC-EC[†]	9.2 ± 1.8
529. Linnoila, 1984	8 (unipolar)	HPLC-EC	19.2 ± 1.7
235. Devanand, 1985	4 (M) (psychotic)	GC-MS	10.8 ± 1.0
	5 (M) (non-psychotic)	GC-MS	12.3 ± 1.6
	7 (F) (psychotic)	GC-MS	21.1 ± 3.2
	13 (F) (non-psychotic)	GC-MS	16.2 ± 2.1
	9 (M) (combined)	GC-MS	11.7 ± 1.0
	20 (F) (combined)	GC-MS	17.9 ± 1.8
562. Mazure, 1987	15 (major (depression)	GC-MS	12.3 ± 1.2
	10 (melancholic)	GC-MS	18.9 ± 2.4
	8 (depressive psychosis)	GC-MS	22.2 ± 6.9
949. Wolkowitz, 1987	18 (all depressed)	HPLC-EC	10.8 ± 2.0
	7 (psychotic)	HPLC-EC	11.4 ± 2.5
	10 (non-psychotic)	HPLC-EC	10.8 ± 3.1
	12 (unipolar)	HPLC-EC	10.7 ± 2.6
	6 (bipolar)	HPLC-EC	11.2 ± 3.8
325. Golden, 1988	10 (unipolar + bipolar)	HPLC-EC	8.4 ± 0.6

Table 152. Unconjugated Homovanillic Acid in CSF of Depressed Subjects

Reference First Author, Year	Number of Subjects	Method of Analysis	Values (ng/mL ± S.E.M.)
231. Dencker, 1966	5	Fl	10 – 50
314. Gerbode, 1968	15 (psychiatric)	Fl	42 ± 8
110. Bowers, 1969	8 (depressed)	Fl	22.7 ± 5.0
	7 (manic)	Fl	22.2 ± 6.2
854. Tamarkin, 1970	9	Fl	19 ± 4.5
892. Van Woert, 1970	31 (psychiatric)	Fl	23 ± 2
490. Korf, 1971	–	Fl[†]	43 ± 13 (S.D.)
619. Nordin, 1971	19 (endogenous)	Fl	21.1 ± 4.3
637. Papeschi, 1971	17 (endogenous)	Fl	19 ± 4
886. Van Praag, 1971	20	Fl	39 ± 3.6
	8 (retarded)	Fl	32 ± 2.8
	12 (non-retarded)	Fl	43 ± 4.9
567. Mendels, 1972	6 (depressed)	Fl	26.5 ± 12.1
	1 (manic)	Fl	44.2
	6 (unipolar)	Fl	27.7 ± 6.8
	5 (psychotic)	Fl	28.6 ± 7.5
	8 (neurotic)	Fl	27.3 ± 9.1
40. Ashcroft, 1973	11 (unipolar)	Fl	20 ± 2
	9 (bipolar-depressed)	Fl	34 ± 4
	11 (bipolar-manic)	Fl	35 ± 4

Table 152.   Unconjugated Homovanillic Acid in CSF of Depressed Subjects

(continued)

Reference First Author, Year	Number of Subjects	Method of Analysis	Values (ng/mL ± S.E.M.)
336. Goodwin, 1973	53 (depressed)	Fl	17.7 ± 3
	16 (hypomanic)	Fl	24.7 ± 5
339. Gordon, 1973	41	Fl	24.6 ± 3.7
671. Post, 1973	9 (depressed)	Fl	16.9 ± 2.8
	9 (simulated mania)	Fl	42.1 ± 5.7
	10 (hypomania)	Fl	18.9 ± 3.2
	49 (depressed)	Fl	15.2 ± 2.1
887. Van Praag, 1973	28 (endogenous)	Fl	42 ± 3.7
	10 (neurotic)	Fl	35 ± 4.1
668. Post, 1974	44 (unipolar + bipolar)	Fl	18.0 ± 10.7
769. Sedvall, 1974	11 (manic)	GC-MS	58.2 ± 5.5
299. Fyrö, 1975	13 (manic)	GC-MS	38.6 ± 5.5
	5 (M)	GC-MS	45.7 ± 6.7
	8 (F)	GC-MS	43.0 ± 4.6
415. Jimerson, 1975	34 (includes schizophrenics)	GC-MS	28.1 ± 3.2
426. Jori, 1975	26 (psychotic)	Fl	30 ± 2
667. Post, 1975	22 (manic)	Fl	20
	69 (depressed)	Fl	20
832. Subrahmanyam, 1975	24 (manic- depressive)	Fl	38.4 ± 3.4

Table 152. Unconjugated Homovanillic Acid in CSF of Depressed Subjects

(continued)

Reference First Author, Year	Number of Subjects	Method of Analysis	Values (ng/mL ± S.E.M.)
889. Van Praag, 1975	20 (endogenous)	–	39 ± 3.6
	8 (retarded)	–	32 ± 2.8
	12 (non-retarded)	–	43 ± 4.9
3. Abrams, 1976	6 (endogenous)	Fl	13.0 ± 2.2
117. Bridges, 1976	10 (severe)	Fl	216 ± 10 (ventricular)
	8 (less severe)	Fl	276 ± 35 (ventricular)
	18 (combined)	Fl	242 ± 24 (ventricular)
187. Curzon, 1976	37 (includes schizophrenics)	Fl	245 ± 15 (ventricular)
473. Kirstein, 1976	10 (unipolar + bipolar)	Fl	104.5 ± 19.9
38. Åsberg, 1977	14 (endogenous)	GC–MS	44.2 ± 5.8
54. Banki, 1977	55 (unipolar)	Fl	24.0 ± 1.5
	16 (bipolar- depressed)	Fl	15.9 ± 2.0
	10 (bipolar-manic)	Fl	44.4 ± 3.8
794. Siwers, 1977	6	GC–MS	50.9 ± 13.5
894. Vestergaard, 1978	29 (before recovery)	GC–ECD	83 ± 6.9
	14 (unipolar)	GC–ECD	88 ± 9.9
	6 (bipolar)	GC–ECD	78 ± 22
	16 (after recovery)	GC–ECD	73 ± 8
	8 (unipolar)	GC–ECD	66 ± 13.4

Table 152.   Unconjugated Homovanillic Acid in CSF of Depressed Subjects

(continued)

Reference First Author, Year	Number of Subjects	Method of Analysis	Values (ng/mL ± S.E.M.)
	4 (bipolar)	GC-ECD	75 ± 19
	4 (manic before)	GC-ECD	115 ± 33
52. Ballenger, 1979	28 (personality disorder)	Fl	34.5 ± 3.8
	10 (alcoholic)	Fl	33.1 ± 5.2
864. Träskman, 1979	28 (endogenous)	GC-MS	38.6 ± 3.2
5. Ågren, 1980	21 (unipolar)	GC-MS	37.0 ± 4.5
	12 (bipolar)	GC-MS	33.3 ± 4.6
75. Berger, 1980	13 (M)	GC-MS	42.0 ± 4.1
	10 (M)	GC-MS	2.2 ± 1.7 (conj.)
188. Curzon, 1980	20 (at worst)	Fl	221 ± 17 (ventricular)
	20 (not at worst)	Fl	272 ± 21 (ventricular)
	4 (agitated, worst)	Fl	274 ± 35 (ventricular)
	10 (other psychiatric)	Fl	200 ± 10 (ventricular)
1. Åberg-Wistedt, 1981	25 (endogenous)	GC-MS	30.3 ± 3.2
58. Banki, 1981; 59. Banki, 1981	33 (severe depression)	Fl	28.6 ± 2.6
106. Bowden, 1981	23 (M) (unipolar)	GC-MS	28.6 ± 2.4
	25 (F) (unipolar)	GC-MS	34.4 ± 2.5
214. Davis, 1981	15 (unipolar + bipolar)	GC-MS	41.3

Table 152.   Unconjugated Homovanillic Acid in CSF of Depressed Subjects

(continued)

Reference First Author, Year	Number of Subjects	Method of Analysis	Values (ng/mL ± S.E.M.)
568. Mendlewicz, 1981	7 (unipolar)	–	52.2 ± 7.5
633. Oreland, 1981	6 (M)	GC–MS	35.0 ± 4.4
	14 (F)	GC–MS	39.8 ± 3.5
	5 (M) (recovered)	GC–MS	40.1 ± 7.1
	6 (F) (recovered)	GC–MS	52.1 ± 9.2
4. Ackenheil, 1982	30 (psychiatric)	HPLC–EC	50
192. Dahl, 1982	25 (endogenous)	GC–MS	40.8 ± 3.6
	9 (M)	GC–MS	40.2 ± 6.2
	16 (F)	GC–MS	40.8 ± 4.6
455. Kasa, 1982	13	Fl[†]	22.3 ± 3.9
	– (unipolar)	Fl	19.6 ± 13.2 (S.D.)
	– (bipolar)	Fl	34.4 ± 14.2 (S.D.)
546. Maas, 1982	40 (F)	–	37.1 ± 2.6
	43 (M) (unipolar + bipolar)	–	30.3 ± 1.7
7. Ågren, 1983	100	GC–MS	31.2 ± 1.6
55. Banki, 1983	43 (includes schizophrenics)	Fl	25.2 ± 1.8
56. Banki, 1983	32	Fl	26.0 ± 4.0
	17 (unipolar)	Fl	27.7 ± 5.7
	9 (bipolar)	Fl	34.4 ± 8.3
493. Koslow, 1983; 548. Maas, 1984	26 (M) (unipolar)	GC–MS	31.8 ± 2.1
	32 (F) (unipolar)	GC–MS	38.4 ± 2.6
	23 (M) (bipolar)	GC–MS	33.1 ± 1.9
	11 (F) (bipolar)	GC–MS	36.9 ± 3.8

Table 152. Unconjugated Homovanillic Acid in CSF of Depressed Subjects

(continued)

Reference First Author, Year	Number of Subjects	Method of Analysis	Values (ng/mL ± S.E.M.)
	9 (M) (manic)	GC-MS	43.7 ± 5.4
	5 (F) (manic)	GC-MS	59.0 ± 10.4
	49 (M) (depressed)	GC-MS	32.4 ± 1.6
	43 (F) (depressed)	GC-MS	38.0 ± 2.1
843. Swann, 1983	14 (mania)	GC-MS	49.1 ± 5.3
36. Åsberg, 1984	58 (melancholic)	GC-MS	36.3 ± 2.0
77. Berrettini, 1984	10 (bipolar)	HPLC-EC	32.4 ± 4.1
98. Bottiglieri, 1984	18	HPLC-EC[†]	29.5 ± 3.2
316. Gerner, 1984	38 (depressed)	HPLC-EC	31.8 ± 2.9
	13 (manic)	HPLC-EC	38.0 ± 5.0
78. Berrettini, 1985	9 (bipolar, euthymic)	HPLC-EC	36.0 ± 5.5
104. Bowden, 1985	34 (M)	GC-MS	30.1 ± 1.7
	26 (F) (unipolar + bipolar)	GC-MS	35.9 ± 2.7
382. Hoffman, 1985	8	HPLC	21.6 ± 2.8
517. Lidberg, 1985	22 (suicide attempters)	GC-MS	34.7 ± 3.6
678. Potter, 1985	11 (unipolar + bipolar)	HPLC-EC[†]	38.2 ± 1.9

Table 152.   Unconjugated Homovanillic Acid in CSF of Depressed Subjects

(continued)

Reference First Author, Year	Number of Subjects	Method of Analysis	Values (ng/mL ± S.E.M.)
726. Roy, 1985	15 (melancholic)	HPLC-EC	20.1 ± 2.7
	8 (major depressive episode)	HPLC-EC	33.1 ± 6.4
	5 (dysthymic disorder)	HPLC-EC	31.3 ± 5.4
8. Ågren, 1986	52	GC-MS	30.7 ± 2.0
	27 (M)	GC-MS	28.0 ± 3.0
	25 (F)	GC-MS	33.6 ± 2.5
688. Redmond, 1986	92 (depressed)	GC-MS	35.1 ± 1.3
	14 (manic)	GC-MS	49.1 ± 5.2
823. Standish-Barry, 1986	15 (severe, endogenous)	Fl	240 ± 13 (ventricular)
322. Gjerris, 1987	33 (endogenous)	GC-MS	43.1
	7 (non-endogenous)	GC-MS	43.0
394. Hsiao, 1987	40 (unipolar + bipolar)	HPLC-EC[†]	31.0 ± 1.6
829. Stokes, 1987	22	GC-MS	31.3 ± 2.5
325. Golden, 1988	6	HPLC-EC	25.1 ± 5.0
723. Roy, 1988	27	HPLC-EC	24.4 ± 2.7
932. Westenberg, 1988	38	HPLC-EC[†]	34.9 ± 0.4
	21 (F)	HPLC-EC[†]	36.2 ± 0.8
	17 (M)	HPLC-EC[†]	33.4 ± 1.0

Table 153. Unconjugated Homovanillic Acid in Urine of Schizophrenic Subjects

Reference First Author, Year	Number of Subjects	Method of Analysis	Values (mg/24h ± S.E.M.)
10. Allegranza, 1965	9	Fl	3.22 ± 0.29
	9	Fl	3.30 ± 0.23
115. Bozzi, 1965	11	Fl	3.20 ± 0.39
125. Bruno, 1965	8	Fl	3.40 ± 0.18
237. Domino, 1979	7 (chronic)	Fl[†]	5.79 ± 0.38
543. Maas, 1988	11 (acute)	GC-MS	6.53 ± 0.60*

* In original paper expressed in μg/3.5 h.

Table 154. Unconjugated Homovanillic Acid in Plasma of Schizophrenic

Subjects

Reference First Author, Year	Number of Subjects	Method of Analysis	Values (ng/mL ± S.E.M.)
554. Markianos, 1976	13 (paranoid)	GC-ECD	79 ± 13 (serum)
190. Cutler, 1982	5	GC-MS	11.2 ± 1.4 (serum)
113. Bowers, 1983	22	GC-MS	16.7 ± 2.1
	12 (F)	GC-MS	20.9 ± 3.4
	10 (M)	GC-MS	11.7 ± 1.2
470. Kirch, 1983	19	GC-MS	10.2
	13 (M) (with tardive dyskinesia)	GC-MS	14.1
	6 (F) (with tardive dyskinesia)	GC-MS	14.2
588. Moore, 1983	61 (with tardive dyskinesia)	GC-MS	14.7
	24 (M) (with tardive dyskinesia)	GC-MS	12.3
	37 (F) (with tardive dyskinesia)	GC-MS	16.3
114. Bowers, 1984	9	GC-MS	12.1 ± 2.0
365. Harris, 1984	13 (psychotic)	HPLC-EC	9.2
660. Pickar, 1984	8	HPLC-EC	13.8 ± 1.1
651. Petty, 1986	6 (M)	HPLC-EC	7.1 ± 1.2
	8 (F)	HPLC-EC	8.4 ± 1.1
659. Pickar, 1986	16	HPLC-EC	13.3 ± 0.9
111. Bowers, 1986	21 (M)	GC-MS	14.9 ± 1.2
	24 (F)	GC-MS	18.3 ± 2.0
112. Bowers, 1987	58 (M)	GC-MS	14.3 ± 0.7
	75 (F)	GC-MS	19.2 ± 1.4
204. Davidson, 1987	28	GC-MS	9.1 ± 0.9

<u>Table 154. Unconjugated Homovanillic Acid in Plasma of Schizophrenic</u>

<u>Subjects (continued)</u>

Reference First Author, Year	Number of Subjects	Method of Analysis	Values (ng/mL ± S.E.M.)
110a.Bowers, 1988	328 (psychotic + depressed)	GC-MS	13.6 ± 0.3 (M) 16.2 ± 0.4 (F)
	22 (psychotic)	GC-MS	29.3 ± 1.4 (M) 36.4 ± 2.5 (F)
203. Davidson, 1988	14 (chronic)	GC-MS	7.1 ± 0.6
206. Davila, 1988	14	HPLC-EC	13.1 ± 1.0
543. Maas, 1988	16 (acute)	GC-MS	13.3 ± 1.2
948. Wolkowitz, 1988	12 (chronic)	HPLC-EC	10.2 ± 0.8
370. Heh, 1989	9 (chronic)	HPLC-EC	10.4 ± 0.8

Table 155. Unconjugated Homovanillic Acid in CSF of Schizophrenic

Subjects

Reference First Author, Year	Number of Subjects	Method of Analysis	Values (ng/mL ± S.E.M.)
648. Persson, 1965	40	Fl	37
649. Persson, 1968	4	Fl	41 ± 7
110. Bowers, 1969	6	Fl	45.5 ± 17.2
662. Pind, 1970	8 (with tardive dyskinesia)	Fl	80 ± 13
341. Gottfries, 1971	40	Fl	44.4 ± 3.1
696. Rimon, 1971	30	Fl	28.0 ± 2.7
	14 (paranoid)	Fl	31.5 ± 3.3
	12 (other paranoid)	Fl	28.5 ± 4.7
	26 (all paranoid)	Fl	30.1 ± 2.8
	16 (non-paranoid)	Fl	24.1 ± 4.1
	15 (other non-paranoid)	Fl	21.3 ± 3.5
	31 (all non-paranoid)	Fl	22.7 ± 2.7
883. Van Praag, 1973	12 (psychiatric)	Fl	42 ± 10
295. Fri, 1974	5	GC-MS	36.9 ± 2.4
296. Fri, 1974	10	GC-MS[†]	39.1 ± 5.2
300. Fyrö, 1974	6 (M)	GC-MS[†]	26.0 ± 5.8
	15 (F)	GC-MS	44.2 ± 3.5
769. Sedvall, 1974	34	GC-MS	34.8 ± 2.5
	11 (M)	GC-MS	26.2 ± 3.1
	23 (F)	GC-MS	38.8 ± 3.1
340. Gordon, 1975	31 (psychiatric)	GC-MS	24.6 ± 2.6
426. Jori, 1975	7	Fl	30 ± 4
667. Post, 1975	20	Fl	21

Table 155.   Unconjugated Homovanillic Acid in CSF of Schizophrenic

Subjects (continued)

Reference First Author, Year	Number of Subjects	Method of Analysis	Values (ng/mL ± S.E.M.)
832. Subrahmanyam, 1975	30 (acute)	Fl	41.4 ± 4.2
	6 (acute, aggressive)	Fl	46.0 ± 2.6
	24 (chronic)	Fl	42.4 ± 4.8
473. Kirstein, 1976	10	Fl[†]	161.2 ± 16.4
554. Markianos, 1976	13 (paranoid)	GC-ECD	66 ± 8
91. Bjerkenstedt, 1977	34 29	GC-MS GC-MS	42.9 ± 3.1 38.2 ± 3.5
440. Karoum, 1977	12	GC-MS	58.2 ± 2.7
416. Jimerson, 1978	– –	GC-MS Fl	37.7 ± 5.2 20.3 ± 5.0
363. Härnryd, 1979	12	GC-MS	33.7 ± 5.5
604. Nagao, 1979	15 12 (with tardive dyskinesia)	Fl Fl	70.8 ± 5.8 87.0 ± 7.7
75. Berger, 1980	9 7	GC-MS GC-MS	45.8 ± 6.1 0.2 ± 0.4 (conj.)
332. Gomes, 1980	10 (acute)	Fl	28.8 ± 2.8
	11 (chronic)	Fl	33.4 ± 3.0
	14 (psycho-organic)	Fl	30.8 ± 2.4
	19 (personality disorder)	Fl	29.7 ± 1.3
770. Sedvall, 1980	11 (with family history)	GC-MS	40.8 ± 4.3
	25 (no family history)	GC-MS	29.5 ± 1.3

Table 155. Unconjugated Homovanillic Acid in CSF of Schizophrenic Subjects

Reference First Author, Year	Number of Subjects	Method of Analysis	Values (ng/mL ± S.E.M.)
767. Sedvall, 1980	8	-	40.2 ± 4.2
976. Zander, 1981	13 (chronic)	GC-ECD	50 ± 8.6
311. Gattaz, 1982	28	HPLC-EC[†]	38.2 ± 17.3
	15 (on neuroleptics)	HPLC-EC	39.0 ± 15.1
	13 (no drugs)	HPLC-EC	37.3 ± 20.2
954. Wood, 1982	9	GC-MS	79.2 ± 12.0
56. Banki, 1983	32 (combined)	Fl	31.7 ± 2.9
	10 (acute)	Fl	38.9 ± 4.1
	6 (catatonic)	Fl	26.9 ± 5.2
	4 (disorganized)	Fl	26.2 ± 8.8
	12 (paranoid)	Fl	38.6 ± 4.7
72. Beckman, 1983	9	HPLC	25.0 ± 4.5
530. Linnoila, 1983	28	HPLC-EC	34.4 ± 2.4
	19 (M)	HPLC-EC	32.4 ± 2.5
	9 (F)	HPLC-EC	37.9 ± 5.3
620. Nybäck, 1983	26	GC-MS	30.0 ± 2.9
880. Van Kammen, 1983	12 (normal brain)	HPLC-EC	38.9 ± 2.4
	6 (atrophied brain)	HPLC-EC	25.1 ± 4.4
316. Gerner, 1984	20	HPLC-EC	31.1 ± 3.7
755. Scheinin, 1984	46 (chronic)	HPLC-EC[†]	23.8 ± 1.2
46. Bagdy, 1985	15 (chronic)	Fl	23.0 ± 2.3

<u>Table 155.   Unconjugated Homovanillic Acid in CSF of Schizophrenic</u>

<u>Subjects (continued)</u>

Reference First Author, Year	Number of Subjects	Method of Analysis	Values (ng/mL ± S.E.M.)
309. Gattaz, 1985	13	HPLC-EC	37.3 ± 5.6
520. Lindstrom, 1985	40	GC-MS	37.7 ± 2.6
392. Houston, 1986	16	HPLC	34.6 ± 2.5
735. Saito, 1986	9 (with Parkinson's disease)	HPLC-EC	69.8 ± 9.0
	9 (with Tardive dyskinesis)	HPLC-EC	64.5 ± 8.4
644. Parnetti, 1987	13	HPLC-Fl[†]	70.4 ± 7.4
543. Maas, 1988	17 (acute)	GC-MS	40.2 ± 2.5
238. Doran, 1989	18 (paranoid)	HPLC-EC	29.9 ± 3.0
	18 (undifferentiated)	HPLC-EC	30.1 ± 2.4
	2 (catatonic)	HPLC-EC	31.6 ± 14.0
	2 (disorganized)	HPLC-EC	26.3 ± 4.5
	6 (schizoaffective)	HPLC-EC	25.0 ± 3.7

Table 156. Homovanillic Acid in Urine of Parkinson's Disease Subjects

Reference First Author, Year	Number of Subjects	Method of Analysis	Values (mg/24h ± S.E.M.)
132. Calne, 1969	14	GC-FID	3.1 ± 0.3
	14	GC-FID	2.7 ± 0.3
927. Weil-Malherbe, 1969	34 (combined)	Fl[†]	2.5 ± 0.2
	20 (M)	Fl	2.4 ± 0.2
	14 (F)	Fl	3.4 ± 0.5
248. Dziedzic, 1973	7	GC-ECD[†]	4.3 mg/g Cr.
	7	GC-ECD	0.06 mg/g Cr. (iso-HVA)

Table 157. Homovanillic Acid in Plasma of Aggressive Subjects

Reference First Author, Year	Number of Subjects	Method of Analysis	Values (ng/mL ± S.E.M.)
974. Yu, 1985	82 (violent)	GC-MS	8.9 ± 0.3
	27 (aggressive)	GC-MS	8.7 ± 0.5

Table 158. Unconjugated Homovanillic Acid in CSF of Parkinson's Disease

Subjects

Reference First Author, Year	Number of Subjects	Method of Analysis	Values (ng/mL ± S.E.M.)
627. Olsson, 1968	8	Fl	20 ± 2
698. Rinne, 1968	22	Fl	54.6 ± 6.5
342. Gottfries, 1969	18	Fl	20 ± 7
928. Weiner, 1969	19	Fl	15
152. Chase, 1970	10	Fl	8.5 ± 1.7
639. Papeschi, 1970	40	Fl	154 ± 19 (ventricular)
682. Pullar, 1970	29	Fl	19 ± 1
892. Van Woert, 1970	10	Fl	<10 ± 1
84. Bertler, 1971	7	Fl	8.8 ± 1.4
186. Curzon, 1971	16	Fl	16 ± 4.8
642. Parkes, 1971	12	Fl	12 ± 2.6
153. Chase, 1972	6	Fl	15 ± 5.5
155. Chase, 1972	15	Fl	15 ± 3.9
412. Jequier, 1972	11 (improved with DOPA)	Fl	30.5 ± 8.6
	10 (not improved)	Fl	82.1 ± 7.6
508. Lakke, 1972	27	Fl	30.4 ± 4.8
638. Papeschi, 1972	13	Fl	166 ± 29 (ventricular)
	5	Fl	15 ± 7 (lumbar)
699. Rinne, 1972	157	Fl	14.4 ± 0.8
	68 (M)	Fl	13.7 ± 1.1
	89 (F)	Fl	15.0 ± 1.2
700. Rinne, 1973	125	Fl	15.8 ± 1.1
643. Parkes, 1974	5 (old)	Fl	10 ± 3
	26 (young)	Fl	14 ± 2
691. Renaud, 1974	4	Fl	17 ± 2

Table 158.   Unconjugated Homovanillic Acid in CSF of Parkinson's Disease

Subjects (continued)

Reference First Author, Year	Number of Subjects	Method of Analysis	Values (ng/mL ± S.E.M.)
202. Davidson, 1977	73	Fl	20 ± 3.5
568. Mendlewicz, 1981	13	–	27.9 ± 3.6
317. Gibson, 1985	21 (combined)	HPLC-EC[†]	27.1 ± 3.0
	4 (mild)	HPLC-EC	24.8 ± 5.1
	8 (moderate)	HPLC-EC	27.0 ± 2.6
	9 (severe)	HPLC-EC	28.2 ± 4.0
822. Stahl, 1985	9 (dystonia)	GC-MS	41.7 ± 7.2
	6 (with Tardive dyskinesia)	GC-MS	43.6 ± 5.9

Table 159. Unconjugated Homovanillic Acid in CSF of Alzheimer's Disease

Subjects

Reference First Author, Year	Number of Subjects	Method of Analysis	Values (ng/mL ± S.E.M.)
342. Gottfries, 1969	18 (senile)	Fl	50 ± 7
	10 (presenile)	Fl	30 ± 6
344. Gottfries, 1973	15	Fl	23 ± 4
643. Parkes, 1974	8	Fl	38 ± 6
107. Bowen, 1981	5	-	29 ± 2
568. Mendlewicz, 1981	40	-	44.4 ± 6.3
814. Soininen, 1981	28 (combined)	Fl	52 ± 6
	9 (less severe)	Fl	72 ± 11
	9 (severe)	Fl	49 ± 8
	10 (very severe)	Fl	37 ± 5
6. Ågren, 1982	16 (combined)	Fl	27.5 ± 1.0
	8 (mild)	Fl	39.1 ± 1.6
	8 (severe)	Fl	14.1 ± 0.6
954. Wood, 1982	11	GC–MS	46.4 ± 7.6
458. Kay, 1984	28	HPLC[†]	26.9 ± 0.4
635. Palmer, 1984	25 (presenile)	HPLC-EC[†]	30.5 ± 3.2
	9 (senile)	HPLC-EC	29.1 ± 5.9
317. Gibson, 1985	32 (combined)	HPLC-EC[†]	33.1 ± 2.8
	17 (mild)	HPLC-EC	35.4 ± 4.5
	10 (moderate)	HPLC-EC	35.2 ± 3.7
	5 (severe)	HPLC-EC	21.2 ± 3.7
816. Sparks, 1985	4	HPLC-EC[†]	32 ± 16

Table 159.   Unconjugated Homovanillic Acid in CSF of Alzheimer's Disease

Subjects (continued)

Reference First Author, Year	Number of Subjects	Method of Analysis	Values (ng/mL ± S.E.M.)
621. Nybäck, 1987	15	GC-MS	40.8 ± 3.8
644. Parnetti, 1987	12	HPLC-Fl[†]	33.7 ± 5.1
701. Risby, 1987	12	HPLC-EC	37.6 ± 4.2
834. Sunderland, 1987	13	HPLC-EC	41.7 ± 3.8
495. Koyama, 1988	6	HPLC-EC[†]	14.8 ± 2.4

Table 160.   Unconjugated Homovanillic Acid in CSF of Aggressive Subjects

Reference First Author, Year	Number of Subjects	Method of Analysis	Values (ng/mL ± S.E.M.)
88. Bioulac, 1978	4	Fl	29.5 ± 11.4
118. Brown, 1979	4 (antisocial)	Fl	36.6 ± 9.6
	4 (explosive)	Fl	16.2 ± 5.0
	5 (immature)	Fl	25.4 ± 8.7
	3 (passive)	Fl	32.1 ± 13.6
	2 (passive-depressed)	Fl	13.5 ± 9.9
	3 (schizoid)	Fl	32.8 ± 5.4
	2 (obsessional-compulsive)	Fl	73.7 ± 8.9
633. Oreland, 1981	5 (M) (suicidal)	GC-MS	27.5 ± 3.4
	10 (F) (suicidal)	GC-MS	36.6 ± 4.2
865. Träskman, 1981	30 (suicide attempts)	GC-MS	36.4 ± 2.7
	8 (depressed)	GC-MS	26.0 ± 2.6
	22 (not depressed)	GC-MS	40.2 ± 3.2
55. Banki, 1983	6 (violent suicide)	Fl	22.8 ± 4.7
	13 (non-violent suicide)	Fl	26.7 ± 4.0
532. Linnoila, 1983	20 (explosive personality)	HPLC	39.5 ± 3.9
	9 (anti-social)	HPLC	33.5 ± 4.9
	9 (paranoid aggressive)	HPLC	46.0 ± 2.8
517. Lidberg, 1985	15 (homicidal)	GC-MS	45.1 ± 4.1

Table 160. Unconjugated Homovanillic Acid in CSF of Aggressive Subjects

(continued)

Reference First Author, Year	Number of Subjects	Method of Analysis	Values (ng/mL ± S.E.M.)
897. Virkkunen, 1987	20 (violent)	HPLC-EC	39.4 ± 3.5

Table 161. Unconjugated 3-Methoxy-4-hydroxyphenylglycol in Urine of

Normal Subjects

Reference First Author, Year	Number of Subjects	Method of Analysis	Values (µg/24h ± S.E.M.)
747. Sapira, 1968	9	Fl[†]	0.90 ± 0.69 µg/g Cr. (S.D.)
783. Shimizu, 1969	5	Fl	208 ± 35 µg/g Cr.
220. Dekirmenjian, 1970	5 (M) 6 (F)	GC-ECD GC-ECD	110 ± 30 90 ± 30
85. Bigelow, 1971	10	Fl[†]	127 ± 16
446. Karoum, 1973	9	GC-MS[†]	49 ± 7
95. Bond, 1974	7 (M) 6 (F)	GC-ECD[†] GC-ECD	150 ± 23 190 ± 45
427. Joseph, 1976	13	GC-ECD	230
839. Swahn, 1976	5	GC-MS[†]	79 ± 2
595. Murray, 1977	10	GC-MS[†]	80 ± 10
253. Edwards, 1979	1	GC-MS[†]	19
498. Krstulovic, 1980	20	HPLC[†]	60 µg/g Cr.
746. Santagostino, 1982	8 (M) 7 (F)	HPLC-EC[†] HPLC-EC	112 ± 11 140 ± 45
655. Peyrin, 1983	28 14 (M) 14 (F)	Fl Fl Fl	133 ± 11 128 ± 11 139 ± 21
656. Peyrin, 1985	23	Fl	120
211. Davis, 1986	10	GC-MS[†]	160
209. Davis, 1987	8	GC-MS[†]	73 ± 12
277. Filser, 1988	11 (M) 21 (F)	HPLC-UV HPLC-UV	158 ± 27 116 ± 24
431. Julien, 1988	6	HPLC-EC[†]	82 ± 12

Table 162.   Conjugated (or Total) 3-Methoxy-4-hydroxyphenylglycol in

Urine of Normal Subjects

Reference First Author, Year	Number of Subjects	Method of Analysis	Values (µg/24h ± S.E.M.)
730. Ruthven, 1965	18	Fl[†]	3000 ± 200
938. Wilk, 1967	35	GC-ECD[†]	860 ± 85
544. Maas, 1968	11	GC-ECD	1517 ± 73
	5 (M)	GC-ECD	1660 ± 85
	6 (F)	GC-ECD	1397 ± 63
439. Karoum, 1969	20	GC-FID	2400 ± 180
615. Nicholas, 1969	10	Fl[†]	1870 ± 190
783. Shimizu, 1969	5	Fl	1210 ± 235 µg/g Cr. (glucuronide)
	5	Fl	1300 ± 180 µg/g Cr. (sulfate)
220. Dekirmenjian, 1970	5 (M)	GC-ECD	1490 ± 350
	6 (F)	GC-ECD	1230 ± 330
24. Antun, 1971	12	Fl[†]	756 ± 134 (total)
	5 (M)	Fl	923 ± 142 (total)
	7 (F)	Fl	637 ± 200 (total)
85. Bigelow, 1971	10	Fl[†]	2293 ± 165
434. Kahane, 1971	7	Fl	3720 ± 270 (total)
453. Karoum, 1971	3	GC-ECD	1577 ± 342 (total)
666. Pollin, 1971	8 (4 pairs of twins)	GC-ECD	1402 µg/g Cr.
967. Youdim, 1971	12	Fl	2576 ± 232 (total)*
94. Bond, 1972	8	GC-ECD[†]	1830 ± 150 (total)
272. Fawcett, 1972	6 (M)	GC-ECD	1660 ± 85 (total)
	5 (F)	GC-ECD	1397 ± 63 (total)
556. Martin, 1972	9	GC-ECD[†]	1944 ± 194 (sulfate)
	6 (M)	GC-ECD	2084 ± 272 (sulfate)
	3 (F)	GC-ECD	1664 ± 146 (sulfate)
679. Prange, 1972	10	GC-ECD	2090 ± 300 (total)

Table 162.   Conjugated (or Total) 3-Methoxy-4-hydroxyphenylglycol in

<u>Urine of Normal Subjects (continued)</u>

Reference First Author, Year	Number of Subjects	Method of Analysis	Values (µg/24h ± S.E.M.)
223. De Leon-Jones, 1973	12	GC-ECD	1300 (total)
446. Karoum, 1973	9	GC-MS[†]	979 ± 84 (glucuronide)
	9	GC-MS	845 ± 74 (sulfate)
95. Bond, 1974	7 (M)	GC-ECD[†]	910 ± 50 (glucuronide)
	6 (F)	GC-ECD	1000 ± 115 (glucuronide)
	7 (M)	GC-ECD	1360 ± 165 (sulfate)
	6 (F)	GC-ECD	1260 ± 190 (sulfate)
191. Cymerman, 1975	6	GC-ECD	710 ± 40 µg/g Cr. (total)
541. Maas, 1975	19 (M)	GC-ECD	1674 ± 117 (total)
	21 (F)	GC-ECD	1348 ± 65 (total)
798. Sjöquist, 1975	11	GC-MS[†]	1560 µg/L (total)
802. Sjöquist, 1975	20	GC-MS[†]	1360 ± 40 µg/L (total)
832. Subrahmanyam, 1975	12	GC-ECD	2090 ± 300 (total)
	12	GC-ECD	2000 ± 200 (total)
427. Joseph, 1976	13	GC-ECD	1490 ± 95 (glucuronide)
	13	GC-ECD	1020 ± 110 (sulfate)
432. Kahane, 1976	8	GC-FID[†]	1955 µg/L (total)
839. Swahn, 1976	5	GC-MS[†]	2980 ± 115 µg/L (total)
910. Wadman, 1976	6	GC-FID[†]	1490 ± 225 (total)
305. Garfinkel, 1977	10	GC-ECD	1600 ± 80 (total)
595. Murray, 1977	10	GC-MS[†]	1050 ± 120 (sulfate)
	10	GC-MS	1300 ± 135 (glucuronide)
778. Sharpless, 1977	11	GC-ECD[†]	1884 ± 178 (total)
	6 (M)	GC-ECD	2105 ± 255 (total)
	5 (F)	GC-ECD	1618 ± 212 (total)
384. Hollister, 1978	11 (M)	GC-ECD	2253 ± 296 (total)
	6 (F)	GC-ECD	1591 ± 71 (total)

Table 162. Conjugated (or Total) 3-Methoxy-4-hydroxyphenylglycol in

Urine of Normal Subjects

Reference First Author, Year	Number of Subjects		Method of Analysis	Values (μg/24h ± S.E.M.)
598. Muskiet, 1978	14		GC-MS[†]	1500 ± 130 μg/g Cr. (total)
661. Pickar, 1978	5		GC-ECD	1630 ± 97 (total)
856. Taube, 1978	10		GC-ECD	1029 ± 93 (total)
173. Coppen, 1979	27		GC-FID	1680 ± 120 (total)
	10	(M)	GC-FID	2190 ± 230 (total)
	17	(F)	GC-FID	1370 ± 80 (total)
253. Edwards, 1979	1		GC-MS[†]	1380
68. Beckmann, 1980	15		GC-ECD	1330 ± 120 (total)
	7	(M)	GC-ECD	1440 ± 210 (total)
	8	(F)	GC-ECD	1230 ± 120 (total)
498. Krstulovic, 1980	20		HPLC-EC[†]	690 μg/g Cr.
12. Alonso, 1981	12		HPLC-EC[†]	2650 ± 200 (total)
596. Muscettola, 1981	10		GC-ECD[†]	2780 ± 475 (total)
6. Ågren, 1982	16		GC-MS	2981 ± 198 (total)
	8	(M)	GC-MS	3478 ± 280 (total)
	8	(F)	GC-MS	2558 ± 280 (total)
387. Hopkinson, 1982	15		HPLC	931 μg/g Cr. (total)
441. Karoum, 1982	5		GC-MS[†]	2350 ± 310 (total)
746. Santagostino, 1982	8	(M)	HPLC-EC[†]	1340 ± 105 (sulfate)
	7	(F)	HPLC-EC	809 ± 117 (sulfate)
	8	(M)	HPLC-EC	1470 ± 150 (glucuronide)
	7	(F)	HPLC-EC	751 ± 117 (glucuronide)
754. Schatzberg, 1982	26		GC-ECD	1921 ± 117 (total)
	13	(M)	GC-ECD	2021 ± 176 (total)
	13	(F)	GC-ECD	1820 ± 157 (total)
935. Wiesel, 1982	33	(M)	GC-MS	2225 ± 106 (total)
	33	(F)	GC-MS	1810 ± 106 (total)
218. De Jong, 1983	7		GC-FID[†]	1790 ± 650 μg/g Cr. (total)

<u>Table 162. Conjugated (or Total) 3-Methoxy-4-hydroxyphenylglycol in</u>

<u>Urine of Normal Subjects (continued)</u>

Reference First Author, Year	Number of Subjects		Method of Analysis	Values (µg/24h ± S.E.M.)
225. De Lisi, 1983	16		GC-MS	1352 ± 164 (total)
361. Hamlin, 1983	11		GC-ECD	1607 ± 181 (total)
489. Kopin, 1983	12		REA[†]	2539 ± 221 (total)
493. Koslow, 1983	36	(M)	GC-ECD	2267 ± 143 (total)
	36	(F)	GC-ECD	1660 ± 121 (total)
555. Markianos, 1983	20		GC-ECD	1454 ± 177 µg/g Cr. (total)
652. Petursson, 1983	5		GC-ECD	1510 ± 180 (total)
655. Peyrin, 1983	28		Fl	702 ± 58 (sulfate)
	14	(M)	Fl	776 ± 80 (sulfate)
	14	(F)	Fl	622 ± 64 (sulfate)
	28		Fl	944 ± 75 (glucuronide)
	14	(M)	Fl	1031 ± 122 (glucuronide)
	14	(F)	Fl	853 ± 84 (glucuronide)
716. Rosenbaum, 1983	22		GC-ECD	1767 ± 117 (total)
255. Eichholtz, 1984	9	(M)	GC-ECD[†]	600 ± 50 µg/g Cr. (sulfate)
	12	(F)	GC-ECD	690 ± 52 µg/g Cr. (sulfate)
597. Muscettola, 1984	27		GC-ECD	1850 ± 120 (total)
781. Shea, 1984	10		HPLC-EC[†]	1260 ± 180 (total)
228. DeMet, 1985	6		GC-ECD	1707 ± 202 (total)
656. Peyrin, 1985	23		Fl	800 ± 68 (sulfate)
	23		Fl	660 ± 61 (glucuronide)
48. Baker, 1986	15	(M)	GC-ECD[†]	1945 ± 304 (total)
	27	(F)	GC-ECD	1626 ± 175 (total)
290. Frankenhaueser, 1986	19	(M)	GC-MS	2200 ± 185 (total)**
	30	(F)	GC-MS	1510 ± 105 (total)**
724. Roy, 1986	25		GC-MS	1564 ± 131 (total)
790. Siever, 1986	18		GC-MS	2760 ± 190 (total)

Table 162. Conjugated (or Total) 3-Methoxy-4-hydroxyphenylglycol in

Urine of Normal Subjects (continued)

Reference First Author, Year	Number of Subjects	Method of Analysis	Values (µg/24h ± S.E.M.)
657. Peyrin, 1987	11	HPLC-EC	1470 ± 230 µg/g Cr. (sulfate)
	11	HPLC-EC	2500 ± 370 µg/g Cr. (glucuronide)
977. Zhou, 1987	21	Fl	1451 ± 103 (sulfate)
1. Abe, 1988	46 (M)	HPLC-Fl[†]	2040 ± 88 (total)
	43 (F)	HPLC-Fl[†]	1410 ± 59 (total)
277. Filser, 1988	7 (F)	HPLC-UV	654 ± 128 (sulfate)
			1055 ± 211 (glucuronide)
			1855 ± 238 (total)
	10 (M)	HPLC-UV	1033 ± 144 (sulfate)
			1746 ± 204 (glucuronide)
			2937 ± 370 (total)
431. Julien, 1988	6	HPLC-EC[†]	2100 ± 245 (total)
488. Kopin, 1988	18	REA	2576 ± 177 (total)
529. Linnoila, 1988	12	GC-MS	2237 ± 171 (total)
877. Van Bemmel, 1988	8 (M)	GC-ECD	1840
	7 (F)	GC-ECD	1690

*   In original paper expressed as µg/3h.
** In original paper expressed as nmol/min.

Table 163. Unconjugated 3-Methoxy-4-hydroxyphenylglycol in

Plasma of Normal Subjects

Reference First Author, Year	Number of Subjects	Method of Analysis	Values (ng/mL ± S.E.M.)
222. Dekirmenjian, 1974	5	GC-ECD[†]	5.4 ± 1.5
798. Sjöquist, 1975	12	GC-MS[†]	6.3 (serum)
356. Halaris, 1977	6	GC-ECD[†]	2.6 ± 0.5
448. Karoum, 1977	10	GC-MS[†]	5.8 ± 0.6
851. Takahashi, 1977	10	GC-MS[†]	4.6 ± 0.3
545. Maas, 1979	6	GC-MS	3.25 ± 0.63 (venous)
	6	GC-MS	2.72 ± 0.61 (arterial)
514. Leckmann, 1980	3	GC-MS	3.5 ± 0.3
599. Muskiet, 1980	21	GC-MS[†]	3.3 ± 0.3 (serum)
842. Swan, 1980	–	GC-MS	3.38 ± 0.83 (S.D.)
414. Jimerson, 1981	25	GC-MS	3.1 ± 0.1
418. Jimerson, 1981	10	GC-MS[†]	3.77 ± 0.39
419. Jimerson, 1981	26 (13 pairs of twins)	GC-MS	2.8 ± 0.2
513. Leckman, 1981	6	GC-MS	3.6 ± 0.2
150. Charney, 1982	12	GC-MS	4.5 ± 0.3
629. Ong, 1982	3	HPLC-EC[†]	4.62 ± 0.79
826. Sternberg, 1982	11	GC-MS	3.8 ± 0.3
261. Elsworth, 1983	9	GC-MS[†]	0.99 ± 0.08
145. Charney, 1984	11	GC-MS	3.5 ± 0.3
148. Charney, 1984	20	GC-MS	3.5 ± 0.2
576. Minegishi, 1984	5	HPLC-EC[†]	5.76 ± 0.57
685. Raskind, 1984	6	GC-MS	3.4 ± 0.3

Table 163. Unconjugated 3-Methoxy-4-hydroxyphenylglycol in

Plasma of Normal Subjects (continued)

Reference First Author, Year	Number of Subjects	Method of Analysis	Values (ng/mL ± S.E.M.)
781. Shea, 1984	7	HPLC-EC[†]	3.34 ± 1.45
235. Devanand, 1985	7 (M) 5 (F)	GC-MS GC-MS	3.2 ± 0.5 3.5 ± 0.9
584. Molyneux, 1985	8	HPLC-EC[†]	3.18 ± 0.35
763. Schinelli, 1985	8 (M) 7 (F)	HPLC-EC[†] HPLC-EC	3.61 ± 0.25 3.43 ± 0.19
144. Charney, 1986	8	GC-ECD	3.6 ± 0.2
211. Davis, 1986	10	GC-MS[†]	3.2
315. Gerhardt, 1986	6	HPLC-EC[†]	4.2 ± 0.7
395. Huber-Smith, 1986	22	HPLC[†]	2.98 ± 0.14
721. Roy, 1986	43	GC-MS	4.2 ± 0.14
790. Siever, 1986	21	GC-MS	3.0 ± 0.1
112. Bowers, 1987	61 (M) 115 (F)	GC-MS GC-MS	3.4 ± 0.9 3.3 ± 1.1
252. Edlund, 1987	21	HPLC-EC	4.41 ± 0.27
702. Rizzo, 1987	1	HPLC-EC[†]	2.12
665. Pohl, 1987	9	GC-MS	3.6 ± 0.5
949. Wolkowitz, 1987	35	HPLC-EC	3.49 ± 0.16
9. Alfredsson, 1988	10	GC-MS	3.18 ± 0.20
134. Candito, 1988	5 6 (supine)	HPLC-EC[†] HPLC-EC[†]	5.39 ± 1.05 2.91 ± 0.75
250. Echizen, 1988	6	HPLC-EC[†]	3.24 ± 0.22
762. Schinelli, 1988	12	HPLC-EC	3.67 ± 0.25
875. Uhde, 1988	12	GC-MS	3.7 ± 0.9

<u>Table 163.   Unconjugated 3-Methoxy-4-hydroxyphenylglycol in</u>

<u>Plasma of Normal Subjects (continued)</u>

Reference First Author, Year	Number of Subjects	Method of Analysis	Values (ng/mL ± S.E.M.)
362. Hariharan, 1989	10 (M)	HPLC-EC[†]	3.57 ± 0.31
	4 (M)	HPLC-EC[†]	2.90 ± 0.34
	10 (F)	HPLC-EC[†]	3.68 ± 0.28
	4 (F)	HPLC-EC[†]	3.24 ± 0.34

Table 164. Conjugated (and total) 3-Methoxy-4-hydroxyphenylglycol in

Plasma of Normal Subjects

Reference First Author, Year	Number of Subjects	Method of Analysis	Values (ng/mL ± S.E.M.)
222. Dekirmenjian, 1974	5	GC-ECD[†]	10.3 ± 2.0
802. Sjöquist, 1975	18	GC-MS[†]	10.3 ± 0.6 (total)
356. Halaris, 1977	6	GC-ECD[†]	5.3 ± 1.0
448. Karoum, 1977	10 10	GC-MS[†] GC-MS	8.3 ± 0.6 (sulfate) 7.9 ± 0.5 (glucuronide)
851. Takahashi, 1977	10	GC-MS[†]	11.9 ± 1.1
414. Jimerson, 1981	25	GC-MS	7.6 ± 0.5
418. Jimerson, 1981	24	GC-MS[†]	6.9 ± 0.5
419. Jimerson, 1981	26 (13 pairs of twins)	GC-MS	8.7 ± 0.7
603. Naber, 1981	14	GC-MS	11.5 ± 0.7
380. Hjemdahl, 1982	13	GC-MS	17.9 ± 2.0
261. Elsworth, 1983	9	GC-MS[†]	2.8 ± 0.2
436. Karege, 1984	– (M) – (F)	HPLC HPLC	18.8 ± 4.5 (total) 15.6 ± 3.1 (total)
228. DeMet, 1985	6	GC-ECD	3.2 ± 0.31 (total)
950. Wolkowitz, 1985	12	HPLC-EC	17.9 ± 0.8 (total)
779. Sharpless, 1986	16 8 (M) 8 (F)	HPLC-EC[†] HPLC-EC HPLC-EC	14.5 ± 1.0 (total) 16.3 ± 1.4 (total) 12.6 ± 1.4 (total)
357. Halbreich, 1987	57 24 (M) 33 (F)	HPLC-EC HPLC-EC HPLC-EC	14.3 ± 0.7 (total) 14.9 ± 0.9 (total) 13.8 ± 0.9 (total)

Table 165. Unconjugated 3-Methoxy-4-hydroxyphenylglycol in CSF of Normal Subjects

Reference First Author, Year	Number of Subjects	Method of Analysis	Values (ng/mL ± S.E.M.)
338. Gordon, 1971	4	GC-ECD[†]	12.5 ± 1.6 (ventricular)
	9	GC-ECD	15.1 ± 2.6 (lumbar)
453. Karoum, 1971	2	GC-ECD	11.0 ± 1.0
937. Wilk, 1971	19	GC-ECD[†]	22 ± 7 (total)
94. Bond, 1972	1	GC-ECD[†]	106
154. Chase, 1973	6	GC-ECD	9.4 ± 3.7 (ventricular)
	22	GC-ECD	10.0 ± 1.0 (lumbar)
339. Gordon, 1973	5	GC-ECD	10.0 ± 2.0 (total)
626. O'Keefe, 1973	11	GC-ECD[†]	11.0 ± 0.9 (total)
	2	GC-ECD	9.8 ± 0.03 (total)
669. Post, 1973	29	GC-ECD	12.2 ± 1.3 (total)
670. Post, 1973	10	GC-ECD	16 ± 2 (total)
	34	GC-ECD	14 ± 1.5 (total)
780. Shaw, 1973	13	GC-ECD	10.8 ± 0.8
784. Shopsin, 1973	24	GC-ECD	16 ± 0.9
785. Shopsin, 1974	18	GC-ECD	15.9
340. Gordon, 1975	13	GC-MS	14.9 ± 3.2 (total)
444. Karoum, 1975	8	GC-MS	11.7 ± 1 (ventricular)
667. Post, 1975	10	GC-ECD	16
798. Sjöquist, 1975	5	GC-MS[†]	9.2 (total)
802. Sjöquist, 1975	16	GC-MS[†]	13.4 ± 1.1 (total)
803. Sjöström, 1975	11	GC-MS	12.1 ± 1.8 (total)
832. Subrahmanyam, 1975	12	GC-ECD	20.6 ± 2.4 (total)
	12	GC-ECD	21.4 ± 3.2 (total)
839. Swahn, 1976	5	GC-MS[†]	6.7 ± 0.2
202. Davidson, 1977	4	GC-ECD	15 ± 3.5 (total)

Table 165. Unconjugated 3-Methoxy-4-hydroxyphenylglycol in

CSF of Normal Subjects (continued)

Reference First Author, Year	Number of Subjects	Method of Analysis	Values (ng/mL ± S.E.M.)
448. Karoum, 1977	5 5	GC-MS[†] GC-MS	11.9 ± 1.2 (ventricular) 11.0 ± 1.2 (lumbar)
748. Saran, 1978	8	Fl	34.1 ± 4.0
894. Vestergaard, 1978	21	GC-ECD	10 ± 0.9
270. Faull, 1979	23	GC-MS[†]	8.9 ± 0.5
550. Major, 1979	7	GC-MS	7.4 ± 0.4
768. Sedvall, 1980	32 (no family history)	GC-MS	7.4 ± 0.2
	28 (family history of psychiatric morbidity)	GC-MS	7.5 ± 0.2
16. Andersen, 1981	5	GC-MS[†]	9.8 ± 0.4
497. Krstulovic, 1981	20	HPLC-EC[†]	5.1 ± 1.0
633. Oreland, 1981	28 (M) 14 (F)	GC-MS GC-MS	8.8 ± 0.3 9.7 ± 0.6
865. Träskman, 1981	45	GC-MS	9.7 ± 0.3
294. Frattini, 1982	28 (M) 20 (F)	HPLC-EC[†] HPLC-EC	7.3 ± 0.4 8.1 ± 0.6
311. Gattaz, 1982	16	HPLC-EC[†]	16.2 ± 4.9
954. Wood, 1982	32	GC-MS	7.2 ± 0.6
261. Elsworth, 1983	4	GC-MS[†]	4.4 ± 0.2
493. Koslow, 1983	61 30 (M) 31 (F)	GC-MS GC-MS GC-MS	8.0 ± 0.2 7.8 ± 0.3 8.1 ± 0.3
620. Nybäck, 1983	43	GC-MS	7.5 ± 1.1
878. Van Bockstaele, 1983	7	HPLC-EC[†]	5.3 ± 0.9
36. Åsberg, 1984	60	GC-MS	9.4 ± 1.3

Table 165. Unconjugated 3-Methoxy-4-hydroxyphenylglycol in

CSF of Normal Subjects (continued)

Reference First Author, Year	Number of Subjects	Method of Analysis	Values (ng/mL ± S.E.M.)
77. Berrettini, 1984	20	HPLC-EC	8.3 ± 1.8
98. Bottiglieri, 1984	9	HPLC-EC[†]	9.4 ± 1.0
316. Gerner, 1984	33	HPLC-EC	7.7 ± 0.4
409. Javors, 1984	7	HPLC-EC[†]	10.7 ± 1.1
635. Palmer, 1984	25	HPLC-EC[†]	7.2 ± 0.5
685. Raskind, 1984	6	GC-MS	7.6 ± 0.9
78. Berrettini, 1985	28	HPLC-EC	8.2 ± 0.3
517. Lidberg, 1985	39	GC-MS	9.4 ± 0.3
816. Sparks, 1985	4	HPLC-EC[†]	32 ± 2
822. Stahl, 1985	36	GC-MS	9.5 ± 0.6
634. Oxenstierna, 1986	30 (monozygotic twins)	GC-MS	8.32± 0.24
	30 (dizygotic twins)	GC-MS	7.97± 0.24
	30 (brothers)	GC-MS	7.91± 0.22
	30 (unrelated men)	GC-MS	7.76± 0.21
688. Redmond, 1986	61	GC-MS	8.0 ± 0.2
322. Gjerris, 1987	15	GC-MS	7.4
621. Nybäck, 1987	18	GC-MS	7.5 ± 0.4
702. Rizzo, 1987	1	HPLC-EC[†]	3.12
834. Sunderland, 1987	7	HPLC-EC	10.0 ± 0.9
9. Alfredsson, 1988	10	GC-MS	7.0 ± 0.5
495. Koyama, 1988	5	HPLC-EC[†]	8.17± 0.40

Table 166.   Conjugated 3-Methoxy-4-hydroxyphenylglycol in

CSF of Normal Subjects

Reference First Author, Year	Number of Subjects	Method of Analysis	Values (ng/mL ± S.E.M.)
453. Karoum, 1971	2	GC-ECD	15.5 ± 2.5
94. Bond, 1972	1	GC-ECD[†]	91
154. Chase, 1973	6	GC	2.7 ± 1.6 (ventricular)
	22	GC	3.7 ± 0.7 (lumbar)
339. Gordon, 1973	5	GC-ECD	5.0 ± 1.8 (sulfate)
444. Karoum, 1975	8	GC-MS	4.6 ± 0.3 (ventricular)
839. Swahn, 1976	5	GC-MS[†]	0.4 ± 0.3
448. Karoum, 1977	5 (ventricular)	GC-MS[†]	1.2 ± 0.3 (sulfate)
	5 (ventricular)	GC-MS	0.3 ± 0.1 (glucuronide)
	5 (lumbar)	GC-MS	1.7 ± 0.5 (sulfate)
	5 (lumbar)	GC-MS	0.2 ± 0.03 (glucuronide)
270. Faull, 1979	23	GC-MS[†]	0.44± 0.15
497. Krstulovic, 1981	12	HPLC-EC[†]	0.24± 0.07
294. Frattini, 1982	28 (M)	HPLC-EC[†]	0.43± 0.03
	20 (F)	HPLC-EC	0.40± 0.03
261. Elsworth, 1983	4	GC-MS[†]	1.3 ± 0.1

Table 167. Unconjugated 3-Methoxy-4-hydroxyphenylglycol in Urine of

Depressed Subjects

Reference First Author, Year	Number of Subjects	Method of Analysis	Values (µg/24h ± S.E.M.)
656. Peyrin, 1985	36	Fl	64
	6 (endogenous)	Fl	62
	19 (neurotic)	Fl	64
	11 (reactive)	Fl	85
277. Filser, 1988	11 (M)	HPLC-UV	136 ± 30
	21 (F)	HPLC-UV	106 ± 16

Table 168. Conjugated (or Total) 3-Methoxy-4-hydroxyphenylglycol in

Urine of Depressed Subjects

Reference First Author, Year	Number of Subjects	Method of Analysis	Values (μg/24h ± S.E.M.)
544. Maas, 1968	16 (severe)	GC-ECD	1087 ± 128
	7 (M)	GC-ECD	1337 ± 106
	9 (F)	GC-ECD	892 ± 146
346. Greenspan, 1970	2 (hypomanic)	GC-ECD	2780 ± 30
	2 (normothymic)	GC-ECD	2605 ± 115
	3 (agitated depression)	GC-ECD	1480 ± 78
96. Bond, 1972	2 (manic)	GC-ECD[†]	2750 ± 150
	2 (depressed)	GC-ECD	1180 ± 90
127. Bunney, 1972	6 (manic)	Fl	2500 ± 340
	6 (depressed)	Fl	2230 ± 220
272. Fawcett, 1972	6 (responder)	GC-ECD	777 ± 159
	6 (non-responder)	GC-ECD	1150 ± 244
679. Prange, 1972	12	GC-ECD	1840 ± 320
223. De Leon-Jones, 1973	1 (manic)	GC-ECD	1182
	1 (depressed)	GC-ECD	805
758. Schildkraut, 1973	1 (schizoaffective)	GC-ECD	870
	5 (manic depressive)	GC-ECD	1240 ± 160
	1 (recurrent endogenous)	GC-ECD	1550
	5 (chronic characterol.)	GC-ECD	1800 ± 90

Table 168. Conjugated (or Total) 3-Methoxy-4-hydroxyphenylglycol in

Urine of Depressed Subjects (continued)

Reference First Author, Year	Number of Subjects	Method of Analysis	Values (μg/24h $\pm$ S.E.M.)
780. Shaw, 1973	11 (depressed)	GC-ECD	1401 $\pm$ 136
	6 (recovered)	GC-ECD	2124 $\pm$ 403
70. Beckmann, 1975	5 (bipolar, history of mania)	GC-ECD	830 $\pm$ 75
	3 (bipolar, manic- depressive)	GC-ECD	1860 $\pm$ 170
	2 (unipolar)	GC-ECD	1590 $\pm$ 250
224. De Leon-Jones, 1975	33 (all)	GC-ECD	1137 $\pm$ 76
	5 (bipolar)	GC-ECD	916 $\pm$ 53
	14 (single episode, unipolar)	GC-ECD	1161 $\pm$ 142
	13 (recurrent unipolar)	GC-ECD	1207 $\pm$ 113
	1 (undiagnosed)	GC-ECD	788
541. Maas, 1975	20 (M)	–	1394 $\pm$ 89
	48 (F)	–	1155 $\pm$ 58
71. Beckmann, 1976	8	GC-ECD	1470 $\pm$ 110
305. Garfinkel, 1977	8 (bipolar)	GC-ECD	1320 $\pm$ 190
592. Murphy, 1977	4	GC-ECD	2880 $\pm$ 520
673. Post, 1977	1 (x84) (depressed)	GC-ECD	1030 $\pm$ 40
	1 (x52) (manic)	GC-ECD	1190 $\pm$ 80
778. Sharpless, 1977	20	GC-ECD[†]	1688 $\pm$ 133
	10 (M)	GC-ECD	2019 $\pm$ 168
	10 (F)	GC-ECD	1357 $\pm$ 147

Table 168. Conjugated (or Total) 3-Methoxy-4-hydroxyphenylglycol in

Urine of Depressed Subjects (continued)

Reference First Author, Year	Number of Subjects	Method of Analysis	Values (μg/24h ± S.E.M.)
661. Pickar, 1978	10 (depressed)	GC-ECD	1184 ± 99
	10 (recovered)	GC-ECD	1794 ± 388
761. Schildkraut, 1978	9 (schizophrenia- related)	GC-ECD	1403 ± 14
	4 (schizoaffective)	GC-ECD	1149 ± 125
	12 (bipolar)	GC-ECD	1209 ± 89
	16 (unipolar, endogenous)	GC-ECD	1950 ± 177
	13 (unipolar, non-endogenous)	GC-ECD	1814 ± 92
	9 (unclassified)	GC-ECD	1815 ± 171
846. Sweeney, 1978	11 (F)	GC-ECD	926 ± 73
847. Sweeney, 1978	7 (unipolar, delusional)	GC-ECD	740 ± 52
	8 (unipolar, non-delusional)	GC-ECD	1094 ± 133
856. Taube, 1978	· 14 (primary affective disorder)	GC-ECD	791 ± 51
	6 (agitated)	GC-ECD	897 ± 78
	8 (non-agitated)	GC-ECD	711 ± 54
167. Cobbin, 1979	35 (unipolar + bipolar)	Fl	1314 ± 181
173. Coppen, 1979	23 (unipolar)	GC-FID	1580 ± 120
	10 (M)	GC-FID	1730 ± 220
	13 (F)	GC-FID	1480 ± 130

Table 168. Conjugated (or Total) 3-Methoxy-4-hydroxyphenylglycol in

Urine of Depressed Subjects (continued)

Reference First Author, Year	Number of Subjects	Method of Analysis	Values (μg/24h ± S.E.M.)
580. Modai, 1979	15 (elderly, bipolar)	–	1125 ± 230
734. Sacchetti, 1979	25 (combined)	GC-FID	910 ± 99
	5 (bipolar)	GC-FID	676 ± 115
	17 (unipolar)	GC-FID	904 ± 126
68. Beckmann, 1980	41 (combined)	GC-ECD	1540 ± 100
	10 (M)	GC-ECD	1680 ± 200
	31 (F)	GC-ECD	1500 ± 100
	11 (combined, bipolar I)	GC-ECD	1090 ± 120
	2 (M) (bipolar)	GC-ECD	1070 ± 120
	9 (F) (bipolar)	GC-ECD	1090 ± 300
	9 (combined, bipolar II)	GC-ECD	1440 ± 200
	2 (M) (bipolar)	GC-ECD	1180 ± 10
	7 (F) (bipolar)	GC-ECD	1510 ± 200
	21 (combined, unipolar)	GC-ECD	1820 ± 120
	6 (M) (unipolar)	GC-ECD	2040 ± 230
	15 (F) (unipolar)	GC-ECD	1730 ± 130
	5 (combined, schizoaffective)	GC-ECD	900 ± 600
	2 (M) (schizoaffective)	GC-ECD	1120 ± 10
	3 (F) (schizoaffective)	GC-ECD	790 ± 10
383. Hollister, 1980	17 (unipolar + bipolar)	GC-ECD	1983 ± 148

Table 168. Conjugated (or Total) 3-Methoxy-4-hydroxyphenylglycol in

Urine of Depressed Subjects (continued)

Reference First Author, Year	Number of Subjects	Method of Analysis	Values (μg/24h ± S.E.M.)
818. Spiker, 1980	18 (unipolar, endogenous)	GC-ECD	2148 ± 194
106. Bowden, 1981	23 (M) (unipolar)	GC-ECD	2282 ± 202
	25 (F) (unipolar)	GC-ECD	2208 ± 221
151. Charney, 1981	5 (endogenous)	GC-MS	1700 ± 375
214. Davis, 1981	30 (unipolar + bipolar)	GC-MS	1945 ± 160
677. Potter, 1981	8 (major affective disorder)	GC-ECD	1700 ± 185
6. Ågren, 1982	19 (M) (unipolar)	GC-MS	3606 ± 241
	29 (F) (unipolar)	GC-MS	3054 ± 222
	8 (M) (bipolar)	GC-MS	3772 ± 631
	11 (F) (bipolar)	GC-MS	2502 ± 205
	27 (M) (combined)	GC-MS	3643 ± 248
	40 (F) (combined)	GC-MS	2907 ± 175
	67 (all depressed)	GC-MS	3202 ± 148
441. Karoum, 1982	6	GC-MS[†]	2300 ± 300
452. Karoum, 1982	6 (unipolar + bipolar)	GC-MS	1444 ± 357
526. Linnoila, 1982; 527. Linnoila, 1982	12 (unipolar + bipolar)	GC-MS	1207 ± 196
525. Linnoila, 1982	4 (rapid cyclers)	GC-MS	1306 ± 128

Table 168. Conjugated (or Total) 3-Methoxy-4-hydroxyphenylglycol in

Urine of Depressed Subjects (continued)

Reference First Author, Year	Number of Subjects	Method of Analysis	Values (μg/24h ± S.E.M.)
523. Linnoila, 1982;	8	GC-MS	1433 ± 254
521. Linnoila, 1986	8 (unipolar + bipolar)	GC-MS	1270 ± 272
754. Schatzberg, 1982	20 (bipolar)	GC-ECD	1373 ± 110
	10 (M)	GC-ECD	1410 ± 186
	10 (F)	GC-ECD	1336 ± 127
	50 (unipolar)	GC-ECD	2147 ± 104
	28 (M)	GC-ECD	2378 ± 133
	22 (F)	GC-ECD	1853 ± 146
7. Ågren, 1983	100	GC-MS	3220 ± 116
225. De Lisi, 1983	27 (major depressive disorder)	GC-MS	1156 ± 109
361. Hamlin, 1983	12 (agoraphobic)	GC-ECD	727 ± 59
493. Koslow, 1983	60 (M) (depressed)	GC-ECD	2273 ± 144
	54 (F) (depressed)	GC-ECD	1968 ± 136
	11 (M) (manic)	GC-ECD	2740 ± 512
	6 (F) (manic)	GC-ECD	1909 ± 751
524. Linnoila, 1983	12 (unipolar + bipolar)	GC-MS	1288 ± 197
591. Mueser, 1983	6 (unipolar)	GC-ECD	856 ± 136
	3 (bipolar, depressed)	GC-ECD	1496 ± 266
	2 (bipolar, manic)	GC-ECD	1647 ± 538
	2 (schizoaffective)	GC-ECD	593 ± 340

Table 168. Conjugated (or Total) 3-Methoxy-4-hydroxyphenylglycol in

Urine of Depressed Subjects (continued)

Reference First Author, Year	Number of Subjects	Method of Analysis	Values (μg/24h $\pm$ S.E.M.)
652. Petursson, 1983	7 (anxiety)	GC-ECD	1050 $\pm$ 95
716. Rosenbaum, 1983	24 (unipolar)	GC-ECD	2081 $\pm$ 143
548. Maas, 1984	114 (unipolar + bipolar)	GC-ECD	2128 $\pm$ 100
597. Muscettola, 1984	19 (bipolar, depressed)	GC-ECD	1440 $\pm$ 100
	13 (bipolar, manic)	GC-ECD	2110 $\pm$ 190
	11 (F) (bipolar, depressed)	GC-ECD	1370 $\pm$ 130
	8 (M) (bipolar, depressed)	GC-ECD	1600 $\pm$ 140
	6 (F) (bipolar, manic)	GC-ECD	1630 $\pm$ 240
	7 (M) (bipolar, manic)	GC-ECD	2510 $\pm$ 200
	28 (unipolar)	GC-ECD	1790 $\pm$ 110
	13 (F) (unipolar)	GC-ECD	1670 $\pm$ 150
	15 (M) (unipolar)	GC-ECD	1890 $\pm$ 150
	38 (F) (combined)	GC-ECD	1530 $\pm$ 70
	28 (M) (combined)	GC-ECD	1810 $\pm$ 110
	66 (all depressed)	GC-ECD	1650 $\pm$ 60
518. Liebowitz, 1985	8 (atypical)	GC-MS	2541 $\pm$ 347

Table 168. Conjugated (or Total) 3-Methoxy-4-hydroxyphenylglycol in
Urine of Depressed Subjects (continued)

Reference First Author, Year	Number of Subjects	Method of Analysis	Values (μg/24h ± S.E.M.)
586. Mooney, 1985	6 (responders to alprazolam)	GC-ECD	2676 ± 237
	6 (non-responders)	GC-ECD	1810 ± 90
656. Peyrin, 1985	36 (F)	Fl	301 ± 40 (sulfate)
	6 (endogenous)	Fl	202 ± 47 (sulfate)
	19 (neurotic)	Fl	260 ± 44 (sulfate)
	11 (reactive)	Fl	420 ± 94 (sulfate)
	36	Fl	463 ± 47 (glucuronide)
	6 (endogenous)	Fl	315 ± 97 (glucuronide)
	19 (neurotic)	Fl	446 ± 50 (glucuronide)
	11 (reactive)	Fl	575 ± 113 (glucuronide)
533. Lôo, 1986	56 (all depressed)	HPLC-EC	1080 ± 80 (total) μg/g Creat.
	24 (M)	HPLC-EC	1080 ± 130 (total) μg/g Creat.
	32 (F)	HPLC-EC	1070 ± 100 (total) μg/g Creat.
724. Roy, 1986	7 (no melancholia)	GC-MS	929 ± 176
	5 (history of melancholia)	GC-MS	1290 ± 296
	8 (with melancholia)	GC-MS	1240 ± 172
	8 (dysthymic disorder)	GC-MS	1437 ± 144
	7 (M)	GC-MS	1748 ± 140
	21 (F)	GC-MS	1049 ± 492

Table 168. Conjugated (or Total) 3-Methoxy-4-hydroxyphenylglycol in

Urine of Depressed Subjects (continued)

Reference First Author, Year	Number of Subjects	Method of Analysis	Values (μg/24h $\pm$ S.E.M.)
790. Siever, 1986	10 (unipolar)	GC-MS	2521 $\pm$ 245
	4 (bipolar)	GC-MS	2429 $\pm$ 359
	14 (combined)	GC-MS	2502 $\pm$ 197
105. Bowden, 1987	57 (unipolar)	GC-ECD	2155 $\pm$ 131
	26 (bipolar)	GC-ECD	2123 $\pm$ 252
	83 (combined)	GC-ECD	2145 $\pm$ 119
307. Garvey, 1987	8 (panic-disorder)	GC-ECD	2439 $\pm$ 235
	17 (no panic-disorder)	GC-ECD	1871 $\pm$ 171
977. Zhou, 1987	7 (bipolar)	Fl	1037 $\pm$ 191 (sulfate)
	25 (unipolar, combined)	Fl	1350 $\pm$ 88 (sulfate)
	16 (unipolar, endogenous)	Fl	1480 $\pm$ 96 (sulfate)
	9 (unipolar, non-endogenous)	Fl	1120 $\pm$ 159 (sulfate)
	32 (all depressed)	Fl	1283 $\pm$ 83 (sulfate)
137. Carr, 1988	20 (unipolar)	GC-MS	1869 $\pm$ 252 (total)
170. Conti, 1988	3 (M)	GC-FID	1725 (total)
	4 (F)	GC-FID	1282 (total)
277. Filser, 1988	11 (M)	HPLC-UV	2424 $\pm$ 320 (total) 1202 $\pm$ 180 (glucuronide) 1086 $\pm$ 196 (sulfate)
	21 (F)	HPLC-UV	1739 $\pm$ 128 (total) 834 $\pm$ 78 (glucuronide) 788 $\pm$ 86 (sulfate)

Table 168. Conjugated (or Total) 3-Methoxy-4-hydroxyphenylglycol in

Urine of Depressed Subjects (continued)

Reference First Author, Year	Number of Subjects	Method of Analysis	Values (μg/24h ± S.E.M.)
534. Lôo, 1988	58 (unipolar + bipolar)	HPLC-EC	1070 ± 75 µg/mg Cr.
	25 (M)	HPLC-EC	1100 ± 125 µg/mg Cr.
	33 (F)	HPLC-EC	1040 ± 90 µg/mg Cr.
539. Lykouras, 1988	18 (delusional)	GC-ECD	2006 ± 217 µg/mg Cr.
	22 (non-delusional)	GC-ECD	1472 ± 145 µg/mg Cr.
587. Mooney, 1988	9	GC-ECD	2530 ± 236 (total)
877. Van Bemmel, 1988	7 (M)	GC-ECD	1900
	8 (F) (melancholia)	GC-ECD	1440

Table 169.   Unconjugated 3-Methoxy-4-hydroxyphenylglycol in

Plasma of Depressed Subjects

Reference First Author, Year	Number of Subjects	Method of Analysis	Values (ng/mL ± S.E.M.)
845. Sweeney, 1980	10 (unipolar + bipolar)	GC-MS	3.3 ± 0.4
151. Charney, 1981	8 (endogenous)	GC-MS	4.1 ± 0.8
150. Charney, 1982	15 (endogenous)	GC-MS	4.4 ± 0.6
149. Charney, 1983	9 (endogenous)	GC-MS	4.2 ± 0.6
479. Ko, 1983	6 (panic, phobia)	GC-MS[†]	4.35 ± 0.42
148. Charney, 1984	39 (panic, phobia)	GC-MS	3.6 ± 0.1
529. Linnoila, 1984	8 (unipolar)	HPLC-EC	5.1 ± 0.7
146. Charney, 1985	14 (anxiety)	GC-MS	3.3 ± 0.2
147. Charney, 1985	18 (agoraphobia, panic)	GC-MS	4.0 ± 0.3
235. Devanand, 1985	5 (M) (melancholic)	GC-MS	3.5 ± 0.3
	4 (M) (melancholic, psychotic)	GC-MS	3.0 ± 0.3
	11 (F) (melancholic)	GC-MS	4.2 ± 0.6
	7 (F) (melancholic, psychotic)	GC-MS	4.0 ± 0.4
	9 (M) (all melancholic)	GC-MS	3.3 ± 0.2
	18 (F) (all melancholic)	GC-MS	4.1 ± 0.4
727. Rubin, 1985	33 (unipolar)	GC-MS	4.14 ± 0.20

Table 169. Unconjugated 3-Methoxy-4-hydroxyphenylglycol in

Plasma of Depressed Subjects (continued)

Reference First Author, Year	Number of Subjects	Method of Analysis	Values (ng/mL ± S.E.M.)
918. Warsh, 1985	18 (unipolar + bipolar)	GC-MS	4.4 ± 0.5
721. Roy, 1986	11 (dysthymic disorder)	GC-MS	2.7 ± 0.2
	40 (major depressive episode)	GC-MS	3.5 ± 0.2
	20 (present melancholia)	GC-MS	3.9 ± 0.5
	16 (unipolar)	GC-MS	4.3 ± 0.6
	4 (bipolar)	GC-MS	2.7 ± 0.4
	8 (past melancholia)	GC-MS	3.7 ± 0.3
	6 (unipolar)	GC-MS	3.7 ± 0.4
	2 (bipolar)	GC-MS	3.7 ± 0.1
	28 (past and present)	GC-MS	3.9 ± 0.4
	22 (unipolar)	GC-MS	4.1 ± 0.4
	6 (bipolar)	GC-MS	3.0 ± 0.4
	12 (unipolar, no melancholia)	GC-MS	2.6 ± 0.2
	40 (all major depressive episode)	GC-MS	3.5 ± 0.2
	34 (unipolar)	GC-MS	3.6 ± 0.3
	6 (bipolar)	GC-MS	3.0 ± 0.4
790. Siever, 1986	17	GC-MS	3.3 ± 0.2
	9 (unipolar)	GC-MS	3.2 ± 0.4
	8 (bipolar)	GC-MS	3.4 ± 0.3

Table 169.   Unconjugated 3-Methoxy-4-hydroxyphenylglycol in

Plasma of Depressed Subjects (continued)

Reference First Author, Year	Number of Subjects	Method of Analysis	Values (ng/mL ± S.E.M.)
252. Edlund, 1987	28 (panic)	HPLC-EC	3.31± 0.20
562. Mazure, 1987	15 (major depression)	GC-MS	3.9 ± 0.2
	10 (melancholia)	GC-MS	5.1 ± 0.6
	8 (depressive psychosis)	GC-MS	4.4 ± 0.6
665. Pohl, 1987	10 (anxiety)	GC-MS	3.3 ± 0.3
949. Wolkowitz, 1987	18	HPLC-EC	3.42± 0.35
	4 (psychotic)	HPLC-EC	3.36± 0.74
	7 (non-psychotic)	HPLC-EC	3.53± 0.65
	8 (unipolar)	HPLC-EC	3.69± 0.62
	4 (bipolar)	HPLC-EC	2.89± 0.28
875. Uhde, 1988	12 (panic attacks)	GC-MS	3.6 ± 0.8
362. Hariharan, 1989	10 (M)	HPLC-EC[†]	2.80± 0.19
	10 (F) (unipolar)	HPLC-EC[†]	3.30± 0.35
	4 (M)	HPLC-EC[†]	3.43± 0.11
	4 (F) (obsessive- compulsive)	HPLC-EC[†]	3.10± 0.42
775. Sevy, 1989	14 (anxiety)	HPLC-EC	7.4 ± 0.6
	14 (major depression)	HPLC-EC	4.0 ± 0.1

Table 170. Conjugated 3-Methoxy-4-hydroxyphenylglycol in Plasma of

Depressed Subjects

Reference First Author, Year	Number of Subjects	Method of Analysis	Values (ng/mL ± S.E.M.)
845. Sweeney, 1980	5	GC-MS	5.5 ± 0.6 (conjugated)
419. Jimerson, 1981	1 (bipolar, manic)	GC-MS	21.1 ± 1.3 (total)
	1 (bipolar, depressed)	GC-MS	13.7 ± 0.6 (total)
	1 (schizoaffective, manic)	GC-MS	24.9 ± 0.7 (total)
	1 (schizoaffective, depressed)	GC-MS	18.8 ± 0.7 (total)
918. Warsh, 1985	8	GC-MS	10.1 ± 0.7 (conjugated)
357. Halbreich, 1987	42	HPLC-EC	16.7 ± 1.2 (total)
	15 (M)	HPLC-EC	16.9 ± 1.8 (total)
	27 (F)	HPLC-EC	16.6 ± 1.5 (total)

Table 171. Unconjugated (or Total) 3-Methoxy-4-hydroxyphenylglycol in

CSF of Depressed Subjects

Reference First Author, Year	Number of Subjects	Method of Analysis	Values (ng/mL ± S.E.M.)
338. Gordon, 1971	7	GC-ECD[†]	7.3 ± 1.0
82. Bertilsson, 1973	14	GC-MS[†]	11.9 ± 0.8
339. Gordon, 1973	16	GC-ECD	9.0 ± 0.9
626. O'Keefe, 1973	22 (unipolar)	GC-ECD[†]	11.9 ± 0.6 (total)
	7 (recovered unipolar)	GC-ECD	10.2 ± 0.7 (total)
	1 (bipolar)	GC-ECD	6.1 (total)
	1 (manic)	GC-ECD	8.8 (total)
670. Post, 1973	9 (manic)	GC-ECD	15.5 ± 3.0 (total)
	25 (depressed)	GC-ECD	8.9 ± 1.1 (total)
671. Post, 1973	9 (simulated mania)	GC-ECD	14.2 ± 3.4
	9 (depressed)	GC-ECD	7.5 ± 2.2
780. Shaw, 1973	22 (unipolar)	GC-ECD	11.9 ± 0.6
784. Shopsin, 1973	1 (depressed)	GC-ECD	18
	4 (manic)	GC-ECD	27.8 ± 5.5
785. Shopsin, 1974	8 (depressed)	GC-ECD	15.8
	13 (manic)	GC-ECD	23
415. Jimerson, 1975	34 (22 depressed)	GC-MS	12.1 ± 1.1
667. Post, 1975	15 (manic)	GC-ECD	15.5
	38 (depressed)	GC-ECD	10.5

Table 171.   Unconjugated (or Total) 3-Methoxy-4-hydroxyphenylglycol in

CSF of Depressed Subjects (continued)

Reference First Author, Year	Number of Subjects	Method of Analysis	Values (ng/mL ± S.E.M.)
832. Subrahmanyam, 1975	24 (manic-depressive)	GC-ECD	14.2 ± 2.6
38. Åsberg, 1977	14	GC-MS	12.5 ± 0.9
794. Siwers, 1977	6	GC-MS	11.9 ± 0.9
882. Van Praag, 1977	8 (endogenous)	GC-ECD	10.2 ± 1.2
894. Vestergaard, 1978	27 (before recovery)	GC-ECD	12 ± 0.8
	13 (unipolar)	GC-ECD	14 ± 1.1
	6 (bipolar)	GC-ECD	15 ± 2.0
	13 (after recovery)	GC-ECD	11 ± 1.1
	6 (unipolar)	GC-ECD	10 ± 1.6
	3 (bipolar)	GC-ECD	12 ± 2.3
	4 (manic, before)	GC-ECD	15 ± 4
864. Träskman, 1979	28 (endogenous)	GC-MS	11.5 ± 0.6
5. Ågren, 1980	21 (unipolar)	GC-MS	10.7 ± 0.4
	12 (bipolar)	GC-MS	10.5 ± 0.5
75. Berger, 1980	13 (M)	GC-MS	9.3 ± 0.6
2. Åberg-Wistedt, 1981	25 (endogenous)	GC-MS	10.8 ± 1.0
106. Bowden, 1981	23 (M) (unipolar)	GC-MS	8.0 ± 0.3
	23 (F) (unipolar)	GC-MS	9.4 ± 0.5
214. Davis, 1981	12 (unipolar + bipolar)	GC-MS	10.3

Table 171. Unconjugated (or Total) 3-Methoxy-4-hydroxyphenylglycol in

CSF of Depressed Subjects (continued)

Reference First Author, Year	Number of Subjects	Method of Analysis	Values (ng/mL ± S.E.M.)
633. Oreland, 1981	6 (M) (depressed)	GC-MS	8.9 ± 0.7
	14 (F) (depressed)	GC-MS	9.7 ± 0.5
	5 (M) (recovered)	GC-MS	8.8 ± 0.4
	6 (F) (recovered)	GC-MS	8.4 ± 0.9
677. Potter, 1981	8 (unipolar + bipolar)	GC-MS	8.7 ± 0.7
708. Roccatagliata, 1981	12 (endogenous)	Fl	17.2 ± 3.8
4. Ackenheil, 1982	30 (psychiatric)	HPLC-EC	9
192. Dahl, 1982	25 (endogenous)	GC-MS	11.2 ± 0.7
	9 (M)	GC-MS	10.7 ± 0.9
	16 (F)	GC-MS	11.6 ± 1.1
546. Maas, 1982	40 (F)	–	9.2 ± 0.4
	43 (M) (unipolar + bipolar)	–	8.1 ± 0.3
7. Ågren, 1983	100	GC-MS	10.9 ± 0.2
493. Koslow, 1983; 843. Swann, 1983; 548. Maas, 1984; 688. Redmond, 1986	99 (depressed)	GC-MS	8.8 ± 0.2
	46 (F)	GC-MS	9.1 ± 0.3
	53 (M)	GC-MS	8.5 ± 0.3
	14 (manic)	GC-MS	11.0 ± 1.0
	5 (F)	GC-MS	11.7 ± 1.5
	9 (M)	GC-MS	10.6 ± 1.3
	61 (unipolar)	GC-MS	8.9 ± 0.3
	38 (bipolar)	GC-MS	8.5 ± 0.3
36. Åsberg, 1984	34 (melancholic)	GC-MS	9.4 ± 0.3

Table 171. Unconjugated (or Total) 3-Methoxy-4-hydroxyphenylglycol in

CSF of Depressed Subjects (continued)

Reference First Author, Year	Number of Subjects	Method of Analysis	Values (ng/mL ± S.E.M.)
77. Berrettini, 1984	10 (bipolar)	HPLC-EC	8.1 ± 0.4
98. Bottiglieri, 1984	18	HPLC-EC[†]	9.4 ± 0.9
316. Gerner, 1984	34 (depressed)	HPLC-EC	8.0 ± 0.4
	14 (manic)	HPLC-EC	8.4 ± 0.4
78. Berrettini, 1985	10 (bipolar, euthymic)	HPLC-EC	7.9 ± 0.4
104. Bowden, 1985	65 37 (M) 28 (F) (unipolar + bipolar)	GC-MS GC-MS GC-MS	8.8 ± 0.3 8.5 ± 0.4 9.1 ± 0.4
517. Lidberg, 1985	22 (suicide attempts)	GC-MS	9.4 ± 0.7
678. Potter, 1985	11 (unipolar + bipolar)	HPLC-EC[†]	8.5 ± 0.6
726. Roy, 1985	15 (melancholic)	HPLC-EC	9.0 ± 0.8
	8 (major depressive episode, no melancholia)	HPLC-EC	8.1 ± 0.4
	5 (dysthymic disorder)	HPLC-EC	7.3 ± 0.5
521. Linnoila, 1986	8 8 (unipolar + bipolar)	HPLC-EC HPLC-EC	8.9 ± 0.7 (total) 9.1 ± 0.7 (total)
322. Gjerris, 1987	33 (endogenous)	GC-MS	8.3
	7 (non-endogenous)	GC-MS	8.5

Table 171. Unconjugated (or Total) 3-Methoxy-4-hydroxyphenylglycol in

CSF of Depressed Subjects (continued)

Reference First Author, Year	Number of Subjects	Method of Analysis	Values (ng/mL ± S.E.M.)
394. Hsiao, 1987	40 (unipolar + bipolar)	HPLC-EC[†]	8.0 ± 0.3
829. Stokes, 1987	25	GC-MS	8.2 ± 0.6
325. Golden, 1988	6 (unipolar + bipolar)	HPLC-EC	6.37± 0.24

Table 172. Conjugated 3-Methoxy-4-hydroxyphenylglycol in CSF of

Depressed Subjects

Reference First Author, Year	Number of Subjects	Method of Analysis	Values (ng/mL ± S.E.M.)
82. Bertilsson, 1973	14	GC-MS[†]	1.5 ± 0.1
339. Gordon, 1973	16	GC-ECD	4.2 ± 1.0 (sulfate)
75. Berger, 1980	11	GC-MS	0.3 ± 0.3

Table 173. Conjugated (or Total) 3-Methoxy-4-hydroxyphenylglycol in

Urine of Schizophrenic Subjects

Reference First Author, Year	Number of Subjects	Method of Analysis	Values (μg/24h ± S.E.M.)
666. Pollin, 1971	30 (15 pairs of twins)	GC-ECD	1480 μg/g Cr.
43. Atsmon, 1972	5 (improved)	Fl	1340 (total)
	4 (not improved)	Fl	290
832. Subrahmanyam, 1975	30 (acute)	GC-ECD	1100 ± 400 (total)
	6 (acute, aggressive)	GC-ECD	3200 ± 800
	24 (chronic)	GC-ECD	1400 ± 400
	24 (manic depressive psychotic)	GC-ECD	1000 ± 400
427. Joseph, 1976	18 (chronic)	GC-ECD	1550 ± 125 (glucuronide)
	18 (chronic)	GC-ECD	1170 ± 90 (sulfate)
	18 (chronic)	GC-ECD	170 (unconjugated)
	6 (low severity)	GC-ECD	1710 (glucuronide)
	6 (low severity)	GC-ECD	1470 (sulfate)
	6 (moderate)	GC-ECD	1630 (glucuronide)
	6 (moderate)	GC-ECD	1250 (sulfate)
	6 (high severity)	GC-ECD	1300 (glucuronide)
	6 (high severity)	GC-ECD	790 (sulfate)
856. Taube, 1978	11	GC-ECD	931 ± 132 (total)
	7 (agitated)	GC-ECD	1161 ± 138 (total)
	4 (non-agitated)	GC-ECD	528 ± 80 (total)

<u>Table 173.   Conjugated (or Total) 3-Methoxy-4-hydroxyphenylglycol in</u>

<u>Urine of Schizophrenic Subjects (continued)</u>

Reference First Author, Year	Number of Subjects	Method of Analysis	Values (μg/24h ± S.E.M.)
428. Joseph, 1979	16 (F)	GC-ECD	3610 ± 360 μg/g Cr. (total)
	16 (F)	GC-ECD	1640 ± 210 μg/g Cr. (sulfate)
	21 (M)	GC-ECD	2140 ± 170 μg/g Cr. (total)
	21 (M)	GC-ECD	1010 ± 90 μg/g Cr. (sulfate)
225. De Lisi, 1983	23 (acute)	GC-MS	1097 ± 110 (total)
	12 (chronic)	GC-MS	1530 ± 250 (total)
555. Markianos, 1983	22 (with tardive dyskinesia)	GC-ECD	1920 ± 110 μg/g Cr. (total)
	20 (no tardive dyskinesia)	GC-ECD	2410 ± 170 μg/g Cr. (total)
591. Mueser, 1983	11	GC-ECD	1598 ± 288
543. Maas, 1988	5 (acute)	GC-MS	3919 ± 389* (total)

* In original paper expressed as μg/3.5 h.

Table 174.   3-Methoxy-4-hydroxyphenylglycol in Plasma of Schizophrenic

Subjects

Reference First Author, Year	Number of Subjects	Method of Analysis	Values (ng/mL ± S.E.M.)
826. Sternberg, 1982	11	GC-MS	4.0 ± 0.5
114. Bowers, 1984	7 (good responders)	GC-MS	5.3 ± 0.6
	4 (poor responders)	GC-MS	3.8 ± 0.7
111. Bowers, 1986	14 (M)	GC-MS	4.4 ± 0.5
	19 (F)	GC-MS	4.4 ± 0.3
112. Bowers, 1987	48 (M)	GC-MS	4.0 ± 0.2
	69 (F)	GC-MS	4.4 ± 0.2
110a. Bowers, 1988	328 (psychotic + depression)	GC-MS GC-MS	3.5 ± 0.1 (M) 3.6 ± 0.1 (F)
	22 (psychotic)	GC-MS GC-MS	6.3 ± 0.3 (M) 7.5 ± 0.7 (F)
480. Ko, 1988	14 (chronic)	GC-MS	3.55± 0.25
543. Maas, 1988	23 (acute)	GC-MS	4.0 ± 0.3
948. Wolkowitz, 1988	12 (chronic)	HPLC-EC	3.07± 0.21

Table 175.   3-Methoxy-4-hydroxyphenylglycol in CSF of Schizophrenic

Subjects

Reference First Author, Year	Number of Subjects	Method of Analysis	Values (ng/mL ± S.E.M.)
784. Shopsin, 1973	8	GC-ECD	20
785. Shopsin, 1974	19	GC-ECD	17.2
340. Gordon, 1975	31 (psychiatric)	GC-MS	12.1 ± 1.1 (total)
667. Post, 1975	17	GC-ECD	16
832. Subrahmanyam, 1975	30 (acute)	GC-ECD	12.6 ± 1.2 (total)
	6 (acute, aggressive)	GC-ECD	21.4 ± 3.2 (total)
	24 (chronic)	GC-ECD	15.2 ± 3.6 (total)
	24 (manic depressive psychotic)	GC-ECD	14.2 ± 2.6 (total)
454. Karoum, 1976	17	GC-MS	10.6 ± 0.8
	17	GC-MS	3.6 ± 0.6 (conjugated)
91. Bjerkenstedt, 1977	34	GC-MS	7.6 ± 0.3
	29	GC-MS	7.7 ± 0.5
363. Härnryd, 1979	12	GC-MS	9.8 ± 0.4
604. Nagao, 1979	15 (no tardive dyskinesia)	Fl	13.2 ± 1.1
	12 (with tardive dyskinesia)	Fl	13.3 ± 1.3
75. Berger, 1980	9	GC-MS	8.2 ± 0.8
	9	GC-MS	-0.2 ± 0.1 (conjugated)
770. Sedvall, 1980	9 (family history)	GC-MS	7.7 ± 0.5
	9 (no family history)	GC-MS	7.2 ± 0.3
767. Sedvall, 1980	8	GC-MS	7.5 ± 0.4
976. Zander, 1981	13 (chronic)	GC-ECD	13.3 ± 1.9

<u>Table 175.   3-Methoxy-4-hydroxyphenylglycol in CSF of Schizophrenic</u>

<u>Subjects (continued)</u>

Reference First Author, Year	Number of Subjects	Method of Analysis	Values (ng/mL ± S.E.M.)
311. Gattaz, 1982	28	HPLC-EC[†]	16.1 ± 4.3
	13 (no drugs)	HPLC-EC	17.8 ± 4.8
	15 (on neuroleptics)	HPLC-EC	14.6 ± 3.4
954. Wood, 1982	9	GC-MS	7.4 ± 0.7
72. Beckmann, 1983	9	HPLC	6.6 ± 1.1
530. Linnoila, 1983	28	HPLC	6.4 ± 0.5
	19 (M)	HPLC	5.6 ± 0.5
	9 (F)	HPLC	8.0 ± 1.0
620. Nybäck, 1983	26	GC-MS	7.9 ± 0.4
316. Gerner, 1984	18	HPLC-EC	8.0 ± 0.4
755. Scheinin, 1984	46 (chronic)	HPLC-EC[†]	6.8 ± 0.2
309. Gattaz, 1985	13	HPLC-EC	17.8 ± 1.3
822. Stahl, 1985	4 (with tardive dyskinesis)	GC-MS	9.8 ± 1.1
644. Parnetti, 1987	13	HPLC-Fl[†]	9.4 ± 0.8
543. Maas, 1988	23 (acute)	GC-MS	9.0 ± 0.5

Table 176. 3-Methoxy-4-hydroxyphenylglycol in Urine and Plasma of

Parkinson's and Alzheimer's Disease Subjects

Reference First Author, Year	Number of Subjects	Method of Analysis	Values (Mean ± S.E.M.)
132. Calne, 1969	9 (Parkinson's)	GC-FID	2.2 ± 0.32 mg/24h(total)
	14 (Parkinson's)	GC-FID	1.4 ± 0.16 mg/24h(total)
685. Raskind, 1984	8 (advanced Alzheimer's)	GC-MS	5.4 ± 0.6 ng/mL (plasma)
	7 (moderate Alzheimer's)	GC-MS	3.5 ± 0.5 ng/mL (plasma)

<u>Table 177.   3-Methoxy-4-hydroxyphenylglycol in CSF of Parkinson's</u>

<u>Disease Subjects</u>

Reference First Author, Year	Number of Subjects	Method of Analysis	Values (ng/mL ± S.E.M.)
338. Gordon, 1971	6	GC-ECD[†]	12.5 ± 1.3
453. Karoum, 1971	4	GC-ECD	12.8 ± 1.5
	2	GC-ECD	19 ± 2 (conjugated)
940. Wilk, 1971	10	GC-ECD	18
94. Bond, 1972	6	GC-ECD[†]	17.0 ± 1.9
	6	GC-ECD	16.2 ± 4.3 (conjugated)
154. Chase, 1973	13	GC	15 ± 2.5
670. Post, 1973	14	GC-ECD	14.8 ± 2.4
202. Davidson, 1977	25	GC-ECD	8 ± 1
317. Gibson, 1985	19	HPLC-EC[†]	7.4 ± 0.6
	4 (mild)	HPLC-EC	7.7 ± 0.8
	6 (moderate)	HPLC-EC	7.1 ± 1.3
	9 (severe)	HPLC-EC	7.6 ± 1.0
822. Stahl, 1985	9 (dystonia)	GC-MS	8.5 ± 0.4

Table 178.   3-Methoxy-4-hydroxyphenylglycol in CSF of Alzheimer's

Disease Subjects

Reference First Author, Year	Number of Subjects	Method of Analysis	Values (ng/mL ± S.E.M.)
626. O'Keeffe, 1973	2 (senile dementia)	GC-ECD[†]	10.6 ± 0.05
443. Karoum, 1975	9 (presenile dementia)	GC-MS[†]	11.7 ± 1 (ventricular)
	9 (presenile dementia)	GC-MS	4.7 ± 1.3 (conjugated, ventricular)
954. Wood, 1982	11	GC-MS	8.8 ± 1.1
635. Palmer, 1984	25 (presenile)	HPLC-EC[†]	8.3 ± 0.4
	4 (senile)	HPLC-EC	6.4 ± 0.5
685. Raskind, 1984	8 (advanced)	GC-MS	10.8 ± 0.9
	7 (moderate)	GC-MS	7.6 ± 0.4
317. Gibson, 1985	29	HPLC-EC[†]	7.2 ± 0.3
	16 (mild)	HPLC-EC	7.0 ± 0.4
	9 (moderate)	HPLC-EC	6.7 ± 0.5
	4 (severe)	HPLC-EC	9.3 ± 0.7
816. Sparks, 1985	4	HPLC-EC[†]	30 ± 9
621. Nybäck, 1987	15	GC-MS	7.4 ± 0.4
644. Parnetti, 1987	12	HPLC-Fl[†]	8.5 ± 0.5
834. Sunderland, 1987	13	HPLC-EC	9.5 ± 0.8
495. Koyama, 1988	6	HPLC-EC[†]	9.90± 0.82

<u>Table 179. 3-Methoxy-4-hydroxyphenylglycol in CSF of Aggressive and</u>

<u>Suicidal Subjects</u>

Reference First Author, Year	Number of Subjects	Method of Analysis	Values (ng/mL ± S.E.M.)
118. Brown, 1979	1 (antisocial)	GC-MS	16.1
	1 (explosive)	GC-MS	13.0
	2 (immature)	GC-MS	13.4 ± 0.2
	1 (hysterical)	GC-MS	8.5
	3 (passive- aggressive)	GC-MS	9.5 ± 4.3
	2 (passive- depressive)	GC-MS	6.6 ± 3.9
	2 (schizoid)	GC-MS	8.8 ± 2.8
	12 (more impulsive, aggressive)	GC-MS	12.9 ± 1.2
	12 (less impulsive, aggressive)	GC-MS	8.5 ± 2.0
	12 (history of suicide)	GC-MS	13.8 ± 1.6
	12 (no history of suicide)	GC-MS	7.9 ± 1.6
633. Oreland, 1981	5 (M) (suicidal)	GC-MS	7.9 ± 0.5
	10 (F) (suicidal)	GC-MS	8.4 ± 0.6
865. Träskman, 1981	29 (suicide attempts)	GC-MS	8.8 ± 0.4
	7 (depressed)	GC-MS	9.8 ± 0.9
	22 (not depressed)	GC-MS	8.5 ± 0.4

Table 179. 3-Methoxy-4-hydroxyphenylglycol in CSF of Aggressive and

Suicidal Subjects (continued)

Reference First Author, Year	Number of Subjects	Method of Analysis	Values (ng/mL ± S.E.M.)
532. Linnoila, 1983	20 (explosive)	HPLC	5.7 ± 0.3
	7 (antisocial)	HPLC	5.0 ± 0.5
	7 (paranoid-aggressive)	HPLC	6.7 ± 1.1
517. Lidberg, 1985	15 (homicidal)	GC-MS	8.8 ± 0.4
897. Virkkunen, 1987	15 (violent)	HPLC-EC	5.3 ± 0.3

Table 180. Unconjugated Vanilmandelic Acid in Urine of Normal Subjects

Reference First Author, Year	Number of Subjects	Method of Analysis	Values (mg/24h ± S.E.M.)
737. Sandler, 1959	11	Fl[†]	11.0 ± 0.7
738. Sandler, 1959	–	Fl	6.1 ± 0.7
909. Von Studnitz, 1959	17	Fl[†]	4.7 mg/g Cr.
320. Gitlow, 1960	15	Fl[†]	1.4 ± 0.1 mg/g Cr.
321. Gitlow, 1960	10	Fl[†]	1.6 ± 0.1 mg/g Cr.
835. Sunderman, 1960	68	Fl[†]	4.0 ± 0.2
908. Von Studnitz, 1960	62	Fl[†]	4.8 ± 0.1
	70	Fl	4.4 ± 0.1 mg/g Cr.
476. Klein, 1961	7	Fl[†]	2.7 ± 0.4 mg/g Cr.
739. Sandler, 1961	15	Fl[†]	3.9 ± 0.2
930. Weise, 1961	10 (M)	Fl[†]	3.7 ± 0.2
	14 (F)	Fl	2.9 ± 0.2
947. Woiwod, 1961	9	Fl[†]	13.6 ± 1.1
549. Mahler, 1962	14	Fl[†]	5.4 ± 0.8
579. Miyake, 1962	20	Fl[†]	3.7 ± 0.9
233. De Quattro, 1964	9	Fl[†]	3.6 ± 0.3*
375. Hermann, 1964	57	Fl[†]	1.9 ± 0.07 mg/g Cr.
185. Curran, 1965	10	Fl	3.21± 0.52
939. Wilk, 1965	21	GC-ECD[†]	1.6 mg/g Cr.
129. Butler, 1967	400	Fl[†]	4.0 ± 0.1
334. Goodman, 1967	5 (fasting)	Fl[†]	n.d.
	27 (regular diet)	Fl	1.3 mg/g Cr.
956. Wybenga, 1967	60	Fl[†]	5.2
747. Sapira, 1968	9	Fl[†]	2.8 ± 1.1 µg/g Cr. (S.D.)

Table 180. Unconjugated Vanilmandelic Acid in Urine of Normal Subjects

(continued)

Reference First Author, Year	Number of Subjects	Method of Analysis	Values (mg/24h ± S.E.M.)
439. Karoum, 1969	20	GC-FID	5.7 ± 0.3
752. Sato, 1969	8	REA[†]	3.7 ± 0.3*
135. Cardon, 1970	7	Fl	3.8
569. Messiha, 1970	8	Fl	2.5 ± 0.9
221. Dekirmenjian, 1971	6	GC-ECD[†]	3.3 ± 0.7
434. Kahane, 1971	7	Fl	4.8 ± 0.3
666. Pollin, 1971	8 (4 pairs of twins)	GC-ECD	1.75 mg/g Cr.
871. Turnbull, 1971	21	–	5.4 ± 0.3
879. Van de Calseyde, 1971	18	GC-FID[†]	3.7 ± 0.3
876. Vahidi, 1971	3	Fl	4.2 ± 0.2
679. Prange, 1972	10	GC-ECD	3.2 ± 0.4
850. Takahashi, 1972	10	Fl[†]	1.6 ± 0.5 mg/g Cr.
130. Buttery, 1973	20	Fl[†]	3.0 ± 0.3
570. Messiha, 1973	12	Fl[†]	3.6 ± 0.3
711. Roginsky, 1974	25	GC-FID[†]	3.4 ± 0.3
191. Cymerman, 1975	6	GC-ECD	2.6 ± 0.2 mg/g Cr.
224. De Leon-Jones, 1975	21	GC-ECD	4.4 ± 0.4
541. Maas, 1975	19 (M) 21 (F)	– –	4.16± 0.65 4.61± 0.41
798. Sjöquist, 1975	11	GC-MS[†]	4.6 mg/L
830. Stott, 1975	123 80 (M) 43 (F)	Fl[†] Fl Fl	3.3 ± 0.08 3.3 ± 0.10 3.3 ± 0.14

Table 180. Unconjugated Vanilmandelic Acid in Urine of Normal Subjects

(continued)

Reference First Author, Year	Number of Subjects	Method of Analysis	Values (mg/24h ± S.E.M.)
832. Subrahmanyam, 1975	12 12	Fl Fl	4.8 ± 0.8 4.4 ± 0.6
427. Joseph, 1976	13	GC-ECD	4.1 ± 0.4
963. Yoshida, 1976	14	HPLC	2.0 ± 0.2
351. Gumboldt, 1977	40	Fl[†]	4.32± 0.79
234. De Schaepdryver, 1978	20	Fl[†]	5.6 ± 0.3
598. Muskiet, 1978	25	GC-MS[†]	1.9 ± 0.2 mg/g Cr.
748. Saran, 1978	7	Fl	4.1 ± 0.5
80. Bertani-Dziedzic, 1979	14 14	HPLC-Fl[†] PC-Fl**	2.86 2.25
713. Rosano, 1979	9	HPLC-Fl[†]	4.9
744. Sandler, 1979	27 10 (M) 17 (F)	GC-FID GC-FID GC-FID	4.61± 0.24 4.55± 0.40 4.65± 0.32
156. Chauhan, 1980	5	GC-ECD[†]	2.75± 0.24
957. Yamada, 1981	10	HPLC-Fl[†]	7.6 ± 0.7 mg/L
441. Karoum, 1982	5	GC-MS[†]	4.1 ± 0.5
218. De Jong, 1983	7	GC-FID[†]	5.43± 0.70 mg/g Cr.
489. Kopin, 1983	12	REA[†]	3.64± 0.24
493. Koslow, 1983	77 36 (M) 41 (F)	GC-ECD GC-ECD GC-ECD	2.72± 0.16 2.72± 0.24 2.72± 0.22
583. Moleman, 1983	7	HPLC-EC[†]	3.54± 0.42
87. Binder, 1984	110	HPLC-EC[†]	3.86± 0.13
471. Kiriike, 1984	31	Fl	5.8 ± 0.5
211. Davis, 1986	10	GC-MS[†]	4.0
485. Kodama, 1986	18	HPLC[†]	3.7 ± 0.3 mg/g Cr.

Table 180. Unconjugated Vanilmandelic Acid in Urine of Normal Subjects

(continued)

Reference First Author, Year	Number of Subjects	Method of Analysis	Values (mg/24h ± S.E.M.)
519. Lindgren, 1986	29	HPLC-Fl[†]	4.24± 0.20
724. Roy, 1986	25	GC-MS	4.75± 0.32 (total)
790. Siever, 1986	18	GC-MS	3.96± 0.22
209. Davis, 1987	8	GC-MS[†]	3.10± 0.26
287. Foti, 1987	14	HPLC-EC	4.0*
	14	Fl	3.9*
628. Ong, 1987	200	HPLC-EC[†]	2.4 ± 0.9
319. Gironi, 1988	120	HPLC-Fl[†]	4.00± 0.14
431. Julien, 1988	6	HPLC-EC	2.8 ± 0.5
488. Kopin, 1988	18	REA	4.14± 0.31
529. Linnoila, 1988	12	GC-MS	4.17± 0.38 (total)
623. Odink, 1988	6 (M)	HPLC-EC[†]	4.67
	6 (F)	HPLC-EC[†]	3.07

* In original paper expressed as μg/h.
** PC = paper chromatography.

Table 181. Vanilmandelic Acid in Plasma of Normal Subjects

Reference First Author, Year	Number of Subjects	Method of Analysis	Values (ng/mL ± S.E.M.)
798. Sjöquist, 1975	12	GC-MS[†]	10.73 (serum)
447. Karoum, 1977	10	GC-MS[†]	12.4 ± 1.3
851. Takahashi, 1977	10	GC-MS[†]	7.0 ± 0.5
853. Takahashi, 1978	5	GC-MS[†]	15.2 ± 1.7
599. Muskiet, 1980	21	GC-MS[†]	5.9 ± 0.5 (serum)
380. Hjemdahl, 1982	11	GC-MS	11.74± 1.90
397. Hunneman, 1983	16	GC-MS[†]	9.01± 1.00
974. Yu, 1985	21 (prisoners)	GC-MS	4.9 ± 0.3
	61 (prisoners)	GC-MS	5.7 ± 0.6
142. Cavanaugh, 1986	9	HPLC-EC[†]	9.0 ± 1.0
209. Davis, 1986	10	GC-MS[†]	5.4
315. Gerhardt, 1986	6	HPLC-EC[†]	9.3 ± 0.6
211. Davis, 1987	14	GC-MS[†]	5.6 ± 0.4
762. Schinelli, 1988	12	HPLC-EC[†]	7.15± 0.88

Table 182. Vanilmandelic Acid in CSF of Normal Subjects

Reference First Author, Year	Number of Subjects	Method of Analysis	Values (ng/mL ± S.E.M.)
14. Andén, 1963	–	Fl	25
415. Jimerson, 1975	8	GC-MS	1.05 ± 0.15
340. Gordon, 1975	13	GC-MS	0.96 ± 0.13
444. Karoum, 1975	5	GC-MS	0.46 ± 0.18 (lumbar)
	8	GC-MS	2.8 ± 0.6 (ventricular)
798. Sjöquist, 1975	5	GC-MS[†]	1.86
803. Sjöström, 1975	11	GC-MS	1.19 ± 0.18
550. Major, 1979	7	GC-MS	2.61 ± 0.95

Table 183. Unconjugated Vanilmandelic Acid in Urine of Depressed Subjects

Reference First Author, Year	Number of Subjects	Method of Analysis	Values (mg/24h ± S.E.M.)
759. Schildkraut, 1964	5	Fl	4.54 ± 0.39
756. Schildkraut, 1965	5 (F) (endogenous)	Fl	4.19 ± 0.85
126. Bunney, 1967	8 (psychotic)	Fl	3.52
	8 (neurotic)	Fl	2.18
849. Takahashi, 1968	1 patient, 8 times	Fl	3.8 ± 0.35
133. Campanini, 1970	7 (manic)	Fl	8.16 ± 0.51 mg/g Cr.
	7 (mixed state)	Fl	4.68 ± 0.29 mg/g Cr.
	7 (normal)	Fl	2.61 ± 0.18 mg/g Cr.
	7 (depressed)	Fl	2.34 ± 0.16 mg/g Cr.
346. Greenspan, 1970	3 (hypomanic)	GC-ECD	6.63 ± 0.71
	2 (normothymic)	GC-ECD	4.35 ± 0.15
	3 (agitated)	GC-ECD	3.83 ± 0.70
569. Messiha, 1970	7 (manic)	Fl	1.8
	6 (depressed)	Fl	1.5
679. Prange, 1972	12	GC-ECD	4.7 ± 0.5
224. De Leon-Jones, 1975	5 (bipolar)	GC-ECD	3.93 ± 0.78
	14 (single episode unipolar)	GC-ECD	4.68 ± 0.51
	13 (recurrent unipolar)	GC-ECD	4.12 ± 0.32
541. Maas, 1975	20 (M) 48 (F)	— —	4.60 ± 0.32 4.38 ± 0.26

Table 183. Unconjugated Vanilmandelic Acid in Urine of Depressed

Subjects (continued)

Reference First Author, Year	Number of Subjects	Method of Analysis	Values (mg/24h ± S.E.M.)
592. Murphy, 1977	4	GC-ECD	4.47 ± 0.68
761. Schildkraut 1978	9 (schizophrenia- related)	GC-ECD	3.63 ± 0.38
	4 (schizoaffective)	GC-ECD	3.81 ± 0.28
	12 (bipolar)	GC-ECD	4.04 ± 0.21
	16 (unipolar, endogenous)	GC-ECD	3.78 ± 0.25
	12 (unipolar, non-endogenous)	GC-ECD	3.54 ± 0.23
	9 (unclassified)	GC-ECD	3.86 ± 0.21
744. Sandler, 1979	23	GC-FID	4.40 ± 0.36
	10 (M)	GC-FID	5.37 ± 0.57
	13 (F)	GC-FID	3.68 ± 0.36
441. Karoum, 1982	6	GC-MS[†]	4.1 ± 0.4
452. Karoum, 1982	6 (unipolar + bipolar)	GC-MS	4.79 ± 1.11
521. Linnoila, 1982; 526. Linnoila, 1982	12 (unipolar + bipolar)	GC-MS	4.17 ± 0.61
525. Linnoila, 1982	4 (rapid cyclers)	GC-MS	4.64 ± 0.85
523. Linnoila, 1982	8	GC-MS	4.93 ± 0.79
	8 (unipolar + bipolar)	GC-MS	3.97 ± 0.81
754. Schatzberg, 1982	20 (bipolar)	GC-ECD	4.04 ± 0.16
	50 (unipolar)	GC-ECD	3.93 ± 0.17

<u>Table 183. Unconjugated Vanilmandelic Acid in Urine of Depressed</u>

<u>Subjects (continued)</u>

Reference First Author, Year	Number of Subjects	Method of Analysis	Values (mg/24h ± S.E.M.)
493. Koslow, 1983; 548. Maas, 1984	112 (depressed)	GC-ECD	3.56 ± 0.20
	62 (M)	GC-ECD	3.54 ± 0.25
	50 (F)	GC-ECD	3.58 ± 0.34
	16 (manic)	GC-ECD	3.55 ± 0.38
	10 (M)	GC-ECD	3.88 ± 0.50
	6 (F)	GC-ECD	2.99 ± 0.56
524. Linnoila, 1983	12 (unipolar + bipolar)	GC-MS	4.18 ± 0.62
583. Moleman, 1983	14	HPLC-EC[†]	4.28 ± 0.23
521. Linnoila, 1986	8 (unipolar + bipolar)	GC-MS	4.87 ± 0.78
	8 (unipolar + bipolar)	GC-MS	4.12 ± 0.85
724. Roy, 1986	7 (no melancholia)	GC-MS	5.27 ± 0.55
	5 (history of melancholia)	GC-MS	6.49 ± 1.33
	8 (with melancholia)	GC-MS	5.84 ± 0.85
	8 (dysthymic disorder)	GC-MS	5.54 ± 0.22
790. Siever, 1986	14	GC-MS	4.55 ± 0.21
	10 (unipolar)	GC-MS	4.65 ± 0.28
	4 (bipolar)	GC-MS	4.30 ± 0.27
105. Bowden, 1987	80	GC-ECD	3.36 ± 0.23
	55 (unipolar)	GC-ECD	3.61 ± 0.49
	25 (bipolar)	GC-ECD	3.44 ± 0.22
587. Mooney, 1988	9	HPLC-EC	4.54 ± 0.26

Table 184. Vanilmandelic Acid in Urine of Schizophrenic Subjects

Reference First Author, Year	Number of Subjects	Method of Analysis	Values (mg/24h ± S.E.M.)
681. Pscheidt, 1964	9	Fl	4.6 ± 0.4
10. Allegranza, 1965	9	Fl	1.5 ± 0.1
	9	Fl	2.1 ± 0.1
115. Bozzi, 1965	11	Fl	2.0 ± 0.2
125. Bruno, 1965	8	Fl	2.3 ± 0.2
666. Pollin, 1971	30 (15 pairs of twins)	GC-ECD	2.0 mg/g Cr.
832. Subrahmanyam, 1975	30 (acute)	Fl	3.6 ± 0.4
	6 (acute, aggressive)	Fl	5.6 ± 0.6
	24 (chronic)	Fl	4.2 ± 0.4
	24 (manic depressive psychotic)	Fl	3.6 ± 0.4
427. Joseph, 1976	18 (chronic)	GC-ECD	4.6 ± 0.4
	6 (low severity)	GC-ECD	5.1
	6 (moderate severity)	GC-ECD	4.7
	6 (high severity)	GC-ECD	4.1

Table 185. Vanilmandelic Acid in CSF of Depressed and Schizophrenic

Subjects

Reference First Author, Year	Number of Subjects	Method of Analysis	Values (ng/mL ± S.E.M.)
340. Gordon, 1975	31 (psychiatric)	GC-MS	1.06 ± 0.23
415. Jimerson, 1975	10 (depressed)	GC-MS	0.60 ± 0.20
	9 (manic)	GC-MS	0.80 ± 0.15
	12 (acute schizophrenic)	GC-MS	1.60 ± 0.45
	7 (recovered schizophrenic)	GC-MS	1.3 ± 0.5
	3 (schizoaffective)	GC-MS	0.7 ± 0.1
440. Karoum, 1977	12 (schizophrenic)	GC-MS	0.66 ± 0.09
644. Parnetti, 1987	13 (schizophrenic)	HPLC-Fl[†]	2.57 ± 0.55

Table 186. <u>Vanilmandelic Acid in Urine, Plasma and CSF of Some Other</u>

<u>Disorders</u>

Reference First Author, Year	Number of Subjects	Method of Analysis	Values (Mean ± S.E.M.)
132. Calne, 1969	14 (Parkinson's disease)	GC–FID	4.6 ± 0.5 mg/24h (urine)
443. Karoum, 1977	9 (Alzheimer's disease)	GC–MS[†]	3.1 ± 6.0 ng/mL (ventricular)
	5 (Alzheimer's disease)	GC–MS	0.46 ± 0.18 ng/mL (lumbar CSF)
644. Parnetti, 1987	12 (Alzheimer's disease)	HPLC–Fl[†]	3.37 ± 1.03 ng/mL (CSF)
974. Yu, 1985	82 (violent prisoners)	GC–MS	5.4 ± 0.5 (plasma)
	27 (aggressive prisoners)	GC–MS	4.9 ± 0.2 (plasma)

Table 187. Unconjugated (and Conjugated) 3,4-Dihydroxyphenylacetic Acid

in Urine of Normal Subjects

Reference First Author, Year	Number of Subjects	Method of Analysis	Values (µg/24h ± S.E.M.)
240. Drujan, 1966	12	Fl[†]	1200 ± 120
927. Weil-Malherbe, 1969	20 (combined M&F)	Fl[†]	1805 ± 182
	17 (M)	Fl	2302 ± 344
	3 (F)	Fl	1830 ± 391
256. Eichorn, 1971	22	Fl[†]	1825 ± 165 µg/g Cr.
808. Smith, 1971	8	Fl	666 ± 66
	8	Fl	1264 ± 64 (conjugated)
895. Vidi, 1972	10	Fl[†]	2600
570. Messiha, 1973	12	Fl[†]	2980 ± 370
922. Weg, 1975	12	GC-ECD[†]	880 ± 90
	12	GC-ECD	910 ± 90 (conjugated)
198. Dalmaz, 1978	34	Fl[†]	2850 ± 300
598. Muskiet, 1978	5	GC-MS[†]	1500 ± 220 µg/g Cr.
441. Karoum, 1982	5	GC-MS[†]	870 ± 90
935. Wiesel, 1982	33 (M)	GC-MS	2020 ± 130 (total)
	33 (F)	GC-MS	1990 ± 180 (total)
218. De Jong, 1983	7	GC-FID[†]	4010 ± 1340 µg/g Cr.
211. Davis, 1986	10	GC-MS[†]	910
724. Roy, 1986	25	GC-MS	1574 ± 94
431. Julien, 1988	6	HPLC-EC[†]	1389 ± 225
623. Odink, 1988	6 (M)	HPLC-EC[†]	1210
	6 (F)	HPLC-EC[†]	1310

Table 188. 3,4-Dihydroxyphenylacetic Acid in Plasma of Normal Subjects

Reference First Author, Year	Number of Subjects	Method of Analysis	Values (ng/mL ± S.E.M.)
447. Karoum, 1977	10	GC-MS[t]	10.3 ± 1.9
860. Thiede, 1981	9	REA[t]	4.77 ± 0.84
941. Wilkes, 1981	6	REA	29 ± 6
407. Izzo, 1983	20	REA[t]	3.27 ± 0.33
331. Goldstein, 1984	9	HPLC-EC[t]	1.38
211. Davis, 1986	10	GC-MS[t]	0.7
217. De Jong, 1986	10	GC-MS[t]	2.96 ± 0.40
258. Eisenhofer, 1986	12	HPLC-EC[t]	0.73 ± 0.12
74. Benedict, 1987	12	HPLC[t]	1.38 ± 0.11

Table 189. Unconjugated (and Conjugated) 3,4-Dihydroxyphenylacetic Acid

in CSF of Normal Subjects

Reference First Author, Year	Number of Subjects	Method of Analysis	Values (pg/mL ± S.E.M.)
14. Andén, 1963	–	Fl	n.d.
682. Pullar, 1970	6	Fl	9000 ± 400
444. Karoum, 1975	5	GC-MS	3000 ± 1600 (lumbar)
	8	GC-MS	9700 ± 1600 (ventricular)
919. Watson, 1975	22	GC-ECD	<1000
337. Gordon, 1976	11	GC-MS	43 ± 42
	11	GC-MS	1880 ± 560 (conjugated)
553. Markey, 1977	5	GC-MS-NCI	11500 ± 4000
	5	GC-MS-EI	6400 ± 3000
270. Faull, 1979	23	GC-MS[†]	400 ± 37
	23	GC-MS	237 ± 91 (conjugated)
550. Major, 1979	7	GC-MS	1890 ± 540
75. Berger, 1980	19	GC-MS	400 ± 0
	17	GC-MS	200 ± 100 (conjugated)
45. Bagdy, 1983	23 (F)	REA	1910 ± 140
	6 (M)	REA	3120 ± 680
77. Berrettini, 1984	20	HPLC-EC	437 ± 34
773. Seppala, 1984	72	HPLC-EC[†]	515 ± 45
78. Berrettini, 1985	25	HPLC-EC	465 ± 42
822. Stahl, 1985	32	GC-MS	490 ± 60
211. Davis, 1986	10	GC-MS[†]	n.d.
217. De Jong, 1986	14	GC-MS[†]	910 ± 90
354. Guthrie, 1986	24	HPLC-EC	356 ± 36
495. Koyama, 1988	5	HPLC-EC[†]	740 ± 100

Table 190. 3,4-Dihydroxyphenylacetic Acid in Urine of Parkinson's

Disease Subjects

Reference First Author, Year	Number of Subjects	Method of Analysis	Values (μg/24h $\pm$ S.E.M.)
132. Calne, 1969	14	GC-FID	<2000
927. Weil-Malherbe, 1969	34 (combined M&F)	Fl[†]	1273 $\pm$ 78
	20 (M)	Fl	1586 $\pm$ 145
	14 (F)	Fl	1813 $\pm$ 200

Table 191. 3,4-Dihydroxyphenylacetic Acid in Urine of Depressed Subjects

Reference First Author, Year	Number of Subjects	Method of Analysis	Values (μg/24h $\pm$ S.E.M.)
126. Bunney, 1967	8 (psychotic)	Fl	1561
	8 (neurotic)	Fl	1020
441. Karoum, 1982	6	GC-MS[†]	850 $\pm$ 150
452. Karoum, 1982	6 (unipolar + bipolar)	GC-MS	4910 $\pm$ 840
528. Linnoila, 1983	7 (unipolar + bipolar)	GC-MS	674 $\pm$ 149
724. Roy, 1986	7 (no melancholia)	GC-MS	1475 $\pm$ 220
	5 (history of melancholia)	GC-MS	1120 $\pm$ 185
	8 (with melancholia)	GC-MS	1100 $\pm$ 250
	8 (dysthymic disorder)	GC-MS	1240 $\pm$ 125

<u>Table 192. Unconjugated (and Conjugated) 3,4-Dihydroxyphenylacetic Acid</u>

<u>in CSF of Depressed Subjects</u>

Reference <u>First Author, Year</u>	Number of <u>Subjects</u>	Method of <u>Analysis</u>	<u>Values (pg/mL ± S.E.M.)</u>
75. Berger, 1980	12	GC-MS	400 ± 900
	9	GC-MS	400 ± 200 (conjugated)
77. Berrettini, 1984	10 (bipolar)	HPLC-EC	386 ± 48
78. Berrettini, 1985	9 (bipolar, euthymic)	HPLC-EC	387 ± 53
726. Roy, 1985	15 (melancholic)	HPLC-EC	230 ± 29
	8 (major depressive disorder)	HPLC-EC	319 ± 45
	5 (dysthymic disorder)	HPLC-EC	329 ± 61
	15 (melancholic)	HPLC-EC	390 ± 48 (conjugated)
	8 (major depressive disorder)	HPLC-EC	538 ± 65 (conjugated)
	5 (dysthymic disorder)	HPLC-EC	625 ± 104 (conjugated)

Table 193. 3,4-Dihydroxyphenylacetic Acid in Urine, Plasma and CSF of

Schizophrenic Subjects

Reference First Author, Year	Number of Subjects	Method of Analysis	Values (pg/mL ± S.E.M.)
554. Markianos, 1976	13 (paranoid)	GC-ECD	132000 ± 17500 (serum)
	13 (paranoid)	GC-ECD	92000 ± 13300 (CSF)
440. Karoum, 1977	12	GC-MS	810 ± 90 (CSF)
75. Berger, 1980	9	GC-MS	500 ± 100 (CSF)
	7	GC-MS	100 ± 100 (conjugated)
755. Scheinin, 1984	46 (chronic)	HPLC-EC[†]	412 ± 23 (CSF)
773. Seppala, 1984	52 (chronic)	HPLC-EC[†]	494 ± 39 (CSF)
46. Bagdy, 1985	15 (chronic)	RIA	2290 ± 380 (CSF)
822. Stahl, 1985	4 (with tardive dyskinesia)	GC-MS	300 ± 40 (CSF)
644. Parnetti, 1987	13	HPLC-Fl[†]	500 ± 230 (CSF)
543. Maas, 1988 (acute)	11	GC-MS µg/24h)	1376 ± 295* (urine,
	15	GC-MS	2.4 ± 0.4 (plasma, ng/mL)
	17	GC-MS	2.0 ± 0.4 (CSF, ng/mL)

* In original paper expressed as µg/3.5 h.

Table 194. 3,4-Dihydroxyphenylacetic Acid in CSF of Subjects with Other

Disorders

Reference First Author, Year	Number of Subjects	Method of Analysis	Values (pg/mL ± S.E.M.)
682. Pullar, 1970	23 (Parkinson's disease)	Fl	6000 ± 350
532. Linnoila, 1983	16 (explosive personality)	HPLC	487 ± 63
	7 (antisocial personality)	HPLC	554 ± 57
	7 (paranoid aggressive)	HPLC	739 ± 139
822. Stahl, 1985	9 (dystonic)	GC-MS	630 ± 130
644. Parnetti, 1987	12 (Alzheimer's disease)	HPLC-Fl[†]	500 ± 200
495. Koyama, 1988	6 (Alzheimer's disease)	HPLC-EC[†]	410 ± 41

Table 195. 3-Methoxy-4-hydroxyphenylethanol in Urine of Normal Subjects

Reference First Author, Year	Number of Subjects	Method of Analysis	Values (μg/24h ± S.E.M.)
446. Karoum, 1973	9	GC-MS[†]	n.d. (unconjugated)
	9	GC-MS	16 ± 4 (glucuronide)
	9	GC-MS	223 ± 46 (sulfate)
598. Muskiet, 1978	4	GC-MS[†]	32 ± 3 μg/g Cr.
218. De Jong, 1983	7	GC-FID[†]	4 ± 2.4 mg/g Cr. (total)

Table 196. 3,4-Dihydroxyphenylethanol and 3,4-Dihydroxyphenylglycol in

Urine of Normal and Depressed Subjects

Reference First Author, Year	Number of Subjects	Method of Analysis	Values (μg/24h $\pm$ S.E.M.)
453. Karoum, 1971	3	GC-ECD	<100 (DHPE)
432. Kahane, 1976	8	GC-FID[†]	637 μg/L (DHPG) (total)
598. Muskiet, 1978	4	GC-MS[†]	16 $\pm$ 5 μg/g Cr. (DHPE)
	7	GC-MS	325 $\pm$ 60 μg/g Cr. (DHPG)
232. Dennis, 1982	7	REA[†]	155 $\pm$ 42 μg/L (DHPG)
	7	REA	584 $\pm$ 133 μg/L (conj. DHPG)
218. De Jong, 1983	7	GC-FID[†]	818 $\pm$1770 μg/g Cr. (total DHPG)
137. Carr, 1988	20 (unipolar depressed)	GC-MS	352 $\pm$ 38 (DHPG)
431. Julien, 1988	6	HPLC-EC[†]	65 $\pm$ 6 (unconj. DHPG)
	6	HPLC-EC[†]	373 $\pm$ 71 (total DHPG)
	6	HPLC-EC[†]	n.d. (DHPE)

Table 197. 3,4-Dihydroxyphenylglycol in Plasma of Depressed Subjects

Reference First Author, Year	Number of Subjects	Method of Analysis	Values (pg/mL ± S.E.M.)
918. Warsh, 1985	23 (unipolar + bipolar)	GC-MS	1790 ± 210
533. Lôo, 1986	56 (all depressed)	HPLC-EC	573 ± 30 (unconjugated)
	24 (M)		596 ± 31
	32 (F)		556 ± 36
	56 (all)	HPLC-EC	821 ± 82 (conjugated)
	24 (M)		966 ± 161
	32 (F)		707 ± 75
753. Scatton, 1986	45 (M+F)	REA	552 ± 48
	45 (M+F)	REA	797 ± 63 (conjugated)
	21 (M)	REA	560 ± 48
	24 (F)	REA	546 ± 50
	21 (M)	REA	807 ± 94 (conjugated)
	24 (F)	REA	789 ± 88 (conjugated)

Table 198. 3,4-Dihydroxyphenylethanol in Plasma of Normal Subjects

Reference First Author, Year	Number of Subjects	Method of Analysis	Values (pg/mL ± S.E.M.)
47. Baker, 1981	13	REA[†]	187 ± 74
860. Thiede, 1981	9	REA[†]	150 ± 56

Table 199. Unconjugated (and Conjugated) 3,4-Dihydroxyphenylglycol in

Plasma of Normal Subjects

Reference First Author, Year	Number of Subjects	Method of Analysis	Values (pg/mL ± S.E.M.)
898. Vlachakis, 1979	16	REA[†]	792 ± 63
47. Baker, 1981	13	REA[†]	973 ± 174
418. Jimerson, 1981	8	GC-MS[†]	3944 ± 187 (total)
860. Thiede, 1981	9	REA[†]	900 ± 50
901. Vlachakis, 1981	36	REA	563 ± 34
232. Dennis, 1982	11	REA[†]	1142 ± 195
	11	REA	1235 ± 128 (conjugated)
	6 (M)	REA	1184 ± 346
	5 (F)	REA	1091 ± 163
261. Elsworth, 1983	9	GC-MS[†]	460 ± 20
	9	GC-MS	1340 ± 20 (conjugated)
407. Izzo, 1983	20	REA[†]	1010 ± 60
900. Vlachakis, 1984	5	REA[†]	810 ± 90
	5	REA	1000 ± 180 (conjugated)
393. Howes, 1985	6	HPLC-EC[†]	877 ± 68
408. Izzo, 1985	13	REA	1020 ± 80
258. Eisenhofer, 1986	12	HPLC-EC[†]	821 ± 96
753. Scatton, 1986	45 (M+F)	REA	814 ± 45
	45 (M+F)	REA	1147 ± 112 (conjugated)
	21 (M)	REA	784 ± 52
	24 (F)	REA	839 ± 73
	21 (M)	REA	1119 ± 140 (conjugated)
	24 (F)	REA	1161 ± 175 (conjugated)
267. Eriksson, 1987	–	HPLC-EC[†]	1360 (total)
329. Goldstein, 1988	19	HPLC-EC	716 ± 56 (arterial)
	19	HPLC-EC	789 ± 56 (venous)

Table 200. 3-Methoxy-4-hydroxyphenylethanol in CSF of Normal and Other

Subjects

Reference First Author, Year	Number of Subjects	Method of Analysis	Values (pg/mL ± S.E.M.)
453. Karoum, 1971	3 (normal)	GC-ECD	5700 ± 900
	2 (normal)	GC-ECD	3300 ± 1000 (conjugated)
	4 (Parkinson's disease)	GC-ECD	2800 ± 800
	2 (Parkinson's disease)	GC-ECD	5700 ± 500 (conjugated)
644. Parnetti, 1987	12 (Alzheimer's disease)	HPLC-Fl[†]	0.0
	13 (schizophrenic)	HPLC-Fl	340 ± 230

Table 201. 3,4-Dihydroxyphenylglycol in CSF of Normal Subjects

Reference First Author, Year	Number of Subjects	Method of Analysis	Values (pg/mL ± S.E.M.)
47. Baker, 1981	8	REA[†]	7170 ± 2720 (DHPG)
	8	REA	1620 ± 860 (DHPE)
901. Vlachakis, 1981	36	REA	950 ± 43
232. Dennis, 1982	5	REA[†]	1470 ± 186
	5	REA	0.0 (conjugated)
261. Elsworth, 1983	4	GC-MS[†]	890 ± 200
	4	GC-MS	310 ± 100 (conjugated)

Table 202. 3,4-Dihydroxymandelic Acid in Urine of Depressed Subjects

Reference First Author, Year	Number of Subjects	Method of Analysis	Values (µg/24h ± S.E.M.)
126. Bunney, 1967	8 (psychotic)	Fl	745
	8 (neurotic)	Fl	389
924. Weil-Malherbe, 1967	41	Fl[†]	82 ± 11

Table 203. 3,4-Dihydroxymandelic Acid in Urine of Normal Subjects

Reference First Author, Year	Number of Subjects	Method of Analysis	Values (µg/24h ± S.E.M.)
579. Miyake, 1962	20 (day)	Fl[†]	990 µg/g Cr.
	20 (night)	Fl	420 µg/g Cr.
233. De Quattro, 1964	9	Fl[†]	355 ± 45*
	9	Fl	168 ± 43* (conjugated)
240. Drujan, 1966	12	Fl[†]	920 ± 90
924. Weil-Malherbe, 1967	32	Fl[†]	98 ± 16
752. Sato, 1969	8	REA[†]	91 ± 17*
570. Messiha, 1973	12	Fl[†]	343 ± 39
598. Muskiet, 1978	4	GC-MS[†]	118 ± 21 µg/g Cr.
218. De Jong, 1983	7	GC-FID[†]	650 ± 815 µg/g Cr.
431. Julien, 1988	6	HPLC-EC[†]	69 ± 12

* In original paper expressed as µg/h.

Table 204. 3,4-Dihydroxymandelic Acid in Plasma (and CSF) of Normal

Subjects

Reference First Author, Year	Number of Subjects	Method of Analysis	Values (pg/mL ± S.E.M.)
14. Andén, 1963	–	Fl	n.d. (CSF)
898. Vlachakis, 1979	16	REA[†]	1946 ± 294
860. Thiede, 1981	9	REA[†]	1780 ± 500
901. Vlachakis, 1981	36	REA	2350 ± 255 (CSF)
	36	REA	1856 ± 170
407. Izzo, 1983	20	REA[†]	2090 ± 720
900. Vlachakis, 1984	5	REA[†]	2000 ± 500
	5	REA	7900 ± 1025 (conjugated)
408. Izzo, 1985	13	REA	2010 ± 200
267. Eriksson, 1987	–	HPLC-EC[†]	368

Table 205. 3,4-Dimethoxyphenylacetic Acid in Urine of Normal and

Schizophrenic Subjects

Reference First Author, Year	Number of Subjects	Method of Analysis	Values (mean ± S.E.M.)
501. Kuehl, 1966	6 (normal)	GC-FID[†]	12.8 ± 4.6 μg/g Cr.
	5 (acute schizophrenia)	GC-FID	19.6 ± 6.1 μg/g Cr.
	8 (sub-acute)	GC-FID	13.1 ± 1.5 μg/g Cr.
	1 (chronic)	GC-FID	27 μg/g Cr.
904. Vogel, 1967	8 (normal)	GC-Tritium[†]	detected
	9 (schizophrenic)	GC-Tritium	detected
424. Jones, 1969	(normal)	GC-FID[†]	detected
	(schizophrenic)	GC-FID	detected

Table 206. 5-Methoxyindoleacetic Acid in Urine and Plasma of Normal

Subjects

Reference First Author, Year	Number of Subjects	Method of Analysis	Values (mean ± S.E.M.)
391. Hoskins, 1978	10	GC-MS[†]	37.5 ± 14.2 μg/24h (urine)
376. Higa, 1985	23	GC-MS[†]	4.8 ± 0.5 μg/24h (urine)
944. Wilson, 1979	3	GC-MS	20-100 pg/mL (plasma)

<u>Table 207. 5-Hydroxytryptophol in CSF of Neurological Subjects</u>

Reference First Author, Year	Number of Subjects	Method of Analysis	Values (pg/mL ± S.E.M.)
852. Takahashi, 1978	15 (neurological)	GC-MS[†]	730 ± 115
	9 (back pain)	GC-MS	850 ± 100

Section 8

References

REFERENCES

1. **Abe, K., and Konaka, R.,** Specific determination of 3-methoxy-4-hydroxyphenylethylene glycol in urine by liquid chromatography with post-column reaction, *Clin. Chem.* (Winston-Salem, N.C.), 34, 87, 1988.

2. **Åberg-Wistedt, A., Jostell, K.-G., Ross, S. B., and Westerlund, D.,** Effects of zimelidine and desipramine on serotonin and noradrenaline uptake mechanisms in relation to plasma concentrations and to therapeutic effects during treatment of depression, *Psychopharmacology,* 74, 297, 1981.

3. **Abrams, R., Essman, W.B., Taylor, M.A., Fink, M.,** Concentration of 5-hydroxyindoleacetic acid, homovanillic acid and tryptophan in the cerebrospinal fluid of depressed patients before and after ECT, *Biol. Psychiatry,* 11, 85, 1976.

4. **Ackenheil, M., Fröhler, M., Goldig, G., Rall, G., and Welter, D.,** Catecholamine detection in blood and CSF by means of high pressure liquid chromatography and electrochemical detector, *Arzneim. Forsch.,* 32, 893, 1982.

5. **Ågren, H.,** Symptom patterns in unipolar and bipolar depression correlating with monoamine metabolites in the cerebrospinal fluid. I. General patterns, *Psychiatry Res.,* 3, 211, 1980.

6. **Ågren, H.,** Depressive symptom patterns and urinary MHPG excretion, *Psychiatry Res.,* 6, 185, 1982.

7. **Ågren, H.,** Depression and altered neurotransmission-states, traits and interactions, in *The Origins of Depression: Current Concepts and Approaches,* Angst, J., Ed., Dahlem Konferenzen 1983, Springer-Verlag, Berlin, Heidelberg, New York, Tokyo, 1983, 297.

8. **Ågren, H., Mefford, I. N., Rudorfer, M. V., Linnoila, M., and Potter, W. Z.,** Interacting neurotransmitter systems. A non-experimental approach to the 5-HIAA-HVA correlation in human CSF, *J. Psychiatr. Res.,* 20, 175, 1986.

9. **Alfredsson, G., Wiesel, F.-A., and Tyler, A.,** Relationships between glutamate and monoamine metabolites in cerebrospinal fluid and serum in healthy volunteers, *Biol. Psychiatr.,* 23, 689, 1988.

10. **Allegranza, A., Bozzi, R., and Bruno, A.,** Urinary excretion of 5-hydroxyindoleacetic, homovanillic and vanilmandelic acid in schizophrenics taking reserpine and chlorpromazine, *J. Nerv. Ment. Dis.,* 140, 207, 1965.

11. **Almay, B. G. L., Häggendal, J., von Knorring, L., and Oreland, L.,** 5-HIAA and HVA in CSF in patients with idiopathic pain disorders. *Biol. Psychiatry,* 22, 403, 1987.

12. **Alonso, R., Gibson, C. J., and McGill, J.,** Determination of 3-methoxy-4-hydroxyphenylglycol in urine by high-performance liquid chromatography with amperometric detection, *Life Sci.,* 29, 1689, 1981.

13. **Andén, N.-E., Roos, B.-E., and Werdinius, B.,** On the occurrence of homovanillic acid in brain and cerebrospinal fluid and its determination by a fluorometric method, *Life Sci.,* 2, 448, 1963.

14. **Andén, N.-E., Roos, B.-E., and Werdinius, B.,** On the occurrence of homovanillic acid and 3-methoxy-4-hydroxymandelic acid in human cerebrospinal fluid. *Experientia,* 19, 359, 1963.

15. **Andersen, H., and Braestrup, C.,** Mass fragmentographic demonstration of low amounts of β-phenylethylamine in human urine, *Scand. J. Clin. Lab. Invest.,* 37, 33, 1977.

16. **Andersen, O., Johansson, B.B., and Svennerholm, L.,** Monoamine metabolites in successive samples of spinal fluid. A comparison between healthy volunteers and patients with multiple sclerosis, *Acta Neurol. Scand.,* 63, 247, 1981.

17. **Anderson, G. M., Durkin, T. A., Morton, J. B., and Cohen, D. J.,** Liquid chromatographic determination of urinary catecholamines after one-step alumina extraction, *J. Chromatogr.,* 424, 373, 1988.

18. **Anderson, G. M., Feibel, F. C., and Cohen, D. J.,** Determination of serotonin in whole blood, platelet-rich plasma, platelet-poor plasma and plasma ultrafiltrate. *Life Sci.,* 40, 1063, 1987.

19. **Anderson, G. M., Gerner, R. H., Cohen, D. J., and Fairbanks, L.,** Central tryptamine turnover in depression, schizophrenia and anorexia. Measurement of indoleacetic acid in cerebrospinal fluid, *Biol. Psychiatry,* 19, 1427, 1984.

20. **Anderson, G. M., Schlicht, K. R., and Cohen, D. J.,** Two-dimensional high performance liquid chromatographic determination of 5-hydroxyindoleacetic acid and homovanillic acid in urine, *Anal. Biochem.,* 144, 27, 1985.

21. **Anderson, G. M., Young, J. G., Jatlow, P. I., and Cohen, D. J.,** Urinary free catecholamines determined by liquid chromatography-fluorometry, *Clin. Chem.* (Winston-Salem, N.C.), 27, 2060, 1981.

22. **Ånggard, E., Sjöquist, B., Fyrö, B., and Sedvall, G.,** Quantitative determination of homovanillic acid in serum by mass fragmentography, *Eur. J. Pharmacol.,* 24, 37, 1973.

23. **Anton, A. H., and Sayre, D. F.,** A study of the factors affecting the aluminum oxide-trihydroxyindole procedure for the analysis of catecholamines, *J. Pharmacol. Exp. Ther.,* 138, 360, 1962.

24. **Antun, F. T., Pullar, I. A., Eccleston, D., and Sharman, D. F.,** A fluorimetric method for the determination of 4-hydroxy-3-methoxyphenylglycol in urine, *Clin. Chim. Acta*, 34, 387, 1971.

25. **Arakawa, Y., Imai, K., and Tamura, Z.,** Determination of catecholamine sulfoconjugate isomers in normal human urine by use of high-performance liquid chromatography with a photochemical detector, *Anal. Biochem.*, 132, 389, 1983.

26. **Arakawa, Y., and Tachibana, S.,** A direct and sensitive determination of histamine in acid-deproteinized biological samples by high-performance liquid chromatography, *Anal. Biochem.*, 158, 20, 1986.

27. **Arendt, J., Bojkowski, C., Franey, C., Wright, J., and Marks, V.,** Immunoassay of 6-hydroxymelatonin sulfate in human plasma and urine: abolition of the urinary 24-hour rhythm with atenolol. *J. Clin. Endocrinol. Metab.*, 60, 1166, 1985.

28. **Arendt, J., Paunier, L., and Sizonenko, P. C.,** Melatonin radioimmunoassay, *J. Clin. Endocrinol. Metab.*, 40, 347, 1975.

29. **Arendt, J., Wetterberg, L., Heyden, T., Sizonenko, P. C., and Paunier, L.,** Radioimmunoassay of melatonin: human serum and cerebrospinal fluid, *Horm. Res.*, 8, 65, 1977.

30. **Arnett, E. L., and Watts, D. T.,** Catecholamine excretion in men exposed to cold. *J. Appl. Physiol.*, 15, 499, 1960.

31. **Aronow, L., Howard, F. A., and Wolff, D.,** Plasma epinephrine and norepinephrine content in mammals, *J. Pharmacol. Exp. Ther.*, 116, 1, 1956.

32. **Aronow, W. S., Harding, P. R., De Quattro, V., and Isbell, M.,** Diurnal variation of plasma catecholamines and systolic time intervals, *Chest,* 63, 722, 1973.

33. **Arterberry, J. D., and Conley, M. P.,** Urinary excretion of serotonin (5-hydroxytryptamine) and related indoles in normal subjects, *Clin. Chim. Acta,* 17, 431, 1967.

34. **Artigas, F., Ortiz, J., Sarrias, M. J., Martinez, E., and Gelpi, E.,** Free 5-hydroxytryptamine in plasma: Fact or artifact? *Clin. Chem.* (Winston-Salem, N. C.), 32, 1985, 1986.

35. **Artigas, F., Sarrias, M. J., Martinez, E., and Gelpi, E.,** Serotonin in body fluids: Characterization of human plasmatic and cerebrospinal fluid pools by means of a new HPLC method. *Life Sci.,* 37, 441, 1985.

36. **Åsberg, M., Bertilsson, L., Martensson, B., Scalia-Tomba, G.-P., Thoren, P., and Träskman-Bendz, L.,** CSF monoamine metabolites in melancholia, *Acta Psychiatr. Scand.,* 69, 201, 1984.

37. **Åsberg, M., Bertilsson, L., Tuck, D., Cronholm, B., and Sjöqvist, F.,** Indoleamine metabolites in the cerebrospinal fluid of depressed patients before and during treatment with nortriptyline. *Clin. Pharmacol. Ther.,* 14, 277, 1973.

38. **Åsberg, M., Ringberger, V.-A., Sjöqvist, F., Thorén, P., Träskman, L., and Tuck, J. R.,** Monoamine metabolites in cerebrospinal fluid and serotonin uptake inhibition during treatment with clorimipramine, *Clin. Pharmacol. Ther.,* 21, 201, 1977.

39. **Åsberg, M., Träskman, L., Thorén, P.,** 5-HIAA in the cerebrospinal fluid. A biochemical suicide prediction? *Arch. Gen. Psychiatry,* 33, 1193, 1976.

40. **Ashcroft, G. W., Blackburn, I. M., Eccleston, D., Glen, A. I. M., Hartley, W., Kinloch, N. E., Lonergan, M., Murray, L. G., and Pullar, I. A.,** Changes on recovery in the concentrations of tryptophan and the biogenic amine metabolites in the cerebrospinal fluid of patients with affective illness, *Psychol. Med.,* 3, 319, 1973.

41. **Ashcroft, G. W., Crawford, T. B. B., Eccleston, D., Sharman, D. F., MacDougall, E. J., Stanton, J. B., and Binns, J. K.,** 5-Hydroxyindole compounds in the cerebrospinal fluid of patients with psychiatric or neurological diseases, *Lancet,* 2, 1049, 1966.

42. **Ashcroft, G. W., and Sharman, D. F.,** 5-Hydroxyindoles in human cerebrospinal fluid, *Nature,* 186, 1050, 1960.

43. **Atsmon, A., Blum, I., Steiner, M., Latz, A., Wijsenbeck, H.,** Further studies with propranolol in psychotic patients. Relation to initial psychiatric state, urinary catecholamines and 3-methoxy-4-hydroxyphenylglycol excretion, *Psychopharmacologia,* 27, 249, 1972.

44. **Baba, S., Utoh, M., Horie, M., and Mori, Y.,** Revised method for the quantitative determination of 5-hydroxytryptamine in human plasma by gas chromatography-mass spectrometry selected ion monitoring, *J. Chromatogr.,* 307, 1, 1984.

45. **Bagdy, G., Arato, M., Baraczka, K., and Fekete, M. I. K.,** Comparative analysis of indices of central dopaminergic functions in man. *Life Sci.,* 32, 2667, 1983.

46. **Bagdy, G., Perenyi, A., Frecska, E., Revai, K., Papp, Z., Fekete, M. I. K., and Arato, M.,** Decrease in dopamine, its metabolites and noradrenaline in cerebrospinal fluid of schizophrenic patients after withdrawal of long-term neuroleptic treatment. *Psychopharmacology,* 85, 62, 1985.

47. **Baker, C. A., and Johnson, G. A.,** Radioenzymatic assay of dihydroxyphenylglycol (DOPEG) and dihydroxyphenylethanol (DOPET) in plasma and cerebrospinal fluid. *Life Sci.,* 29, 165, 1981.

48. **Baker, G. B., Coutts, R. T., Bornstein, R. A., Dewhurst, W. G., Douglass, A. B., and MacDonald, R.N.,** An electron-capture gas chromatographic method for analysis of urinary 3-methoxy-4-hydroxyphenylethylene glycol (MHPG), *Res. Commun. Chem. Pathol. Pharmacol.,* 54, 141, 1986.

49. **Baker, G. B., Rao, T. S., and Coutts, R. T.,** Gas chromatography-electron-capture detection and analysis of β-phenylethylamine in tissues and body fluids using pentafluorobenzenesulfonyl chloride for derivatization. *J. Chromatogr.,* 381, 211, 1986.

50. **Baker, G. B., Yeragani, V. K., Dewhurst, W. G., Coutts, R. T., MacDonald, R.N., and Wong, T. F. J.,** Simultaneous analysis of urinary *m*- and *p*-hydroxyphenylacetic acid, homovanillic acid and 5-hydroxyindole-3-acetic acid using electron-capture gas chromatography, *Biochem. Arch.,* 3, 257, 1987.

51. **Baldessarini, R. J., and Fischer, J. E.,** Substitute and alternative neurotransmitters in neuropsychiatric illness. *Arch. Gen. Psychiatry,* 34, 958, 1977.

52. **Ballenger, J. C., Goodwin, F. K., Major, L. F., and Brown, G. L.,** Alcohol and central serotonin metabolism in man, *Arch. Gen. Psychiatry,* 36, 224, 1979.

53. **Banister, E. W., and Griffiths, J.,** Blood levels of adrenergic amines during exercise, *J. Appl. Physiol.,* 33, 674, 1972.

54. **Banki, C. M.,** Correlation between cerebrospinal fluid amine metabolites and psychomotor activity in affective disorders, *J. Neurochem.,* 28, 255, 1977.

55. **Banki, C. M., and Arato, M.,** Amine metabolites, neuroendocrine findings, and personality dimensions as correlates of suicidal behavior, *Psychiatry Res.,* 10, 253, 1983.

56. **Banki, C. M., Arato, M., and Papp, Z.,** Cerebrospinal fluid biochemical examinations: Do they reflect clinical or biological differences? *Biol. Psychiatry,* 18, 1033, 1983.

57. **Banki, C. M., and Molnar, G.,** Cerebrospinal fluid 5-hydroxy-indoleacetic acid as an index of central serotonergic processes, *Psychiatry Res.,* 5, 23, 1981.

58. **Banki, C. M., and Molnar, G.,** The influence of age, height and body weight on cerebrospinal fluid amine metabolites and tryptophan in women, *Biol. Psychiatry,* 16, 753, 1981.

59. **Banki, C. M., Molnar, G., and Fekete, I.,** Correlation of individual symptoms and other clinical variables with cerebrospinal fluid amine metabolites and tryptophan in depression, *Arch. Psychiatr. Nervenkr.,* 229, 345, 1981.

60. **Barbeau, A., Murphy, G. F., and Sourkes, T. L.,** Excretion of dopamine in diseases of the basal ganglia, *Science,* 133, 1706, 1961.

61. **Barbeito, L., Lista, A., Silveira, R., and Dajas, F.,** Resting urinary catecholamine excretion in schizophrenics: Methodology and interpretation of results, *Biol. Psychiatry,* 19, 1419, 1984.

62. **Bareggi, S. R., Franceschi, M., Bonini, L., Zecca, L., and Smirne, S.,** Decreased CSF concentrations of homovanillic acid and γ-aminobutyric acid in Alzheimer's disease. Age- or disease-related modifications, *Arch. Neurol.,* 39, 709, 1982.

63. **Barnes, P. J., Ind, P. W., and Brown, M. J.,** Plasma histamine and catecholamines in stable asthmatic subjects, *Clin. Sci.,* 62, 661, 1982.

64. **Baxter, L. R., Kelly, R. C., Peter, J. B., Liston, E. H., and Touserkani, S.,** Urinary phenylacetate and response to methylphenidate, *J. Psychiatr. Res.,* 22, 131, 1988.

65. **Beall, G. N.,** Histamine in human urine, *Int. Arch. Allergy Appl. Immunol.,* 26, 1, 1965.

66. **Beaven, M. A., Jacobsen, S., and Horakova, Z.,** Modification of the enzymatic isotopic assay of histamine and its application to measurement of histamine in tissues, serum and urine. *Clin. Clin. Acta,* 37, 91, 1972.

67. **Beck, O., and Faull, K. F.,** Extractive acylation and mass spectrometric assay of 3-methoxytyramine, normetanephrine, and metanephrine in cerebrospinal fluid, *Anal. Biochem.,* 149, 492, 1985.

68. **Beckmann, H., and Goodwin, F. K.,** Urinary MHPG in subgroups of depressed patients and normal controls, *Neuropsychobiology,* 6, 91, 1980.

69. **Beckmann, H., Reynolds, G. P., Sandler, M., Waldmeier, P., Lauber, J., Riederer, P., and Gattaz, W. F.,** Phenylethylamine and phenylacetic acid in CSF of schizophrenics and healthy controls, *Arch. Psychiatr. Nervenkr.,* 232, 463, 1982.

70. **Beckmann, H., St.-Laurent, J., and Goodwin, F. K.,** The effect of lithium on urinary MHPG in unipolar and bipolar depressed patients. *Psychopharmacologia,* 42, 277, 1975.

71. **Beckmann, H., Van Kammen, D. P., Goodwin, F. K., and Murphy, D. L.,** Urinary excretion of 3-methoxy-4-hydroxyphenylglycol in depressed patients: Modifications by amphetamine and lithium, *Biol. Psychiatry,* 11, 377, 1976.

72. **Beckmann, H., Waldmeier, P., Lauber, J., and Gattaz, W. F.,** Phenylethylamine and monoamine metabolites in CSF of schizophrenics: Effects of neuroleptic treatment, *J. Neural Transm.,* 57, 103, 1983.

73. **Benassi, C. A., Benassi, P., Allegri, G., and Ballarin, P.,** Tryptophan metabolism in schizophrenic patients, *J. Neurochem.,* 7, 264, 1961.

74. **Benedict, C. R.,** Simultaneous measurement of urinary and plasma norepinephrine, epinephrine, dopamine, dihydroxyphenylalanine, and dihydroxyphenylacetic acid by coupled-column high-performance liquid chromatography on C_8 and C_{18} stationary phases, *J. Chromatogr.,* 385, 369, 1987.

75. **Berger, P. A., Faull, K. F., Kilkowski, J., Anderson, P. J., Kraemer, H., Davis, K. L., Barchas, J. D.,** CSF monoamine metabolites in depression and schizophrenia, *Am. J. Psychiatry,* 137, 174, 1980.

76. **Berlet, H. H., Pscheidt, G. R., Spaide, J. K., and Himwich, H. E.,** Variations of urinary creatinine and its correlation to tryptamine excretion in schizophrenic patients. *Nature,* 203, 1198, 1964.

77. **Berrettini, W. H., Goldin, L. R., Nurnberger, J. I., and Gershon, E. S.,** Genetic factors in affective illness, *J. Psychiatr. Res.,* 18, 329, 1984.

78. **Berrettini, W. H., Nurnberger, J. I., Scheinin, M., Seppala, T., Linnoila, M., Narrow, W., Simmons-Alling, S., and Gershon, E. S.,** Cerebrospinal fluid and plasma monoamines and their metabolites in euthymic bipolar patients, *Biol. Psychiatry,* 20, 257, 1985.

79. **Bertani, L. M., Dziedzic, S. W., Clarke, D. D., and Gitlow, S. E.,** A gas-liquid chromatographic method for the separation and quantitation of normetanephrine and metanephrine in human urine, *Clin. Chim. Acta,* 30, 227, 1970.

80. **Bertani-Dziedzic, L. M., Krstulovic, A. M., Ciriello, S., and Gitlow, S. E.,** Routine reversed-phase high-performance liquid chromatographic measurement of urinary vanillylmandelic acid in patients with neuronal crest tumors, *J. Chromatogr.,* 164, 345, 1979.

81. **Bertani-Dziedzic, L. M., Krstulovic, A. M., Dziedzic, S. W., Gitlow, S. E., and Cerqueira, S.,** Analysis of urinary metanephrines by reversed-phase high-performance liquid chromatography and electrochemical detection, *Clin. Chim. Acta,* 110, 1, 1981.

82. **Bertilsson, L.,** Quantitative determination of 4-hydroxy-3-methoxyphenyl glycol and its conjugates in cerebrospinal fluid by mass fragmentography, *J. Chromatogr.,* 87, 147, 1973.

83. **Bertilsson, L., and Palmer, L.,** Indole-3-acetic acid in human cerebrospinal fluid: Identification and quantification by mass fragmentography, *Science,* 177, 74, 1972.

84. **Bertler, A., Jeppsson, P. G., Nordgren, L., and Rosengren, E.,** Serial determinations of homovanillic acid in the cerebrospinal fluid of Parkinson patients treated with L-DOPA, *Acta Neurol. Scand.,* 47, 393, 1971.

85. **Bigelow, L. B., Neal, S., and Weil-Malherbe, H.,** A spectrophotometric method for the estimation of 3-methoxy-4-hydroxyphenyl glycol in urine, *J. Lab. Clin. Med.,* 77, 677, 1971.

86. **Bigelow, L. B., and Weil-Malherbe, H.,** A simplified method for the differential estimation of metanephrine and normetanephrine in urine, *Anal. Biochem.,* 26, 92, 1968.

87. **Binder, S. R., and Sivorinovsky, G.,** Measurement of urinary vanilmandelic acid and homovanillic acid by high-performance liquid chromatography with electrochemical detection following extraction by ion-exchange and ion-moderated partition, *J. Chromatogr.,* 336, 173, 1984.

88. **Bioulac, B., Benezech, M., Renaud, B., Roche, D., and Noel, B.,** Biogenic amines in 47, XYY syndrome, *Neuropsychobiology,* 4, 366, 1978.

89. **Bischoff, F., and Torres, A.,** Fluorimetric determination of urinary adrenaline, *J. Appl. Physiol.,* 14, 237, 1959.

90. **Bischoff, F., and Torres, A.,** Determination of urinary dopamine, *Clin. Chem.* (Winston-Salem, N. C.), 8, 370, 1962.

91. **Bjerkenstedt, L., Gullberg, B., Härnryd, C., and Sedvall, G.,** Monoamine metabolite levels in cerebrospinal fluid of psychotic women treated with melperone or thiothixene, *Arch. Psychiatr. Nervenkr.,* 224, 107, 1977.

92. **Blau, K., Claxton, I. M., Ismahan, G., and Sandler, M.,** Urinary phenylethylamine excretion: Gas chromatographic assay with electron-capture detection of the pentafluorobenzoyl derivative, *J. Chromatogr.,* 163, 135, 1979.

93. **Bojkowski, C. J., Arendt, J., Shih, M. C., and Markey, S. P.,** Melatonin secretion in humans assessed by measuring its metabolite, 6-sulfatoxymelatonin, *Clin. Chem.* (Winston-Salem, N. C.), 33, 1343, 1987.

94. **Bond, P. A.,** The determination of 4-hydroxy-3-methoxyphenylethylene glycol in urine and CSF using gas chromatography, *Biochem. Med.,* 6, 36, 1972.

95. **Bond, P. A., and Howlett, D. R.,** Measurement of the two conjugates of 3-methoxy-4-hydroxyphenylglycol in urine, *Biochem. Med.,* 10, 219, 1974.

96. **Bond, P. A., Jenner, F. A., and Sampson, G. A.,** Daily variations of the urine content of 3-methoxy-4-hydroxyphenylglycol in two manic-depressive patients, *Psychol. Med.,* 2, 81, 1972.

97. **Bondy, B., Ackenheil, M., Birzle, W., Elbers, R., and Fröhler, M.,** Catecholamines and their receptors in blood: Evidence for alterations in schizophrenia, *Biol. Psychiatry,* 19, 1377, 1984.

98. **Bottiglieri, T., Lim, C. K., and Peters, T. J.,** Isocratic analysis of 3-methoxy-4-hydroxyphenyl glycol, 5-hydroxyindole-3-acetic acid and 4-hydroxy-3-methoxyphenylacetic acid in cerebrospinal fluid by high-performance liquid chromatography with amperometric detection, *J. Chromatogr.,* 311, 354, 1984.

99. **Boulton, A. A.,** The pink spot in parkinsonism, in *Progress in Neurogenetics,* Vol. 1 of the Proceedings of the 2nd International Congress of Neuro-genetics and Neuro-ophthalmology (Montréal, September, 1967), Excerpta Medica International Congress Series No. 175, 1968, 437.

100. **Boulton, A. A., Davis, B. A., Yu, P. H., Wormith, J. S., and Addington, D.,** Trace acid levels in the plasma and MAO activity in the platelets of violent offenders, *Psychiatry Res.,* 8, 19, 1983.

101. **Boulton, A. A., and Marjerrison, G. L.,** Effect of L-dopa therapy on urinary *p*-tyramine excretion and EEG changes in Parkinson's disease, *Nature,* 236, 76, 1972.

102. **Boulton, A. A., and Milward, L.,** Separation, detection and quantitative analysis of urinary β-phenylethylamine, *J. Chromatogr.,* 57, 287, 1971.

103. **Boulton, A. A., Pollit, R. J., and Majer, J. M.,** Identity of a urinary "pink spot" in schizophrenia and Parkinson's disease, *Nature,* 215, 132, 1967.

104. **Bowden, C. L., Koslow, S. H., Hanin, I., Maas, J. W., Davis, J. M., and Robins, E.,** Effects of amitriptyline and imipramine on brain amine neurotransmitter metabolites in cerebrospinal fluid, *Clin. Pharmacol. Ther.,* 37, 316, 1985.

105. **Bowden, C. L., Koslow, S., Maas, J. W., Davis, J. M., Garver, D. L., and Hanin, I.,** Changes in urinary catecholamines and their metabolites in depressed patients treated with amitryptyline or imipramine, *J. Psychiatr. Res.,* 21, 111, 1987.

106. **Bowden, C. L., Redmond, D. E., Swann, A., and Maas, J. W.,** Pretreatment amine neurotransmitter system interrelationships in depression, *Psychopharmacol. Bull.,* 17(1), 70, 1981.

107. **Bowen, D. M., Sims, N. R., Benton, J. S., Curzon, G., Davison, A. N., Neary, D., and Thomas, D. J.,** Treatment of Alzheimer's disease: A cautionary note, *New Engl. J. Med.,* 305, 1016, 1981.

108. **Bowers, M. B.,** Clinical measurements of central dopamine and 5-hydroxytryptamine metabolism: Reliability and interpretation of cerebrospinal fluid acid monoamine metabolite measures, *Neuropharmacology,* 11, 101, 1972.

109. **Bowers, M. B.,** Cerebrospinal fluid 5-hydroxyindoleacetic acid (5HIAA) and homovanillic acid (HVA) following probenecid in unipolar depressives treated with amitriptyline, *Psychopharmacologia,* 23, 26, 1972.

110. **Bowers, M. B., Heninger, G. R., and Gerbode, F.,** Cerebrospinal fluid 5-hydroxyindoleacetic acid and homovanillic acid in psychiatric patients, *Int. J. Neuropharmacol.,* 8, 255, 1969.

110a. **Bowers, M. B., Swigar, M. E., Hoffman, F. J., and Giocoechea, N.,** Characteristics of patients with the highest plasma catecholamine metabolite levels, *Am. J. Psychiatry,* 145, 246, 1988.

111. **Bowers, M. B., Swigar, M. E., Jatlow, P. I., Hoffman, F., and Giocoechea, N.,** Early neuroleptic response in psychotic men and women: Correlation with plasma HVA and MHPG, *Compr. Psychiatry,* 27, 181, 1986.

112. **Bowers, M. B., and Swigar, M. E.,** Acute psychosis and plasma catecholamine metabolites, *Arch. Gen. Psychiatry,* 44, 190, 1987.

113. **Bowers, M. B., Swigar, M. E., and Jatlow, P. I.,** Sex differences in plasma homovanillic acid in acute psychosis, *New Engl. J. Med.,* 308, 845, 1983.

114. **Bowers, M. B., Swigar, M. E., Jatlow, P. I., and Giocoechea, N.,** Plasma catecholamine metabolites and early response to haloperidol, *J. Clin. Psychiatry,* 45, 248, 1984.

115. **Bozzi, R., Bruno, A., and Allegranza, A.,** Urinary metabolites of some monoamines and clinical effects under reserpine and chlorpromazine. *Br. J. Psychiatry,* 111, 176, 1965.

116. **Branchy, L., Weinberg, U., Branchey, M., Linkowski, P., and Mendlewicz, J.,** Simultaneous study of 24-hour patterns of melatonin and cortisol secretion in depressed patients, *Neuropsychobiology* 8, 225, 1982.

117. **Bridges, P. K., Bartlett, J. R., Sepping, P., Kantamaneni, B. D., and Curzon, G.,** Precursors and metabolites of 5-hydroxytryptamine and dopamine in the ventricular cerebrospinal fluid of psychiatric patients, *Psychol. Med.,* 6, 399, 1976.

118. **Brown, G. L., Ballanger, J. C., Minichiello, M. D., and Goodwin, F. K.,** Human aggression and its relationship to cerebrospinal fluid 5-hydroxyindoleacetic acid, 3-methoxy-4-hydroxyphenylglycol, and homovanillic acid, in *Psychopharmacology of Aggression*, Sandler, M., Ed., Raven Press, New York, 1979, 131.

119. **Brown, H. H., Rhindress, M. C., and Griswold, R. E.,** Automated liquid chromatographic determination of 5-hydroxyindoleacetic acid in urine, *Clin. Chem.* (Winston-Salem, N.C.), 17, 92, 1971.

120. **Brown, M. J., Ind, P. W., Barnes, P. J., Jenner, D. A., and Dollery, C. T.,** A sensitive and specific radiometric method for the measurement of plasma histamine in normal individuals, *Anal. Biochem.,* 109, 142, 1980.

121. **Bruce, C., Weatherstone, R., Seaton, A., and Taylor, W. H.,** Histamine levels in plasma, blood and urine in severe asthma and the effect of corticosteroid treatment, *Thorax,* 31, 724, 1976.

122. **Brune, G. G., and Himwich, H. E.,** Indole metabolites in schizophrenic patients, *Arch. Gen. Psychiatry,* 6, 324, 1962.

123. **Brune, G. G., and Pflughaupt, K. W.,** Effects of L-DOPA treatment on indole metabolism in Parkinson's disease, *Experientia,* 27, 516, 1971.

124. **Brune, G. G., and Pscheidt, G. R.,** Correlations between behavior and urinary excretion of indole amines and catecholamines in schizophrenic patients as affected by drugs, *Fed. Proc., Fed. Am. Soc. Exp. Biol.,* 20, 889, 1961.

125. **Bruno, A., and Allegranza, A.,** The effect of haloperidol on the urinary excretion of dopamine, homovanillic and vanilmandelic acids in schizophrenics, *Psychopharmacologia,* 8, 60, 1965.

126. **Bunney, W. E., Davis, J. M., Weil-Malherbe, H., and Smith, E. R. B.**, Biochemical changes in psychotic depression, *Arch. Gen. Psychiatry,* 16, 448, 1967.

127. **Bunney, W. E., Goodwin, F. K., Murphy, D. L., House, K. M., and Gordon, E. K.**, The "switch process" in manic-depressive illness. II. Relationship to catecholamines, REM sleep and drugs, *Arch. Gen. Psychiatry,* 27, 304, 1972.

128. **Bunney, W. E., Murphy, D. L., Goodwin, F. K., and Borge, G. F.**, The switch process from depression to mania: The relationship to drugs which alter brain amines, *Lancet,* 1, 1022, 1970.

129. **Butler, T. J.**, Electrophoretic determination of vanilmandelic acid (VMA) in urine by direct application to cellulose acetate, *Clin. Chem. (Winston-Salem, N. C.),* 13, 488, 1967.

130. **Buttery, J. E., and DeWitt, G. F.**, A simple and rapid method for the determination of 4-hydroxy-3-methoxymandelic acid (HMMA) in urine. *Clin. Chim. Acta,* 44, 179, 1973.

131. **Buu, N. T., and Kuchel, O.**, A new method for the hydrolysis of conjugated catecholamines, *J. Lab. Clin. Med.,* 90, 680, 1977.

132. **Calne, D. B., Karoum, F., Ruthven, C. R. J., and Sandler, M.**, The metabolism of orally administered L-DOPA in Parkinsonism, *Br. J. Pharmacol.,* 37, 57, 1969.

133. **Campanini, T., Catalano, A., DeRisio, C., and Mardighian, G.**, Vanilmandelicaciduria in the different clinical phases of manic depressive psychosis, *Br. J. Psychiatry,* 116, 435, 1970.

134. **Candito, M., Lapalus, P., and Chambon, P.**, Determination of free and sulfate-conjugated 3-methoxy-4-hydroxyphenylethyleneglycol in human plasma by liquid chromatography with electrochemical detection, *J. Chromatogr.,* 430, 198, 1988.

135.   **Cardon, P. V., and Guggenheim, F. G.,** Effects of large variations in diet on free catecholamines and their metabolites in urine, *J. Psychiatr. Res.,* 7, 263, 1970.

136.   **Carpenter, W. T., Fink, E. B., Narasimhachari, N., and Himwich, H. E.,** A test of the transmethylation hypothesis in acute schizophrenic patients, *Am. J. Psychiatry,* 132, 1067, 1975.

137.   **Carr, V., Edwards, J., and Prior, M.,** Urinary MHPG, platelet ^{3}H-imipramine binding and symptomatology in depression: An exploratory study of clinical heterogeneity, *Biol. Psychiatry,* 23, 560, 1988.

138.   **Castellani, S., Ziegler, M. G., Van Kammen, D. P., Alexander, P. E., Siris, S. G., and Lake, C. R.,** Plasma norepinephrine and dopamine-β-hydroxylase activity in schizophrenia.   *Arch. Gen. Psychiatry,* 39, 1145, 1982.

139.   **Causon, R. C., and Brown, M. J.,** Measurement of tyramine in human plasma, utilizing ion-pair extraction and high-performance liquid chromatography with amperometric detection, *J. Chromatogr.,* 310, 11, 1984.

140.   **Causon, R. C., and Carruthers, M. E.,** Measurement of catecholamines in biological fluids by high-performance liquid chromatography. A comparison of fluorimetric with electrochemical detection, *J. Chromatogr.,* 229, 301, 1982.

141.   **Causon, R. C., Carruthers, M. E., and Rodnight, R.,** Assay of plasma catecholamines by liquid chromatography with electrochemical detection. *Anal. Biochem.,* 116, 223, 1981.

142.   **Cavanaugh, S. T., Hughes, J. D., and Hoeldtke, R. D.,** Measurement of plasma vanillylmandelic acid by liquid chromatography with electrochemical detection. *J. Chromatogr.,* 381, 13, 1986.

143. **Cazzullo, C. L., Mangoni, A., and Mascherpa**, G., Tryptophan metabolism in affective psychoses, *Br. J. Psychiatry*, 112, 157, 1966.

144. **Charney, D. S., Breier, A., Jatlow, P. I., and Heninger, G. R.**, Behavioral, biochemical, and blood pressure responses to alprazolam in healthy subjects: Interactions with yohimbine, *Psychopharmacology*, 88, 133, 1986.

145. **Charney, D. S., Galloway, M. P., and Heninger, G. R.**, The effects of caffeine on plasma MHPG, subjective anxiety, autonomic symptoms and blood pressure in healthy humans, *Life Sci.*, 35, 135, 1984.

146. **Charney, D. S., and Heninger, G. R.**, Noradrenergic function and the mechanism of action of antianxiety treatment. I. The effect of long-term alprazolam treatment, *Arch. Gen. Psychiatry*, 42, 458, 1985.

147. **Charney, D. S., and Heninger, G. R.**, Noradrenergic function and the mechanism of action of antianxiety treatment. II. The effect of long-term imipramine treatment, *Arch. Gen. Psychiatry*, 42, 473, 1985.

148. **Charney, D. S., Heninger, G. R., and Breier, A.**, Noradrenergic function in panic anxiety. Effects of yohimbine in healthy subjects and patients with agoraphobia and panic disorder, *Arch. Gen. Psychiatry*, 41, 751, 1984.

149. **Charney, D. S., Heninger, G. R., and Sternberg, D. E.**, Alpha 2 adrenergic receptor sensitivity and the mechanism of action of antidepressant therapy. The effect of long-term amitriptyline treatment, *Br. J. Psychiatry*, 142, 265, 1983.

150. **Charney, D. S., Heninger, G. R., Sternberg, D. E., Hafstad, K. M., Giddings, S., and Landis, D. H.**, Adrenergic receptor sensitivity in depression. Effects of clonidine in depressed patients and healthy subjects, *Arch. Gen. Psychiatry*, 39, 290, 1982.

151. **Charney, D. S., Heninger, G. R., Sternberg, D. E., and Roth, R. H.**, Plasma MHPG in depression: Effects of acute and chronic desipramine treatment, *Psychiatry Res.*, 5, 217, 1981.

152. **Chase, T. N.**, Cerebrospinal fluid monoamine metabolites and peripheral decarboxylase inhibitors in parkinsonism, *Neurology*, 20(Part 2), 36, 1970.

153. **Chase, T. N.**, Serotonergic mechanisms in Parkinson's disease, *Arch. Neurol.*, 27, 354, 1972.

154. **Chase, T. N., Gordon, E. K., and Ng, L. K. Y.**, Norepinephrine metabolism in the central nervous system of man: Studies using 3-methoxy-4-hydroxyphenylethylene glycol levels in cerebrospinal fluid, *J. Neurochem.*, 21, 581, 1973.

155. **Chase, T. N., and Ng L. K. Y.**, Central monoamine metabolism in Parkinson's disease, *Arch. Neurol.*, 27, 486, 1972.

156. **Chauhan, J., and Darbre, A.**, Determination of homovanillic, isohomovanillic and vanillylmandelic acids in human urine by means of glass capillary gas-liquid chromatography with temperature-programmed electron-capture detection, *J. Chromatogr.*, 183, 391, 1980.

157. **Chodakowska, J., Nazar, K., Wocial, B., Jarecki, M., and Skorka, B.**, Plasma catecholamines and renin activity in response to exercise in patients with essential hypertension, *Clin. Sci. Mol. Med.*, 49, 511, 1975.

158. **Christensen, N. J.**, A sensitive assay for the determination of dopamine in plasma, *Scand. J. Clin. and Lab. Invest.*, 31, 343, 1973.

159. **Christensen, N. J.**, Plasma noradrenaline and adrenaline in patients with thyrotoxicosis and myxoedema, *Clin. Sci. Mol. Med.*, 45, 163, 1973.

160. **Christensen, N. J.,** Plasma norepinephrine and epinephrine in untreated diabetics, during fasting and after insulin administration, *Diabetes,* 23, 1, 1974.

161. **Christensen, N. J., Mathias, C. J., and Frankel, H. L.,** Plasma and urinary dopamine: Studies during fasting and exercise and in tetraplegic man, *Eur. J. Clin. Invest.,* 6, 403, 1976.

162. **Christensen, N. J., Vestergaard, P., Sorensen, T., and Raphaelson, O. J.,** Cerebrospinal fluid adrenaline and noradrenaline in depressed patients, *Acta Psychiatr. Scand.,* 61, 178, 1980.

163. **Christiansen, S. T., Benington, F., Morin, R. D., and Corbett, L.,** Gas-liquid chromatographic separation and identification of biologically important indolealkylamines from human cerebrospinal fluid, *Biochem. Med.,* 14, 191, 1975.

164. **Chryssanthopoulos, C., Barboriak, J. J., Fink, J. N., Stekiel, W. J., and Maksud, M. G.,** Adrenergic responses of asthmatic and normal subjects to submaximal and maximal work levels, *J. Allergy Clin. Immunol.,* 61, 17, 1978.

165. **Clarke, D. D., Wilk, S., Gitlow, S. E., and Franklin, M. J.,** Gas chromatographic determination of dopamine at the nanogram level, *J. Gas Chromatogr.,* 5, 307, 1967.

166. **Claustre, J., Serusclat, P., and Peyrin, L.** Glucuronide and sulfate catecholamine conjugates in rat and human plasma, *J. Neural Transm.,* 56, 265, 1983.

167. **Cobbin, D. M., Requin-Blow, B., Williams, L. R., and Williams, W. O.,** Urinary MHPG levels and tricyclic antidepressant drug selection. A preliminary communication on improved drug selection in clinical practice, *Arch. Gen. Psychiatry,* 36, 1111, 1979.

168. **Cohen, G., and Goldenberg, M.,** The simultaneous fluorimetric determination of adrenaline and noradrenaline in plasma - II, *J. Neurochem.,* 2, 71, 1957.

169. **Comoy, E., and Bohuon, C.,** Iso-homovanillic acid determination in human urine, *Clin. Chim. Acta,* 35, 369, 1971.

170. **Conti, G., Vita, A., and Sacchetti, E.,** Interepisode reliability of urinary MHPG excretion in major depression, *Biol. Psychiatry,* 24, 240, 1988.

171. **Coppen, A.,** Indoleamines and affective disorders, *J. Psychiatr. Res.,* 9, 163, 1972.

172. **Coppen, A., Prange, A. J., Whybrow, P. C., and Noguera, R.,** Abnormalities of indoleamines in affective disorders, *Arch. Gen. Psychiatry,* 26, 474, 1972.

173. **Coppen, A., Rama Rao, V. A., Ruthven, C. R. J., Goodwin, B. L., and Sandler, M.,** Urinary 4-hydroxy-3-methoxyphenylglycol is not a predictor for clinical response to amitriptyline in depressive illness, *Psychopharmacology,* 64, 95, 1979.

174. **Coppen, A., Shaw, D. M., Malleson, A., Eccleston, E., and Gundy, G.,** Tryptamine metabolism in depression, *Br. J. Psychiatry,* 111, 993, 1965.

175. **Corona, G. L., Cucchi, M. L., Santagostino, G., Frattini, P., Zerbi, F., Fenoglio, L., and Savoldi, F.,** Blood noradrenaline and 5HT levels in depressed women during amitriptyline or lithium treatment, *Psychopharmacology,* 77, 236, 1982.

176. **Coutts, R. T., Baker, G. B., LeGatt, D. F., McIntosh, G. J., Hopkinson, G., and Dewhurst, W. G.,** Screening for amines of psychiatric interest in urine using gas chromatography with electron-capture detection, *Prog. Neuro-Psychopharmacol.,* 5, 565, 1981.

177. **Coward, R. F., and Smith, P.,** Recovery of total metanephrines from urine and their estimation by paper chromatography, *Clin. Chim. Acta,* 14, 672, 1966.

178. **Crawford, N.,** Plasma free serotonin (5-hydroxytryptamine), *Clin. Chim, Acta,* 8, 39, 1963.

179. **Crawford, N.,** Systemic venous platelet-bound and plasma free serotonin levels in non-carcinoid malignancy, *Clin. Chim. Acta,* 12, 274, 1965.

180. **Creveling, C. R., and Daly, J. W.,** Identification of 3,4-dimethoxyphenethylamine from schizophrenic urine by mass spectrometry, *Nature,* 216, 190, 1967.

181. **Cryer, P. E., Haymond, M. W., Santiago, J. V., and Shah, S. D.,** Norepinephrine and epinephrine release and adrenergic mediation of smoking-associated hemodynamic and metabolic events, *New Engl. J. Med.,* 295, 573, 1976.

182. **Cryer, P. E., Santiago, J. V., and Shah, S.,** Measurement of norepinephrine and epinephrine in small volumes of human plasma by a single isotope derivative method: Response to the upright posture, *J. Clin. Endocrinol. Metab.,* 39, 1025, 1974.

183. **Cuche, J.-L., Kuchel, O., Barbeau, A., Langlois, Y., Boucher, R., and Genest, J.,** Autonomic nervous system and benign essential hypertension in man, *Circ. Res.,* 35, 281, 1974.

184. **Cuche, J.-L., Prinseau, J., Selz, F., Ruget, G., Tual, J.-L., Reingeissen, L., Devoisin, M., Baglin, A., Guédon, J., and Fritel, D.,** Oral load of tyrosine or L-DOPA and plasma levels of free and sulfoconjugated catecholamines in healthy men, *Hypertension,* 7, 81, 1985.

185. **Curran, D. A., Hinterberger, H., Lance, J. W., and Joffe, A. D.,** Total plasma serotonin, 5-hydroxyindoleacetic acid and *p*-hydroxy-*m*-methoxymandelic acid excretion in normal and migrainous subjects, *Brain,* 88, 997, 1965.

186. **Curzon, G., Gumpert, E. J. W., and Sharpe, D. M.,** Amine metabolites in the lumbar cerebrospinal fluid of humans with restricted flow of cerebrospinal fluid, *Nature* (London), *New Biology,* 231, 189, 1971.

187. **Curzon, G., Kantamaneni, B. D., Bartlett, J. R., and Bridges, P. K.,** Transmitter precursors and metabolites in human ventricular cerebrospinal fluid, *J. Neurochem.,* 26, 613, 1976.

188. **Curzon, G., Kantamaneni, B. D., Van Boxel, P., Gillman, P. K., Bartlett, J. R., and Bridges, P. K.,** Substances related to 5-hydroxytryptamine in plasma and in lumbar and ventricular fluids of psychiatric patients, *Acta Psychiatr. Scand.,* Suppl. 280, 3, 1980.

189. **Curzon, G., Theaker, P., and Phillips, B.,** Excretion of 5-hydroxyindolyl acetic acid (5HIAA) in migraine, *J. Neurol. Neurosurg. Psychiatry,* 29, 85, 1966.

190. **Cutler, N. R., Jeste, D. V., Karoum, F., and Wyatt, R. J.,** Low-dose apomorphine reduces serum homovanillic acid concentrations in schizophrenic patients, *Life Sci.,* 30, 753, 1982.

191. **Cymerman, A., and Francesconi, R. F.,** Alteration of circadian rhythmicities of urinary 3-methoxy-4-hydroxyphenylglycol (MHPG) and vanilmandelic acid (VMA) in man during cold exposure, *Life Sci.,* 16, 225, 1975.

192. **Dahl, L.-E., Lundin, L., LeFèvré, Honoré P., and Dencker, S. J.,** Antidepressant effect of femoxetine and desipramine and relationship to the concentration of amine metabolites in cerebrospinal fluid. A double-blind evaluation, *Acta Psychiatr. Scand.,* 66, 9, 1982.

193. **Dailey, J. W., and Ånggard, E.,** The determination of homovanillic acid in human and rat urine using gas chromatography with flame ionization and mass spectrometric detection, *Biochem. Pharmacol.,* 22, 2591, 1973.

194. **Dajas, F., Barbeito, L., Martinez-Pesquera, G., Lista, A., Puppo, D., Puppo-Touriz, H.,** Plasma noradrenaline and clinical psychotherapy in schizophrenia. A correlation analysis, *Neuropsychobiology,* 10, 70, 1983.

195. **Dajas, F., Lista, A., and Barbeito, L.,** High urinary norepinephrine excretion in major depressive disorders: Effects of a new type of MAO inhibitor (moclobemide, RO 11-1163), *Acta Psychiatr. Scand.,* 70, 432, 1984.

196. **Dajas, F., Nin, A., and Barbeito, L.,** Urinary norepinephrine excretion in panic and phobic disorders, *J. Neural. Transm.,* 65, 75, 1986.

197. **Dalmaz, Y., and Peyrin, L.,** Specific ion-exchange chromatography and fluorimetric assay for urinary 3-0-methyldopamine, *J. Chromatogr.,* 116, 379, 1976.

198. **Dalmaz, Y., and Peyrin, L.,** Rapid procedure for chromatographic isolation of DOPA, DOPAC, epinephrine, norepinephrine and dopamine from a single urinary sample at endogenous levels, *J. Chromatogr.,* 145, 11, 1978.

199. **Da Prada, M.,** Concentration, dynamics and functional meaning of catecholamines in plasma and urine, *Trends Pharmacol. Sci.,* 1(1), 157, 1980.

200. **Da Prada, M., and Zürcher, G.,** Simultaneous radioenzymatic determination of plasma and tissue adrenaline, noradrenaline within the femtomole range, *Life Sci.,* 19, 1161, 1976.

201. **Davidson, D. F., and Williamson, J.,** Improved assay for urinary 5-hydroxyindoleacetic acid by HPLC with electrochemical detection, *Clin. Chem.* (Winston-Salem, N. C.), 34, 768, 1988.

202. **Davidson, D. L. W., Yates, C. M., Mawdsley, C., Pullar, I. A., and Wilson, H.,** CSF studies on the relationship between dopamine and 5-hydroxytryptamine in Parkinsonism and other movement disorders, *J. Neurol. Neurosurg. Psychiatry,* 40, 1136, 1977.

203. **Davidson, M., and Davis, K. L.,** A comparison of plasma homovanillic acid concentrations in schizophrenic patients and normal controls, *Arch. Gen. Psychiatry,* 45, 561, 1988.

204. **Davidson, M., Giordani, A. B., Mohs, R. C., Horvath, T. B., Davis, B. M., Powchik, P., and Davis, K. L.,** Shortterm haloperidol administration acutely elevates human plasma homovanillic acid concentration, *Arch. Gen. Psychiatry,* 44, 189, 1987.

205. **Davidson, M., Losonczy, M. F., Mohs, R. C., Lesser, J. C., Powchik, P., Freed, L. B., Davis, B. M., Mykytyn, V. V., and Davis, K. L.,** Effects of debrisoquin and haloperidol on plasma homovanillic acid concentration in schizophrenic patients, *Neuropsychopharmacology,* 1, 17, 1987.

206. **Davila, R., Manero, E., Zumarraga, M., Andia, I., Schweitzer, J. W., and Friedhoff, A. J.,** Plasma homovanillic acid as a predictor of response to neuroleptics, *Arch. Gen. Psychiatry,* 45, 564, 1988.

207. **Davis, B. A., and Boulton, A.A.,** Longitudinal urinary excretion of some "trace" acids in a human male, *J. Chromatogr.,* 222, 161, 1981.

208. **Davis, B. A., and Boulton, A.A.,** Excretion of *m*-hydroxymandelic acid in human urine, *J. Chromatogr.,* 222, 271, 1981.

209. **Davis, B. A., Dawson, B., Boulton, A.A., Yu, P. H., and Durden, D. A.,** Investigation of some biological trait markers in migraine: Deuterated tyramine challenge test, monoamine oxidase, phenolsulfotransferase and plasma and urinary biogenic amine and acid metabolite levels, *Headache,* 27, 384, 1987.

210. **Davis, B. A., Durden, D. A., and Boulton, A.A.,** Plasma concentrations of *p*- and *m*-hydroxyphenylacetic acid and phenylacetic acid in humans: Gas chromatographic-high resolution mass spectrometric analysis, *J. Chromatogr.,* 230, 219, 1982.

211. **Davis, B. A., Durden, D. A., and Boulton, A.A.,** Simultaneous analysis of twelve biogenic amine metabolites in plasma, cerebrospinal fluid and urine by capillary column gas chromatography-high resolution mass spectrometry with selected ion monitoring, *J. Chromatogr.,* 374, 227, 1986.

212. **Davis, B. A., Yu, P. H., Boulton, A.A., Wormith, J. S., and Addington, D.,** Correlative relationship between biochemical activity and aggressive behaviour, *Prog. Neuro-Psychopharmacol. Biol. Psychiatry,* 7, 529, 1983.

213. **Davis, B. A., Yu, P. H., Carlson, K., O'Sullivan, K., and Boulton, A.A.,** Plasma levels of phenylacetic acid, *m*- and *p*-hydroxyphenylacetic acid, and platelet monoamine oxidase activity in schizophrenic and other patients, *Psychiatry Res.*, 6, 97, 1982.

214. **Davis, K. L., Hollister, L. E., Mathé, A. A., Davis, B. M., Rothpearl, A. B., Faull, K. F., Hsieh, J. Y. K., Barchas, J. D., and Berger, P. A.,** Neuroendocrine and neurochemical measurements in depression, *Am. J. Psychiatry,* 138, 1555, 1981.

215. **Davis, R. B.,** The concentration of serotonin in normal human serum as determined by an improved method, *J. Lab. Clin. Med.,* 54, 344, 1959.

216. **Davis, V. E., Huff, J. A., and Brown, H.,** Free and conjugated serotonin excretion in carcinoid syndrome, *J. Lab. Clin. Med.,* 66, 390, 1965.

217. **De Jong, A. P. J. M., Kok, R. M., Cramers, C. A., and Wadman, S. K.,** Determination of acidic catecholamine metabolites in plasma and cerebrospinal fluid using gas chromatography-negative ion mass spectrometry, *J. Chromatogr.,* 382, 19, 1986.

218. **De Jong, E. B. M., Horsten, B. P. M., and Goldschmidt, H. M. J.,** Determination of nine catecholamine metabolites and 5-hydroxyindoleacetic acid in urine by capillary gas chromatography, *J. Chromatogr.,* 279, 563, 1983.

219. **De Jong, J., Tjaden, U. R., Visser, E., Meijer, W. H.,** Determination of serotonin and 5-hydroxyindoleacetic acid in urine by reversed-phase ion-pair partition chromatography with fluorimetric detection, *J. Chromatogr.,* 419, 85, 1987.

220. **Dekirmenjian, H., and Maas, J. W.,** An improved procedure of 3-methoxy-4-hydroxyphenylethylene glycol determination by gas-liquid chromatography, *Anal. Biochem.,* 35, 113, 1970.

221. **Dekirmenjian, H., and Maas, J. W.,** Determination of urinary 3-methoxy-4-hydroxymandelic acid by gas-liquid chromatography as vanillyl alcohol, *Clin. Chim. Acta,* 32, 310, 1971.

222. **Dekirmenjian, H., and Maas, J. W.,** 3-Methoxy-4-hydroxyphenyl-ethylene glycol in plasma, *Clin. Chim. Acta,* 52, 203, 1974.

223. **De Leon-Jones, F., Maas, J. W., Dekirmenjian, H., and Fawcett, J. A.,** Urinary catecholamine metabolites during behavioral changes in a patient with manic depressive cycles, *Science,* 179, 300, 1973.

224. **De Leon-Jones, F., Maas, J. W., Dekirmenjian, H., and Sanchez, J.,** Diagnostic subgroups of affective disorders and their urinary excretion of catecholamine metabolites, *Am. J. Psychiatry,* 132, 1141, 1975.

225. **De Lisi, L. E., Karoum, F., Targum, S., Byrnes, S., and Wyatt, R. J.,** The determination of urinary 3-methoxy-4-hydroxyphenylglycol excretion in acute schizophreniform and depressed patients, *Biol. Psychiatry,* 18, 1189, 1983.

226. **De Lisi, L. E., Murphy, D. L., Karoum, F., Mueller, E., Targum, S., and Wyatt, R. J.,** Phenylethylamine excretion in depression, *Psychiatry Res.,* 13, 193, 1984.

227. **Demassieux, S., Corneille, L., Lachance, S., and Carriere, S.,** Determination of free and conjugated catecholamines and L-3,4-dihydroxyphenylalanine in plasma and urine: Evidence for a catechol-O-methyltransferase inhibitor in uraemia, *Clin. Chim. Acta,* 115, 377, 1981.

227a. **De Met, E. M., Halaris, A. E., and Bhatarakamol, S.,** Indoleamine compartmentation in human blood, *Clin. Chim. Acta,* 89, 285, 1978.

228. **De Met, E. M., Halaris, A. E., Gwirtsman, H. E., and Reno, R. M.,** Diurnal rhythm of 3-methoxy-4-hydroxyphenylglycol (MHPG): Relationship between plasma and urinary levels, *Life Sci.,* 37, 1731, 1985.

229. **Demisch, K., Demisch, L., Nickelsen, T., Rieth, R.,** The influence of acute and subchronic administration of various antidepressants on early morning melatonin plasma levels in healthy subjects: Increases following fluvoxamine, *J. Neural Transm.,* 68, 257, 1987.

230. **Dencker, S. J., Häggendal, J., and Malm, U.,** Noradrenaline content of cerebrospinal fluid in mental disease, *Lancet,* 2, 754, 1966.

231. **Dencker, S. J., Malm, U., Roos, B.-E., Werdinius, B.,** Acid monoamine metabolites of cerebrospinal fluid in mental depression and mania, *J. Neurochem.,* 13, 1545, 1966.

232. **Dennis, T., and Scatton, B.,** A radioenzymatic technique for the measurement of free and conjugated 3,4-dihydroxyphenylethyleneglycol in brain tissue and biological fluids, *J. Neurosci. Meth.,* 6, 369, 1982.

233. **De Quattro, V., Wybenga, D., Von Studnitz, W., and Brunjes, S.,** Determination of urinary 3,4-dihydroxymandelic acid, *J. Lab. Clin. Med.,* 63, 864, 1964.

234. **De Schaepdryver, A. F., and Moerman, E. J.,** Simultaneous quantitation of catecholamines and metabolites in urine, *Clin. Chim. Acta,* 84, 321, 1978.

235. **Devanand, D. P., Bowers, M. B., Hoffman, F. J., and Nelson, J. C.,** Elevated plasma homovanillic acid in depressed females with melancholia and psychosis, *Psychiatry Res.,* 15, 1, 1985.

236. **Dimsdale, J. E., and Moss, J.,** Plasma catecholamines in stress and exercise, *J. Am. Med. Assoc.,* 243, 340, 1980.

237. **Domino, E. F., Mathews, B. N., and Tait, S. K.,** Urinary neurotransmitter metabolites in drug-free chronic schizophrenic patients measured by gas chromatography selected positive ion monitoring, *Biomed. Mass Spectrom.,* 6, 331, 1979.

238. **Doran, A. R., Rubinow, D. R., Wolkowitz, O. M., Roy, A., Breier, A., and Pickar, D.,** Fluphenazine treatment reduces CSF somatostatin in patients with schizophrenia: Correlations with CSF HVA, *Biol. Psychiatry,* 25, 431, 1989.

239. **Doshi, P. S., and Edwards, D. J.,** Use of 2,6-dinitro-4-trifluoromethylbenzenesulfonic acid as a novel derivatizing agent for the analysis of catecholamines, histamines and related amines by gas chromatography with electron-capture detection, *J. Chromatogr.,* 176, 359, 1979.

240. **Drujan, B. D., Alvarez, N., and Diaz-Borges, J. M.,** A method for determination of 3,4-dihydroxyphenylacetic acid and 3,4-dihydroxymandelic acid in urine, *Anal. Biochem.,* 15, 8, 1966.

241. **Duke, P. S., and Demopoulos, H. B.,** One-dimensional paper chromatographic method for determination of urinary homovanillic acid, *Clin. Chem.* (Winston-Salem, N. C.), 14, 212, 1968.

242. **Dunér, H., Liljedahl, S. O., and Pernow, B.,** Does the urinary excretion of imidazole acetic acid reflect the endogenous histamine metabolism in man? *Acta Physiol. Scand.,* 51, 41, 1961.

243. **Dunér, H., and Pernow, B.,** Urinary excretion of histamine in healthy human subjects, *Scand. J. Clin. Lab. Invest.,* 8, 296, 1956.

244. **Dunne, J. W., Davidson, L., Vandongen, R., Beilin, L. J., and Rogers, P.,** The effect of ascorbic acid on plasma sulfate conjugated catecholamines after eating bananas, *Life Sci.,* 33, 1511, 1983.

245. **Durden, D. A., Juorio, A. V., and Davis, B. A.,** Analysis of *p*-synephrine and related β-hydroxyphenylethylamines by direct probe high resolution mass spectrometry, in *Quantitative Mass Spectrometry in Life Sciences II,* De Leenheer, A. P., Roncucci, R. R., and Van Peteghem, C., Eds., Elsevier Scientific Publishing Co., Amsterdam, 1978, 389.

246. **Dyer, J., Warren, K., Merlin, S., Metcalfe, D. D., Kaliner, M.,** Measurement of plasma histamine: Description of an improved method and normal values, *J. Allergy Clin. Immunol.,* 70, 82, 1982.

247. **Dziedzic, S. W., Bertani, L. M., Clarke, D. D., and Gitlow, S. E.,** A new derivative for the gas-liquid chromatographic determination of homovanillic acid, *Anal. Biochem.,* 47, 592, 1972.

248. **Dziedzic, S. W., Bertani-Dziedzic, L., and Gitlow, S. E.,** Separation and determination of urinary homovanillic acid and iso-homovanillic acid by gas-liquid chromatography and electron capture detection, *J. Lab. Clin. Med.,* 82, 829, 1973.

249. **Dziedzic, S. W., and Gitlow, S. E.,** Cerebrospinal fluid homovanillic acid and iso-homovanillic acid: A gas-liquid chromatographic method, *J. Neurochem.,* 22, 333, 1974.

250. **Echizen, H., Itoh, R., and Ishizaki, T.,** Microassay of free 3-methoxy-4-hydroxyphenylglycol in plasma using high-performance liquid chromatography with electrochemical detection, *J. Chromatogr.,* 426, 351, 1988.

251. **Echizen, H., Itoh, R., and Ishizaki, T.,** Adenosine and dopamine simultaneously determined in urine by reversed-phase HPLC with on line measurement of ultraviolet absorbance and electrochemical detection, *Clin. Chem.* (Winston-Salem, N. C.), 35, 64, 1989.

252. **Edlund, M. J., Swann, A. C., and Davis, C. M.,** Plasma MHPG in untreated panic disorder, *Biol. Psychiatry,* 22, 1491, 1987.

253. **Edwards, D. J., Rizk, M., and Neil, J.,** Simultaneous analysis of phenyglycols and phenylethanols in human urine by gas chromatography-mass spectrometry, *J. Chromatogr.,* 164, 407, 1979.

254. **Ehrhardt, J. D., and Schwartz, J.,** A gas chromatography-mass spectrometry assay of human plasma catecholamines, *Clin. Chim. Acta,* 88, 71, 1978.

255. **Eichholtz, P. C. N., Binkhuyzen, D., and Thieme, R. E.,** Direct determination of 3-methoxy-4-sulphonyloxyphenylglycol (MHPG sulphate) in urine using gas-liquid chromatography, *J. Chromatogr.,* 305, 438, 1984.

256. **Eichorn, F., Rutenberg, A., and Kott, E.** Fluorometric method for quantitatively estimating urinary dihydroxyphenylethylamine (dopamine), dihydroxyphenylalanine (DOPA) and dihydroxyphenylacetic acid (DOPAC), *Clin. Chem.* (Winston-Salem, N. C.), 17, 296, 1971.

257. **Eisenhofer, G.,** Analytical differences between the determination of plasma catecholamines by liquid chromatography with electrochemical detection and by radioenzymatic assay, *J. Chromatogr.,* 377, 328, 1986.

258. **Eisenhofer, G., Goldstein, D. S., Stull, R., Keiser, H. R., Sunderland, T., Murphy, D. L., and Kopin, I. J.,** Simultaneous liquid-chromatographic determination of 3,4-dihydroxyphenylglycol, catecholamines, and 3,4-dihydroxyphenylalanine in plasma, and their responses to inhibition of monoamine oxidase, *Clin. Chem.* (Winston-Salem, N. C.), 32, 2030, 1986.

259. **Elchisak, M. A., and Carlson, J. H.,** Assay of free and conjugated catecholamines by high-performance liquid chromatography with electrochemical detection, *J. Chromatogr.*, 233, 79, 1982.

260. **Elchisak, M. A., and Carlson, J. H.,** Method for analysis of dopamine sulfate isomers by high performance liquid chromatography, *Life Sci.*, 30, 2325, 1982.

261. **Elsworth, J. D., Roth, R. H., and Redmond, D. E.,** Relative importance of 3-methoxy-4-hydroxyphenylglycol and 3,4-dihydroxy-phenylglycol as norepinephrine metabolites in rat, monkey and humans, *J. Neurochem.*, 41, 786, 1983.

262. **Emanuelsson, B.-M., Widerlöv, E., Walléus, H., and Paalzow, L. K.,** Determinations of 5-hydroxyindoleacetic acid and homovanillic acid in human CSF with monitoring of probenecid levels in CSF and plasma, *Psychopharmacology,* 92, 144, 1987.

263. **Endert, E.,** Determination of noradrenaline and adrenaline in plasma by a radioenzymatic assay using high pressure liquid chromatography for the separation of the radiochemical products, *Clin. Chim. Acta,* 96, 233, 1979.

264. **Engbaek, F., and Voldby, B.,** Radioimmunoassay of serotonin (5-hydroxytryptamine) in cerebrospinal fluid, plasma and serum, *Clin. Chem.* (Winston-Salem, N. C.), 28, 624, 1982.

265. **Engelman, K., and Portnoy, B.,** A sensitive double-isotope derivative assay for norepinephrine and epinephrine, *Circ. Res.,* 26, 53, 1970.

266. **Eriksson, B. M., Gustafsson, S., and Persson, B.-A.,** Determination of catecholamines in urine by ion-exchange liquid chromatography with electrochemical detection, *J. Chromatogr.,* 278, 255, 1983.

267. **Eriksson, B. M., and Persson, B.-A.,** Liquid chromatographic method for the determination of 3,4-dihydroxyphenylethylene glycol and 3,4-dihydroxymandelic acid in plasma, *J. Chromatogr.,* 386, 1, 1987.

268. **Evans, E., and Nicholls, P. J.,** A method for the gas chromatographic determination of urinary 1,4-methylimidazoleacetic acid, *J. Chromatogr.,* 82, 394, 1973.

269. **Fanget, F., Claustrat, B., Dalery, J., Brun, J., Terra, J.-L., Marie-Cardine, M., and Guyotat, J.,** Nocturnal plasma melatonin levels in schizophrenia patients, *Biol. Psychiatry,* 25, 499, 1989.

270. **Faull, K. F., Anderson, P. J., Barchas, J. D., and Berger, P. A.,** Selected ion monitoring assay for biogenic amine metabolites and probenecid in human lumbar cerebrospinal fluid, *J. Chromatogr.,* 163, 337, 1979.

271. **Faurbye, A., and Pind, K.,** Investigation on the occurrence of the dopamine metabolite 3,4-dimethoxyphenylethylamine in the urine of schizophrenics, *Acta Psychiatr. Scand.,* 40, 240, 1964.

272. **Fawcett, J., Maas, J. W., and Dekirmenjian, H.,** Depression and MHPG excretion, *Arch. Gen. Psychiatry,* 26, 246, 1972.

273. **Feldstein, A., Hoagland, H., and Freeman, H.,** On the relationship of serotonin to schizophrenia, *Science,* 128, 358, 1958.

274. **Feldstein, A., Hoagland, H., and Freeman, H.,** Blood and urinary serotonin and 5-hydroxyindoleacetic acid levels in schizophrenic patients and normal subjects, *J. Nerv. Ment. Dis.,* 129, 62, 1959.

275. **Fellenberg, A. J., Phillipou, G., and Seamark, R. F.,** Specific quantitation of urinary 6-hydroxymelatonin sulfate by gas chromatography mass spectrometry, *Biomed. Mass Spectrom.,* 7, 84, 1980.

276. **Fellows, L. E., King, G. S., Pettit, B. R., Goodwin, B. L., Ruthven, C. R. J., and Sandler, M.,** Phenylacetic acid in human cerebrospinal fluid and plasma: Selected ion monitoring assay, *Biomed. Mass Spectrom.,* 5, 508, 1978.

277. **Filser, J. G., Spira, J., Fischer, M., Gattaz, W. F., and Müller, W. E.,** The evaluation of 4-hydroxy-3-methoxyphenylglycol sulfate as a possible marker of central norepinephrine turnover. Studies in healthy volunteers and depressed patients, *J. Psychiatr. Res.,* 22, 171, 1988.

278. **Fiorica, V., and Moses, R.,** Automated differential fluorometric analysis of norepinephrine and epinephrine in blood plasma and urine, *Biochem. Med.,* 5, 483, 1971.

279. **Fischer, E., Heller, B., and Miró, A. H.,** β-Phenylethylamine in urine, *Arzneim. Forsch.,* 18, 1486, 1968.

280. **Fischer, E., and Spatz, H.,** Determination of bufotenin in the urine of schizophrenics, *Int. J. Neuropsychiatry,* 3, 226, 1967.

281. **Fischer, E., Spatz, H., Fernandez Labriola, R. S., Rodriguez Casanova, E. M., and Spatz, N.,** Quantitative gas-chromatographic determination and infrared spectrographic identification of urinary phenethylamine, *Biol. Psychiatry,* 7, 161, 1973.

282.   **Fischer, E., Spatz, H., Saavedra, J. M., Reggiani, H., Miró, A. H., and Heller, B.,** Urinary elimination of phenethylamine, *Biol. Psychiatry,* 5, 139, 1972.

283.   **Fischer, J. E., and Baldessarini, R. J.,** False neurotransmitters and hepatic failure, *Lancet,* 2, 75, 1971.

284.   **Fornstedt, N.,** Determination of 5-hydroxyindole-3-acetic acid in urine by high performance liquid chromatography, *Anal. Chem.,* 50, 1342, 1978.

285.   **Fornstedt, N.,** High performance liquid chromatographic determination of 5-hydroxyindole-3-acetic acid in urine using Sephadex G-10 for isolation, *J. Chromatogr.,* 181, 456, 1980.

286.   **Fotherby, K., Ashcroft, G. W., Affleck, J. W., Forrest, A. D.,** Studies on sodium transfer and 5-hydroxyindoles in depressive illness, *J. Neurol. Neurosurg. Psychiatry,* 26, 71, 1963.

287.   **Foti, A., Kimura, S., De Quattro, V., and Lee, D.,** Liquid chromatographic measurement of catecholamines and metabolites in plasma and urine, *Clin. Chem.* (Winston-Salem, N. C.), 33, 2209, 1987.

288.   **Fram, D. H., and Green, J. D.,** The presence and measurement of methylhistamine in urine, *J. Biol. Chem.,* 240, 2036, 1965.

289.   **Franco-Morselli, R., Elghozi, J. L., Joly, E., Di Giulio, S., and Meyer, P.,** Increased plasma adrenaline concentrations in benign essential hypertension, *Br. Med. J.,* 2, 1251, 1977.

290.   **Frankenhaeuser, M., Lundberg, U., von Wright, M. R., von Wright, J., and Sedvall, G.,** Urinary monoamine metabolites as indices of mental stress in healthy males and females, *Pharmacol. Biochem. Behav.,* 24, 1521, 1986.

291. **Franzen, F., and Gross, H.,** Tryptamine, *N,N*-dimethyltryptamine, *N,N*-dimethyl-5-hydroxytryptamine and 5-methoxytryptamine in human blood and urine, *Nature,* 206, 1052, 1965.

292. **Fraser, S., Cowen, P., Franklin, M., Franey, C., and Arendt, J.,** Direct radioimmunoassay for melatonin in plasma, *Clin. Chem. (Winston-Salem, N. C.),* 29, 396, 1983.

293. **Frattini, P., Cucchi, M. L., Santagostino, G., and Corona, G. L.,** A sensitive fluorimetric method for determination of platelet-bound and plasma free serotonin, *Clin. Chim. Acta,* 92, 353, 1979.

294. **Frattini, P., Santagostino, G., Cucchi, M. L., Corona, G. L., and Schinelli, S.,** 3-Methoxy-4-hydroxyphenylglycol in human cerebrospinal fluid, *Clin. Chim. Acta,* 125, 97, 1982.

295. **Fri, C.-G., Wiesel, F.-A., and Sedvall, G.,** Simultaneous quantification of homovanillic acid and 5-hydroxyindoleacetic acid in cerebrospinal fluid by mass fragmentography, *Life Sci.,* 14, 2469, 1974.

296. **Fri, C.-G., Wiesel, F.-A., and Sedvall, G.,** Mass fragmentographic analysis of homovanillic acid and its homoiso analogue in cerebrospinal fluid using the α-dideutero acid as internal standard, *Psychopharmacologia,* 35, 295, 1974.

297. **Friedhoff, A. J., Park, S., Schweitzer, J. W., Burdock, E. I., and Armour, M.,** Excretion of 3,4-dimethoxyphenethylamine (DMPEA) by acute schizophrenics and controls, *Biol. Psychiatry,* 12, 643, 1977.

298. **Friedman, M. J., Krstulovic, A. M., Colin, H., Guiochon, G., and Pajer, K.,** Serum indole-3-acetic acid in control subjects and newly abstinent alcoholics after an oral loading with L-tryptophan: A preliminary study using liquid chromatography with amperometric detection, *Anal. Biochem.,* 142, 480, 1984.

299. **Fyrö, B., Petterson, W., and Sedvall, G.,** The effect of lithium treatment on manic symptoms and levels of monoamine metabolites in cerebrospinal fluid of manic depressive patients, *Psychopharmacologia,* 44, 99, 1975.

300. **Fyrö, B., Wode-Helgodt, B., Borg, S., and Sedvall, G.,** The effect of chlorpromazine on homovanillic acid levels in cerebrospinal fluid of schizophrenic patients, *Psychopharmacologia,* 35, 287, 1974.

301. **Gaffney, F. A., Fenton, B. J., Lane, L. D., and Lake, C. R.,** Hemodynamics, ventilatory, and biochemical responses of panic patients and normal controls with sodium lactate infusion and spontaneous panic attacks, *Arch. Gen. Psychiatry,* 45, 53, 1988.

302. **Garden, J. W.,** Plasma and sweat histamine concentrations after heat exposure and physical exercise, *J. Appl. Physiol.,* 21, 631, 1966.

303. **Garelis, E., and Sourkes, T. L.,** Sites of origin in the central nervous system of monoamine metabolites measured in human cerebrospinal fluid, *J. Neurol. Neurosurg. Psychiatry,* 36, 625, 1973.

304. **Garfinkel, P. E., Warsh, J. J., and Stancer, H. C.,** Depression: New evidence in support of biological differentiation, *Am. J. Psychiatry,* 136, 535, 1979.

305. **Garfinkel, P. E., Warsh, J. J., Stancer, H. C., and Godse, D. D.,** CNS monoamine metabolism in bipolar affective disorder. Evaluation using a peripheral decarboxylase inhibitor, *Arch. Gen. Psychiatry,* 34, 735, 1977.

306.   **Garnier, J. P., Bousquet, B., and Dreux, C.,** Determination of 5-hydroxyindoleacetic acid in urine by high-performance liquid chromatography: A fully automated method, *J. Chromatogr.,* 204, 225, 1981.

307.   **Garvey, M. J., Tollefson, G. D., and Orsulak, P. J.,** Elevations of urinary MHPG in depressed patients with panic attacks, *Psychiatry Res.,* 20, 183, 1987.

308.   **Gashkoff, P., Matalon, R., Papa, V., and Sebasta, D.,** Analysis of the pentafluorobenzoyl derivative of phenylethylamine utilizing negative ion chemical ionization and gas chromatography/mass spectrometry, *Biomed. Environ. Mass Spectrom.,* 16, 327, 1988.

309.   **Gattaz, W. F., Gasser, T., and Beckmann, H.,** Multidimensional analysis of the concentrations of 17 substances in the CSF of schizophrenics and controls, *Biol. Psychiatry,* 20, 360, 1985.

310.   **Gattaz, W. F., Riederer, P., Reynolds, G. P., Gattaz, D., and Beckmann, H.,** Dopamine and noradrenaline in the cerebrospinal fluid of schizophrenic patients, *Psychiatry Res.,* 8, 243, 1983.

311.   **Gattaz, W. F., Waldmeier, P., and Beckmann, H.,** CSF monoamine metabolites in schizophrenic patients, *Acta Psychiatr. Scand.,* 66, 350, 1982.

312.   **Geffen, L. B., Rush, R. A., Louis, W. J., and Doyle, A. E.,** Plasma dopamine-β-hydroxylase and noradrenaline amounts in essential hypertension, *Clin. Sci.,* 44, 617, 1973.

313.   **Geissbühler, F.,** Dosage fluorométrique de l'acide homovanillic dans le liquide céphalorachidien, l'urine et le sang, *Clin. Chim. Acta,* 26, 231, 1969.

314. **Gerbode, F. A., and Bowers, M. B.**, Measurement of acid monoamine metabolites in human and animal cerebrospinal fluid, *J. Neurochem.*, 15, 1053, 1968.

315. **Gerhardt, G. A., Drebing, C. J., and Freedman, R.**, Simultaneous determination of free homovanillic acid, (3-methoxy-4-hydroxyphenyl)ethylene glycol, and vanilmandelic acid in human plasma by high-performance liquid chromatography coupled with dual-electrode coulometric electrochemical detection, *Anal. Chem.*, 58, 2879, 1986.

316. **Gerner, R. H., Fairbanks, L., Anderson, G. M., Young, J. G., Scheinin, M., Linnoila, M., Hare, T. A., Shaywitz, B. A., and Cohen, D. J.**, CSF neurochemistry in depressed, manic and schizophrenic patients compared with that of normal controls, *Am. J. Psychiatry*, 141, 1533, 1984.

317. **Gibson, C. J., Logue, M., Growdon, J. H.**, CSF monoamine metabolite levels in Alzheimer's and Parkinson's disease, *Arch. Neurol.*, 42, 489, 1985.

318. **Gilbert, H. S., Warner, R. R. P., and Wasserman, L. R.**, A study of histamine in myeloproliferative disease, *Blood*, 28, 795, 1966.

319. **Gironi, A., Seghieri, G., Niccolai, M., and Mammini, P.**, Simultaneous liquid-chromatographic determination of urinary vanillylmandelic acid, homovanillic acid, and 5-hydroxyindoleacetic acid, *Clin. Chem.* (Winston-Salem, N. C.), 34, 2504, 1988.

320. **Gitlow, S. E., Mendlowitz, M., Khassis, S., Cohen, G., and Sha, J.**, The diagnosis of pheochromocytoma by determination of urinary 3-methoxy-4-hydroxymandelic acid, *J. Clin. Invest.*, 39, 221, 1960.

321. **Gitlow, S. E., Ornstein, L., Mendlowitz, M., Khassis, S., and Kruk, E.,** A simple colorimetric test for pheochromocytoma, *Am. J. Med.,* 28, 921, 1960.

322. **Gjerris, A., Werdelin, L., Gjerris, F., Sorensen, P. S., Rafaelsen, O. J., and Alling, C.,** CSF amine metabolites in depression, dementia and in controls, *Acta Psychiatr. Scand.,* 75, 619, 1987.

323. **Godwin-Austen, R. B., Kantamaneni, B. D., and Curzon, G.,** Comparison of benefit from L-DOPA in Parkinsonism with increase of amine metabolites in the CSF, *J. Neurol. Neurosurg. Psychiatry,* 34, 219, 1971.

324. **Golden, R. N., Markey, S. P., Risby, E. D., Rudorfer, M. V., Cowdry, R. W., and Potter, W. Z.,** Antidepressants reduce whole-body norepinephrine turnover while enhancing 6-hydroxymelatonin output, *Arch. Gen. Psychiatry,* 45, 150, 1988.

325. **Golden, R. N., Rudorfer, M. V., Sherer, M. A., Linnoila, M., and Potter, W. Z.,** Bupropion in depression. I. Biochemical effects and clinical response, *Arch. Gen. Psychiatry,* 45, 139, 1988.

326. **Goldenberg, H.,** Specific photometric determination of 5-hydroxy-indoleacetic acid in urine, *Clin. Chem.* (Winston-Salem, N. C.), 19, 38, 1973.

327. **Goldfien, A., Zileli, S., Goodman, D., and Thorn, G. W.,** The estimation of epinephrine and norepinephrine in human plasma, *J. Clin. Endocrinol. Metab.,* 21, 281, 1961.

328. **Goldstein, D. S.,** Modified sample preparation for high-performance liquid chromatographic-electrochemical assay of urinary catecholamines, *J. Chromatogr.,* 275, 174, 1983.

329. **Goldstein, D. S., Eisenhofer, G., Stull, R., Folio, C. J., Keiser, H. R., and Kopin, I. J.,** Plasma dihydroxyphenylglycol and the intraneuronal disposition of norepinephrine in humans, *J. Clin. Invest.,* 81, 213, 1988.

330. **Goldstein, D. S., Feuerstein, G., Izzo, J. L., Kopin, I. J., and Keiser, H. R.,** Validity and reliability of liquid chromatography with electrochemical detection for measuring plasma levels of norepinephrine and epinephrine in man, *Life Sci.,* 28, 467, 1981.

331. **Goldstein, D. S., Stull, R., Zimlichman, R., Levinson, P. D., Smith, H., and Keiser, H. R.,** Simultaneous measurement of DOPA, DOPAC, and catecholamines in plasma by liquid chromatography with elctrochemical detection, *Clin. Chem.* (Winston-Salem, N. C.), 30, 815, 1984.

332. **Gomes, U. C. R., Shanley, B. C., Potgieter, L., and Roux, J. T.,** Noradrenergic overactivity in chronic schizophrenia: Evidence based on cerebrospinal fluid noradrenaline and cyclic nucleotide concentrations, *Br. J. Psychiatry,* 137, 346, 1980.

333. **González-Sastre, F., Mora, J., Guillamat, R., Queralto, J. M., Alvarez, E., Udina, C., and Massana, J.,** Urinary phenylacetic acid excretion in depressive patients, *Acta Psychiatr. Scand.,* 78, 208, 1988.

334. **Goodman, I., Olenczak, A. P., and Hiatt, R. B.,** 4-Hydroxy-3-methoxymandelic acid (HMMA) in the urine of normal and fasting subjects and in patients with colitis, *Clin. Chim. Acta,* 16, 245, 1967.

335. **Goodwin, B. L., Ruthven, C. R. J., and Sandler, M.,** Gas chromatographic assay of phenylacetic acid in biological fluids, *Clin. Chim. Acta,* 62, 443, 1975.

336. **Goodwin, F. K., Post, R. M., Dunner, D. L., and Gordon, E. K.,** Cerebrospinal fluid amine metabolites in affective illness: The probenecid technique, *Am. J. Psychiatry,* 130, 73, 1973.

337. **Gordon, E. K., Markey, S. P., Sherman, R. L., and Kopin, I. J.,** Conjugated 3,4-dihydroxyphenylacetic acid (DOPAC) in human and monkey cerebrospinal fluid and rat brain and the effects of probenecid treatment, *Life Sci.,* 18, 1285, 1976.

338. **Gordon, E. K. and Oliver, J.,** 3-Methoxy-4-hydroxyphenylethylene glycol in human cerebrospinal fluid, *Clin. Chim. Acta,* 35, 145, 1971.

339. **Gordon, E. K., Oliver, J., Goodwin, F. K., Chase, T. N., and Post, R. M.,** Effect of probenecid on free 3-methoxy-4-hydroxyphenylethylene glycol (MHPG) and its sulfate in human cerebrospinal fluid, *Neuropharmacology,* 12, 391, 1973.

340. **Gordon, E. K., Oliver, J., and Kopin, I. J.,** The effect of probenecid on catecholamine metabolites in human cerebrospinal fluid analyzed by mass fragmentography, *Life Sci.,* 16, 1527, 1975.

341. **Gottfries, C. G., Gottfries, I., Johansson, B., Olsson, R., Person, T., Roos, B.-E., and Sjöstrom, R.,** Acid monoamine metabolites in human cerebrospinal fluid and their relations to age and sex, *Neuropharmacology,* 10, 665, 1971.

342. **Gottfries, C. G., Gottfries, I., and Roos, B.-E.,** Homovanillic acid and 5-hydroxyindoleacetic acid in the cerebrospinal fluid of patients with senile dementia, presenile dementia, and parkinsonism, *J. Neurochem.,* 16, 1341, 1969.

343. **Gottfries, C. G., Gottfries, I., and Roos, B.-E.,** Homovanillic acid and 5-hydroxyindoleacetic acid in cerebrospinal fluid related to rated mental and motor impairment in senile and presenile dementia, *Acta Psychiatr. Scand.,* 46, 99, 1970.

344. **Gottfries, C. G., and Roos, B.-E.,** Acid monoamine metabolites in cerebrospinal fluid from patients with presenile dementia (Alzheimer's Disease), *Acta Psychiatr. Scand.,* 49, 257, 1973.

345. **Graham, H., Scarpellini, J. A. D., Hubka, B. P., and Lowry, O. H.,** Measurement and normal range of free histamine in human blood plasma, *Biochem. Pharmacol.,* 17, 2271, 1968.

346. **Greenspan, K., Schildkraut, J. J., Gordon, E. K., Baer, L., Aronoff, M. S., and Durell, J.,** Catecholamine metabolism in affective disorders. III. MHPG and other catecholamine metabolites in patients treated with lithium carbonate, *J. Psychiatr. Res.,* 7, 171, 1970.

347. **Griffiths, J. C., Leung, F. Y. T., and McDonald, T. J.,** Fluorimetric determination of plasma catecholamines: Normal human epinephrine and norepinephrine levels, *Clin. Chim. Acta,* 30, 395, 1970.

348. **Guilbault, G. G., and Froehlich, P. M.,** New assay for tryptophan and its 5-hydroxyindole metabolites in blood, *Clin. Chem.* (Winston-Salem, N. C.), 20, 812, 1974.

349. **Guillemin, A., Troupel, S., and Galli, A.,** Determination of catecholamines in plasma by high-performance liquid chromatography, *Clin. Chem.* (Winston-Salem, N. C.), 34, 1913, 1988.

350. **Guilloux, L., Hartmann, D., and Ville, G.,** Enzymatic isotopic assay for human plasma histamine, *Clin. Chim. Acta,* 116, 269, 1981.

350a. **Gullestad, L., Øystein Dolva, L., Kjeldsen, S. E., Eide, I., and Kjekshus, J.,** The effects of naloxone and timolol on plasma catecholamine levels during short-term dynamic exercise, *Scand. J. Clin. Lab. Invest.,* 47, 847, 1987.

351. **Gumboldt, G.,** Colorimetric method for the rapid and quantitative determination of 4-hydroxy-3-methoxymandelic acid (vanilmandelic acid) in human urine, *Clin. Chem.* (Winston-Salem, N. C.), 23, 1949, 1977.

352. **Gupta, R. N., Price, D., Keane, P. M.,** Modified Pisano method for estimating urinary metanephrines, *Clin. Chem.* (Winston-Salem, N. C.), 19, 611, 1973.

353. **Gusovsky, F., Sabelli, H., Fawcett, J., Edwards, J., and Javaid, J. I.,** Gas-liquid chromatographic determination of total phenylacetic acid in urine, *Anal. Biochem.,* 136, 202, 1984.

354. **Guthrie, S. K., Berrettini, W., Rubinow, D. R., Nurnberger, J. I., Bartko, J. J., and Linnoila, M.,** Different neurotransmitter metabolite concentrations in CSF samples from inpatient and outpatient normal volunteers, *Acta Psychiatr. Scand.,* 73, 315, 1986.

355. **Häggendal, J.,** An improved method for fluorimetric determination of small amounts of adrenaline and noradrenaline in plasma and tissues, *Acta Physiol. Scand.,* 59, 242, 1963.

356. **Halaris, A. E., De Met, E. M., and Halari, M. E.,** Determination of plasma 3-methoxy-4-hydroxyphenylglycol by pulsed electron capture gas chromatography, *Clin. Chim. Acta,* 78, 285, 1977.

357. **Halbreich, U., Sharpless, N., Asnis, G. M., Endicott, J., Goldstein, S., Vital-Herne, J., Eisenberg, J., Zander, K., Kang, B.-J., Shindledecker, R., and Yeh, C.-M.,** Afternoon continuous plasma levels of 3-methoxy-4-hydroxyphenylglycol and age Distinctive biologic subgroups of endogenous depression? *Arch. Gen. Psychiatry,* 44, 804, 1987.

358. **Halbrügge, T., Gerhardt, T., Ludwig, J., Heidbreder, E., and Graefe, K.-H.,** Assay of catecholamines and dihydroxyphenylethylene-glycol in human plasma and its application in orthostasis and mental stress, *Life Sci.,* 43, 19, 1988.

359. **Hallman, H., Farnebo, L.-O., Hamberger, B., and Jonsson, G.,** A sensitive method for the determination of plasma catecholamines using liquid chromatography with electrochemical detection, *Life Sci.,* 23, 1049, 1978.

360. **Hamaji, M., and Seki, T.,** Estimation of catecholamines in human plasma by ion-exchange chromatography coupled with fluorimetry, *J. Chromatogr.,* 163, 329, 1979.

361. **Hamlin, C. L., Lydiard, R. B., Martin, D., Dackis, C. A., Pottash, A. C., Sweeney, D., and Gold, M. S.,** Urinary excretion of noradrenaline metabolite decreased in panic disorder, *Lancet,* 2, 740, 1983.

362. **Hariharan, M., Van Noord, T., Cameron, O. G., Curtis, G. C., and Ostrow, D. G.,** Free 3-methoxy-4-hydroxyphenylglycol determined in plasma by liquid chromatography with coulometric detection, *Clin. Chem.* (Winston-Salem, N. C.), 35, 202, 1989.

363. **Härnryd, C., Bjerkenstedt, L., Grimm, V. E., and Sedvall, G.,** Reduction of MOPEG levels in cerebrospinal fluid of psychotic women after electroconvulsive treatment, *Psychopharmacology,* 64, 131, 1979.

364. **Harris, P. Q., Bacopoulos, N. G., and Brown, S. J.,** Measurement of homovanillic acid in human plasma by high performance liquid chromatography with electrochemical detection, *J. Chromatogr.,* 309, 379, 1984.

365. **Harris, P. Q., Brown, S. J., Friedman, M. J., and Bacopoulos, N. G.,** Plasma, drug and homovanillic acid levels in psychotic patients receiving neuroleptics, *Biol. Psychiatry,* 19, 849, 1984.

366. **Harris, J., Davis, B. A., Krahenbuhl, G. S., and Boulton, A. A.,** Trace amines/metabolite responses in stress, in *Neuropsychopharmacology of the Trace Amines,* Boulton, A. A., Maitre, L., Bieck, P., and Reiderer, P., Eds., Humana Press Inc., New Jersey, 1985, 395.

367. **Harsing, L. G., Nagashima, H., Duncalf, D., Vizi, E. S., and Goldiner, P. L.,** Determination of histamine concentration in plasma by liquid chromatography/electrochemistry, *Clin. Chem.* (Winston-Salem, N. C.), 32, 1823, 1986.

368. **Hathaway, P. W., Jakoi, L., Troyer, W. G., and Bogdonoff, M. D.,** A method for semiautomatic differential analysis of urinary catecholamines, *Anal. Biochem.,* 20, 466, 1967.

369. **Haverback, B. J., Sjoerdsma, A., and Terry, L. L.,** Urinary excretion of the serotonin metabolite, 5-hydroxyindoleacetic acid, in various clinical conditions, *New Engl. J. Med.,* 255, 270, 1956.

370. **Heh, C. W. C., Potkin, S. G., Pickar, D., Costa, J., Herrara, J., Sramek, J., and De Met, E.,** Serum homovanillic acid concentrations in carbamazine-treated chronic schizophrenics, *Biol. Psychiatry,* 25, 639, 1989.

371. **Heller, B., and Fischer, E.,** Diminution of phenethylamine in the urine of Parkinson patients, *Arzneim. Forsch.,* 23, 884, 1973.

372. **Hempel, K., Ullrich, H., and Philippu, G.,** Quantitative investigation on the urinary excretion and metabolism of 3,4-dimethoxyphenylethylamine in schizophrenics and normal individuals, *Biol. Psychiatry,* 17, 49, 1982.

373. **Henry, D. P., Starman, B. J., Johnson, D. G., and Williams, R. H.**, A sensitive radioenzymatic assay for norepinephrine in tissues and plasmas, *Life Sci.*, 16, 375, 1975.

374. **Herkert, E. E., and Keup, W.**, Excretion patterns of tryptamine, indoleacetic acid, and 5-hydroxyindoleacetic acid, and their correlation with mental changes in schizphrenic patients under medication with *alpha*-methyldopa, *Psychopharmacologia*, 15, 48, 1969.

375. **Hermann, G. A.**, The determination of urinary 3-methoxy-4-hydroxymandelic (vanilmandelic) acid by means of electrophoresis with cellulose acetate membrane, *Am. J. Clin. Pathol.*, 41, 373, 1964.

376. **Higa, S., and Markey, S. P.**, Identification and quantification of 5-methoxyindole-3-acetic acid in human urine, *Anal. Biochem.*, 144, 86, 1985.

377. **Higa, S., Suzuki, T., Hayashi, A., Tsuge, I., and Yamamura, Y.**, Isolation of catecholamines in biological fluids by boric acid gel, *Anal. Biochem.*, 77, 18, 1977.

378. **Hindberg, I.**, An improved specific and sensitive radioenzymatic method for determination of serotonin concentrations in biological fluids (radioenzymatic serotonin method), *Scand. J. Clin. Lab. Invest.*, 44, 47, 1984.

379. **Hiramatsu, M., Fujimoto, N., and Mori, A.**, Catecholamine level in cerebrospinal fluid of epileptics, *Neurochem. Res.*, 7, 1299, 1982.

380. **Hjemdahl, P., Sjöquist, B., Daleskog, M., and Eliasson, K.**, A comparison of noradrenaline, HMPG and VMA in plasma as indicators of sympathetic nerve activity in man, *Acta Physiol. Scand.*, 115, 507, 1982.

381. **Hoeldtke, R. D., and Sloan, J. W.**, Acid hydrolysis of urinary catecholamines, *J. Lab. Clin. Med.*, 75, 159, 1970.

382.   **Hoffmann, G., Linkowski, P., Kerkhofs, M., Desmedt, D., and Mendlewicz, J.,** Effects of ECT on sleep and CSF biogenic amines in affective illness, *Psychiatry Res.,* 16, 199, 1985.

383.   **Hollister, L. E., Davis, K. L., and Berger, P. A.,** Subtypes of depression based on excretion of MHPG and response to nortriptyline, *Arch. Gen. Psychiatry,* 37, 1107, 1980.

384.   **Hollister, L. E., Davis, K. L., Overall, J. E., and Anderson, T.,** Excretion of MHPG in normal subjects. Implications for biological classification of affective disorders, *Arch. Gen. Psychiatry,* 35, 1410, 1978.

385.   **Holly, J. M. P., and Makin, H. L. J.,** The estimation of catecholamines in human plasma, *Anal. Biochem.,* 128, 257, 1983.

386.   **Honegger, C. G., Burri, R., Langemann, H., Kempf, A.,** Determination of neurotransmitter systems in human cerebrospinal fluid and rat nervous tissue by high-performance liquid chromatography with on-line data evaluation, *J. Chromatogr.,* 309, 53, 1984.

387.   **Hopkinson, G., Baker, G. B., Douglass, A. B., McKim, H. R., and Dewhurst, W. G.,** Analysis of urinary excretion patterns of bioactive amines and their metabolites in normal control subjects, *Prog. Neuro-Psychopharmacol. Biol. Psychiatry,* 6, 495, 1982.

388.   **Horakova, Z., Keiser, H. R., and Beaven, M. A.,** Blood and urine histamine levels in normal and pathological states as measured by a radiochemical assay, *Clin. Chim. Acta,* 79, 447, 1977.

389.   **Hörtnagl, H., Benedict, C. R., Grahame-Smith, D. G., and McGrath, B.,** A sensitive radioenzymatic assay for adrenaline and noradrenaline in plasma, *Br. J. Clin. Pharmacol.,* 4, 553, 1977.

390. **Hoskins, J. A., and Pollitt, R. J.,** Quantitative aspects of urinary indole-3-acetic acid and 5-hydroxyindole-3-acetic acid excretion, *J. Chromatogr.*, 109, 436, 1975.

391. **Hoskins, J. A., Pollitt, R. J., and Evans, S.,** The determination of 5-methoxyindole-3-acetic acid in human urine by mass fragmentography, *J. Chromatogr.*, 145, 285, 1978.

392. **Houston, J. P., Maas, J. W., Bowden, C. L., Contreras, S. A., McIntyre, K. L., and Javors, M. A.,** Cerebrospinal fluid HVA, central brain atrophy and clinical state in schizophrenia, *Psychiatry Res.*, 19, 207, 1986.

393. **Howes, L. G., Miller, S., and Reid, J. L.,** Simultaneous assay of 3,4-dihydroxyphenylethylene glycol and norepinephrine in human plasma by high-performance liquid chromatography with electrochemical detection, *J. Chromatogr.*, 338, 401, 1985.

394. **Hsiao, J. K., Ågren, H., Bartko, J. J., Rudorfer, M. V., Linnoila, M., and Potter, W. Z.,** Monoamine neurotransmitter interactions and the prediction of antidepressant response, *Arch. Gen. Psychiatry,* 44, 1078, 1987.

395. **Huber-Smith, M. J., Nesse, R., Mazhar, M., and McCann, D. S.,** Evaluation of plasma 3-methoxy-4-hydroxyphenylglycol, *J. Chromatogr.*, 377, 91, 1986.

396. **Huebert, N. D., and Boulton, A. A.,** Longitudinal urinary trace amine excretion in a human male, *J. Chromatogr.*, 162, 169, 1979.

397. **Hunneman, D. H.,** Mass fragmentographic determination of homovanillic and 4-hydroxy-3-methoxymandelic acids in 50 µL plasma, *Clin. Chim. Acta,* 135, 169, 1983.

397a.   **Hussain, M. N., and Benedict, C. R.,** Radioenzymatic assay for picogram quantities of serotonin or acetylserotonin in biological fluids and tissues, *Biochem. Med. Metab. Biol.,* 37, 314, 1987.

398.   **Hussain, M. N., and Sole, M. J.,** A simple, specific radioenzymatic assay for picogram quantities of serotonin or acetylserotonin in biological fluids and tissues, *Anal. Biochem.,* 111, 105, 1981.

399.   **Ibrahim, K. E., Couch, M. W., Williams, C. M., Budd, M. B., Yost, R. A., and Midgley, J. M.,** Quantitative measurement of octopamines and synephrines in urine using capillary column gas chromatography negative ion chemical ionization mass spectrometry, *Anal. Chem.,* 56, 1695, 1984.

400.   **Imai, Y., Ito, S., Maruta, K., and Fujita, K.,** Simultaneous determination of catecholamines and serotonin by liquid chromatography after treatment with boric acid gel, *Clin. Chem.* (Winston-Salem, N. C.), 34, 528, 1988.

401.   **Imai, Y., and Tamura, Z.,** Liquid chromatographic determination of urinary dopamine and norepinephrine as fluorescamine derivatives, *Clin. Chim. Acta,* 85, 1, 1978.

402.   **Imai, K., Wang, M.-T., Yoshiue, S., and Tamura, Z.,** Determination of catecholamines in the plasma of patients with essential hypertension and of normal persons, *Clin. Chim. Acta,* 43, 145, 1973.

403.   **Imamura, I., Maeyama, K., Wada, H., Watanabe, T.,** Determination of imidazole acetic acid and its conjugate(s) levels in urine, serum and tissues of rats: Studies on changes in their levels under various conditions, *Br. J. Pharmacol.,* 82, 701, 1984.

404.   **Ind, P. W., Barnes, P. J., Brown, M. J., Causon, R., Dollery, C. T.,** Measurement of plasma histamine in asthma, *Clin. Allergy,* 13, 61, 1983.

405. **Inwang, E. E., Madubuike, P. U., and Mosnaim, A. D.,** Evidence for the excretion of 2-phenylethylamine glucuronide in human urine, *Experientia,* 29, 1080, 1973.

406. **Ishimitsu, T., and Hirose, S.,** Simultaneous assay of 3,4-dihydroxyphenylalanine, catecholamines and *O*-methylated metabolites in human plasma using high-performance liquid chromatography, *J. Chromatogr.,* 337, 239, 1985.

407. **Izzo, J. L., and Greulich, D.,** Radioenzymatic assay for plasma dihydroxyphenylglycol (DHPG), dihydroxymandelic acid (DOMA) and dihydroxyphenylacetic acid (DOPAC), *Life Sci.,* 33, 483, 1983.

408. **Izzo, J. L., Thompson, D. A., and Horwitz, D.,** Plasma dihydroxyphenylglycol (DHPG) in the *in vivo* assessment of human neuronal norepinephrine metabolism, *Life Sci.,* 37, 1033, 1985.

409. **Javors, M. A., Bowden, C. L., and Maas, J. W.,** 3-Methoxy-4-hydroxyphenylglycol, 5-hydroxyindoleacetic acid, and homovanillic acid in human cerebrospinal fluid. Storage and measurement by reversed-phase high-performance liquid chromatography and coulometric detection using 3-methoxy-4-hydroxyphenyllactic acid as an internal standard, *J. Chromatogr.,* 336, 259, 1984.

410. **Jepson, J. B.,** Indolylacetyl-glutamine and other indole metabolites in Hartnup disease, *Biochem. J.,* 64, 14P, 1956.

411. **Jepson, J. B., Lovenberg, W., Zaltzman, P., Oates, J. A., Sjoerdsma, A., and Udenfriend, S.,** Amine metabolism studied in normal and phenylketonuric humans by monoamine oxidase inhibition, *Biochem. J.,* 74, 5P, 1960.

412. **Jéquier, E., and Dufresne, J. J.,** Biochemical investigations in patients with Parkinson's disease treated with L-DOPA, *Neurology,* 22, 15, 1972.

413.   **Jeste, D. V., Doongaji, D. R., Panjwani, D., Datta, M., Potkin, S. G., Karoum, F., Thatte, S., Sheth, A. S., Apte, J. S., and Wyatt, R. J.,** Cross-cultural study of a biochemical abnormality in paranoid schizophrenia, *Psychiatry Res.,* 3, 341, 1980.

414.   **Jimerson, D. C., Ballenger, J. C., Lake, C. R., Post, R. M., Goodwin, F. K., and Kopin, I. J.,** Plasma and CSF MHPG in normals, *Psychopharmacol. Bull.,* 17(1), 86, 1981.

415.   **Jimerson, D. C., Gordon, E. K., Post, R. M., and Goodwin, F. K.,** Vanillylmandelic acid in CSF, *Brain Res.,* 99, 434, 1975.

416.   **Jimerson, D. C., Gordon, E. K., Post, R. M., and Goodwin, F. K.,** Homovanillic acid in human CSF: Comparison of fluorimetry and gas chromatography-mass spectrometry, *Commun. Psychopharmacol.,* 2, 343, 1978.

417.   **Jimerson, D. C., Lynch, H. J., Post, R. M., Wurtman, R. J., and Bunney, W.E.,** Urinary melatonin rhythms during sleep deprivation in depressed patients and normals, *Life Sci.,* 20, 1501, 1977.

418.   **Jimerson, D. C., Markey, S. P., Oliver, J. A., and Kopin, I. J.,** Simultaneous measurement of plasma 4-hydroxy-3-methoxy-phenylethylene glycol and 3,4-dihydroxyphenylethylene glycol by gas chromatography-mass spectrometry, *Biomed. Mass Spectrom.,* 8, 256, 1981.

419.   **Jimerson, D. C., Nurnberger, J. I., Post, R. M., Gershon, E. S., and Kopin, I. J.,** Plasma MHPG in rapid cyclers and healthy twins, *Arch. Gen. Psychiatry,* 38, 1287, 1981.

420.   **Johansson, B., and Roos, B.-E.,** Concentrations of monoamine metabolites in human lumbar and cisternal cerebrospinal fluid, *Acta Neurol. Scand.,* 52, 137, 1975.

421. **Johnson, G. A., Baker, C. A., and Smith, R. T.,** Radioenzymatic assay of sulfate conjugates of catecholamines and DOPA in plasma, *Life Sci.,* 26, 1591, 1980.

422. **Jonassen, F., Granerus, G., and Wetterqvist, H.,** Histamine metabolism during the mestrual cycle, *Acta Obstet. Gynecol. Scand.,* 55, 297, 1976.

423. **Jones, D. H., Hamilton, C. A., and Reid, J. L.,** Plasma noradrenaline, age and blood pressure: A population study, *Clin. Sci. Mol. Med.,* 55, 73s, 1978.

424. **Jones, R. L., Bory, P., Brown, W. T., and McGeer, P. L.,** Failure to detect *p*-methoxyphenylethylamine derivatives in human urine, *Can. J. Biochem.,* 47, 185, 1969.

425. **Jonsson, J., and Lewander, T.,** A method for the simultaneous determination of 5-hydroxy-3-indole-acetic acid (5-HIAA) and 5-hydroxytryptamine (5-HT) in brain tissue and cerebrospinal fluid, *Acta Physiol. Scand.,* 78, 43, 1970.

426. **Jori, A., Dolfini, E., Casati, C., and Argenta, G.,** Effect of ECT and imipramine treatment on the concentration of 5-hydroxy-indoleacetic acid (5-HIAA) and homovanillic acid (HVA) in the cerebrospinal fluid of depressed patients, *Psychopharmacologia,* 44, 87, 1975.

427. **Joseph, M. H., Baker, H. F., Johnstone, E. C., and Crow, T. J.,** Determination of 3-methoxy-4-hydroxyphenylglycol conjugates in urine. Application to the study of central noradrenaline metabolism in unmedicated chronic schizophrenic patients, *Psychopharmacology,* 51, 47, 1976.

428. **Joseph, M. H., Baker, H. F., Johnstone, E. C., and Crow, T. J.**, 3-Methoxy-4-hydroxyphenylglycol excretion in acutely schizophrenic patients during a controlled clinical trial of the isomers of flupenthixol, *Psychopharmacology*, 64, 35, 1979.

429. **Joyce, D. A., Beilin, L. J., Vandongen, R., and Davidson, L.**, Plasma free and sulfate conjugated catecholamine levels during acute physiological stimulation in man, *Life Sci.*, 30, 447, 1982.

430. **Jouve, J., Mariotte, N., Sureau, C., and Muh, J. P.**, High-performance liquid chromatography with electrochemical detection for the simultaneous determination of the methoxylated amines, normetanephrine, metanephrine and 3-methoxytyramine in urine, *J. Chromatogr.*, 274, 53, 1983.

431. **Julien, C., Rodriguez, C., Sacquet, J., Cuisinaud, G., and Sassard, J.**, Liquid-chromatographic determination of free and total 3,4-dihydroxyphenylglycol and 3-methoxy-4-hydroxyphenylglycol in urine, *Clin. Chem. (Winston-Salem, N. C.)*, 34, 966, 1988.

432. **Kahane, Z., Jindal, S. P., and Vestergaard, P.**, Gas chromatographic estimation of 3,4-dihydroxyphenylglycol in urine as the diacetylphenyl-bis (tri-methyl) silyl ether, *Clin. Chim. Acta*, 73, 203, 1976.

433. **Kahane, Z., and Vestergaard, P.**, Fluorimetric assay for metanephrine and normetanephrine in urine, *J. Lab. Clin. Med.*, 70, 333, 1967.

434. **Kahane, Z., and Vestergaard, P.**, The quantitative estimation of urinary 3-methoxy-4-hydroxyphenylacetic acid (homovanillic acid), *Clin. Chim. Acta*, 35, 49, 1971.

435. **Kangasniemi, P. K., Sonninen, V., and Rinne, U. K.,** Excretion of free and conjugated 5-HIAA and VMA in urine and concentration of 5-HIAA and HVA in CSF during migraine attacks and free intervals, *Headache,* 12, 62, 1972.

436. **Karege, F.,** Method for total 3-methoxy-4-hydroxyphenylglycol extraction from urine, plasma and brain tissue using bonded-phase materials: Comparison with the ethyl acetate extraction method, *J. Chromatogr.,* 311, 361, 1984.

437. **Kärki, N. T.,** The urinary excretion of noradrenaline and adrenaline in different age groups, its diurnal variation and the effect of muscular work on it, *Acta Physiol. Scand.,* 39 (Suppl. 132), 1, 1956.

438. **Kärkkäinen, J., Räisänen, M., Naukkarinen, H., Spoov, J., and Rimon, R.,** Urinary excretion of free bufotenin by psychiatric patients, *Biol. Psychiatry,* 24, 441, 1988.

439. **Karoum, F., Anah, C. O., Ruthven, C. R. J., and Sandler, M.,** Further observations on the gas chromatographic measurement of urinary phenolic and indolic metabolites, *Clin. Chim. Acta,* 24, 341, 1969.

440. **Karoum, F., Bunney, W., Gillin, J. C., Jimerson, D., Van Kammen, D., and Wyatt, R. J.,** Effect of probenecid on the concentration of the lumbar cerebrospinal fluid acidic metabolites of tyramine, octopamine, dopamine and norepinephrine, *Biochem. Pharmacol.,* 26, 629, 1977.

441. **Karoum, F., Chuang, L.-W., Eisler, T., Calne, D. B., Liebowitz, M. R., Quitkin, F. M., Klein, D. F., and Wyatt, R. J.,** Metabolism of (-)deprenyl to amphetamine and methamphetamine may be responsible for deprenyl's therapeutic benefit: A biochemical assessment, *Neurology,* 32, 503, 1982.

442. **Karoum, F., Chuang, L.-W., Mosnaim, A. D., Staub, R. A., and Wyatt, R. J.,** Plasma and cerebrospinal fluid concentration of phenylacetic acid in humans and monkeys, *J. Chromatogr. Sci.,* 21, 546, 1983.

443. **Karoum, F., Gillin, J. C., McCullough, D., and Wyatt, R. J.,** Vanilmandelic acid (VMA) free and conjugated 3-methoxy-4-hydroxyphenylglycol (MHPG) in human ventricular fluid, *Clin. Chim. Acta,* 62, 451, 1975.

444. **Karoum, F., Gillin, J. C., Wyatt, R. J. and Costa, E.,** Mass fragmentography of nanogram quantities of biogenic amine metabolites in human cerebrospinal fluid and whole rat brain, *Biomed. Mass Spectrom.,* 2, 183, 1975.

445. **Karoum, F., Karson, C. N., Bigelow, L. B., Lawson, W. B., and Wyatt, R. J.,** Preliminary evidence of reduced combined output of dopamine and its metabolites in chronic schizophrenia, *Arch. Gen. Psychiatry,* 44, 604, 1987.

446. **Karoum, F., Lefèvre, H., Bigelow, L. B., and Costa, E.,** Urinary excretion of 4-hydroxy-3-methoxyphenylglycol and 4-hydroxy-3-methoxyphenylethanol in man and rat, *Clin. Chim. Acta,* 43, 127, 1973.

447. **Karoum, F., Moyer-Schwing, J., Potkin, S. G., and Wyatt, R. J.,** Plasma concentrations of some acidic and alcoholic metabolites derived from *m-* and *p-*tyramine, octopamine and catecholamines in humans, *Commun. Psychopharmacol.,* 1, 343, 1977.

448. **Karoum, F., Moyer-Schwing, J., Potkin, S. G., and Wyatt, R. J.,** Presence of free, sulfate and glucuronide conjugated 3-methoxy-4-hydroxyphenylglycol (MHPG) in human brain, cerebrospinal fluid and plasma, *Brain Res.,* 125, 333, 1977.

449. **Karoum, F., Nasrallah, H., Potkin, S., Chuang, L., Moyer-Schwing, J., Phillips, I., and Wyatt, R. J.,** Mass fragmentography of phenylethylamine, *m-* and *p*-tyramine and related amines in plasma, cerebrospinal fluid, urine and brain, *J. Neurochem.,* 33, 201, 1979.

450. **Karoum, F., Potkin, S. G., Chuang, L. W., Murphy, D. L., Liebowitz, M. R., and Wyatt, R. J.,** Phenylacetic acid excretion in schizophrenia and depression: The origins of PAA in man, *Biol. Psychiatry,* 19, 165, 1984.

451. **Karoum, F., Potkin, S. G., Murphy, D. L., and Wyatt, R. J.,** Quantitation and metabolism of phenylethylamine and tyramine's three isomers in humans, in *Noncatecholic Phenylethylamines Part 2. Phenylethanolamine, Tyramines and Octopamine,* Mosnaim, A. D., and Wolf, M. E., Eds., Marcel Dekker, New York, 1980, 177.

452. **Karoum, F., Linnoila, M., Potter, W. Z., Chuang, L. W., Goodwin, F. K., and Wyatt, R. J.,** Fluctuating high urinary phenylethylamine excretion rates in some bipolar affective disorder patients, *Psychiatry Res.,* 6, 215, 1982.

453. **Karoum, F., Ruthven, C. R. J., and Sandler, M.,** Gas chromatographic assay of phenolic alcohols in biological material using electron capture detection, *Biochem. Med.,* 5, 505, 1971.

454. **Karoum, F., Van Kammen, D. P., Bunney, W. E., Gillin, J. C., Jimerson, D. C., Post, R. M., and Wyatt, R. J.,** The effect of probenecid on the free and conjugated 3-methoxy-4-hydroxyphenylglycol (MHPG) in lumbar cerebrospinal fluid, *Psychopharmacol. Commun.,* 2, 141, 1976.

455. **Kasa, K., Otsuki, S., Yamamoto, M., Sato, M., Kuroda, H., and Ogawa, N.,** Cerebrospinal fluid γ-aminobutyric acid and homovanillic acid in depressive disorders, *Biol. Psychiatry,* 17, 877, 1982.

456. **Käser, H., and Thomke, E.,** Quantitative fluorimetric determination of urinary 3-methoxytyramine, *Clin. Chim. Acta,* 27, 203, 1970.

457. **Kawabata, M., Kobayashi, K., and Shohmori, T.,** Determination of phenylacetic acid in cerebrospinal fluid by gas chromatography-mass spectrometry, *Acta Med. Okayama,* 40, 271, 1986.

458. **Kay, A. D., Milstien, S., Kaufman, S., Rapoport, S. I., and Cutler, N. R.,** 5-HIAA and HVA in the CSF of patients with Alzheimer's disease, *Neurology,* 34, (Suppl. 1), 161, 1984.

459. **Kelvin, A. S.,** A further method of eliminating interfering compounds in the gas chromatographic determination of urinary methylimidazoleacetic acids, *Br. J. Pharmacol.,* 38, 466P, 1970.

460. **Kemali, D., Del Vecchio, M., and Maj, M.,** Increased noradrenaline levels in CSF and plasma of schizophrenic patients, *Biol. Psychiatry,* 17, 711, 1982.

461. **Kemerer, V. F., Lichtenfeld, K. M., and Koch, T. R.,** A column chromatographic method for the determination of 5-hydroxytryptamine (serotonin) and 5-hydroxyindoleacetic acid in cerebrospinal fluid, *Clin. Chim. Acta,* 92, 81, 1979.

462. **Keyzer, J. J., Breukelman, H., Elzinga, H., Koopman, B. J., Wolthers, B. G., and Bruins, A. P.,** Determination of histamine by chemical ionization mass spectrometry: Application to human urine, *Biomed. Mass Spectrom.,* 10, 480, 1983.

463. **Keyzer, J. J., Wolthers, B. G., Breukelman, H., Kauffman, H. F., and de Monchy, J. G. R.,** Determination of N^τ-methyl-imidazoleacetic acid (a histamine metabolite) in urine by gas chromatography using nitrogen-phosphorus detection, *Clin. Chim. Acta,* 121, 379, 1982.

464. **Keyzer, J. J., Wolthers, B. G., Muskiet, F. A. J., Breukelman, H., Kauffman, H. F., and de Vries, K.,** Measurement of plasma histamine by stable isotope dilution gas chromatography-mass spectrometry: Methodology and normal values, *Anal. Biochem.,* 139, 474, 1984.

465. **Keyzer, J. J., Wolthers, B. G., Muskiet, F. A. J., Kauffman, H. F., and Groen, A.,** Determination of N^τ-methylhistamine in plasma and urine by isotope dilution mass fragmentography, *Clin. Chim. Acta,* 113, 165, 1981.

466. **Khandelwal, J. K., Hough, L. B., and Green, J. P.,** Histamine and some of its metabolites in human body fluids, *Klin. Wochenschr.,* 60, 914, 1982.

467. **Khandelwal, J. K., Hough, L. B., Pazhenchevsky, B., Morrishow, A. M., and Green, J. P.,** Presence and measurement of methylimidazoleacetic acids in brain and body fluids, *J. Biol. Chem.,* 257, 12815, 1982.

468. **Khandelwal, J. K., Kline, T., and Green, J. P.,** Measurement of imidazoleacetic acid in urine by gas chromatography-mass spectrometry, *J. Chromatogr.,* 343, 249, 1985.

469. **King, G. S., Goodwin, B. L., Ruthven, C. R. J., and Sandler, M.,** Urinary excretion of *o*-tyramine, *Clin. Chim. Acta,* 51, 105, 1974.

470.   **Kirch, D., Hattox, S., Bell, J., Murphy, R., and Freedman, R.,** Plasma homovanillic acid and tardive dyskinesia during neuroleptic maintenance and withdrawal, *Psychiatry Res.,* 9, 217, 1983.

471.   **Kiriike, N., Uete, T., Motomura, K., Enomoto, M., and Murata, K.,** Urinary excretion of catecholamines and their metabolites in chronic schizophrenics treated with oxypertine and chlorpromazine, *Biol. Psychiatry,* 19, 417, 1984.

472.   **Kirschberg, G. J., Cote, L. J., Lowe, Y. H., and Ginsburg, S.,** Interference with the fluorometric assay for homovanillic acid caused by acid metabolites of catecholamines, *J. Neurochem.,* 19, 2873, 1972.

473.   **Kirstein, L., Bowers, M. B., and Heninger, G.,** CSF amine metabolites, clinical symptoms, and body movement in psychiatric patients, *Biol. Psychiatry,* 11, 421, 1976.

474.   **Kissinger, P. T., Riggin, R. M., Alcorn, R. L., and Rau, L.-D.,** Estimation of catecholamines in urine by high performance liquid chromatography with electrochemical detection, *Biochem. Med.,* 13, 299, 1975.

475.   **Klaniecki, T. S., Corder, C. N., McDonald, R. H., and Feldman, J. A.,** High-performance liquid chromatographic radioenzymatic assay for plasma catecholamines, *J. Lab. Clin. Med.,* 90, 604, 1977.

476.   **Klein, D., and Chernaik, J. M.,** Determination of urinary 3-methoxy-4-hydroxymandelic acid (vanillylmandelic acid) by paper elctrophoresis, *Clin. Chem.* (Winston-Salem, N. C.), 7, 257, 1961.

477.   **Knoll, E., and Wisser, H.,** Radioimmunologische Bestimmung von 3,4-Dimethoxyphenyläthylamin im Urin, *Clin. Chim. Acta,* 68, 327, 1976.

478. **Knoll, E., Wisser, H., and Emrich, H. M.,** 3,4-Dimethoxyphenyl-ethylamine excretion of normals and schizophrenics, behavior during total fasting, *Clin. Chim. Acta,* 89, 493, 1978.

479. **Ko, G. N., Elsworth, J. D., Roth, R. H., Rifkin, B. G., Leigh, H., and Redmond, D. E.,** Panic-induced elevation of plasma MHPG levels in phobic-anxious patients. Effects of clonidine and imipramine, *Arch. Gen. Psychiatry,* 40, 425, 1983.

480. **Ko, G. N., Jimerson, D. C., Wyatt, R. J., and Bigelow, L. B.,** Plasma 3-methoxy-4-hydroxyphenylglycol changes associated with clinical state and schizophrenic subtype, *Arch. Gen. Psychiatry,* 45, 842, 1988.

481. **Kobayashi, K., De Quattro, V., Kolloch, R., Miano, L.,** A radioenzymatic assay for plasma normetanephrine in man and patients with pheochromocytoma, *Life Sci.,* 26, 567, 1980.

482. **Kobayashi, K., Koide, Y., Shohmori, T.,** Determination of *p*-hydroxyphenylacetic acid in cerebrospinal fluid by high-performance liquid chromatography with electrochemical detection, *Clin. Chim. Acta,* 123, 161, 1982.

483. **Koch, D. D., and Kissinger, P. T.,** Determination of tryptophan and several of its metabolites in physiological samples by reversed-phase liquid chromatography with electrochemical detection, *J. Chromatogr.,* 164, 441, 1979.

484. **Koch, D. D., and Kissinger, P. T.,** Determination of serotonin in serum and plasma by liquid chromatography with precolumn sample enrichment and electrochemical detection, *Anal. Chem.,* 52, 27, 1980.

485. **Kodama, K., Yamanaka, K., Nakata, T., and Aoyama, M.,** Liquid-chromatographic assay of urinary vanillylmandelic acid and homovanillic acid, with clean-up by on-column injection of acetonitrile or methanol, *Clin. Chem.* (Winston-Salem, N. C.), 32, 1944, 1986.

486. **Kopin, I. J.,** Tryptophan loading and excretion of 5-hydroxyindoleacetic acid in normal and schizophrenic subjects, *Science,* 129, 835, 1959.

487. **Kopin, I. J., Lake, R. C., and Ziegler, M.,** Plasma levels of norepinephrine, *Ann. Int. Med.,* 88, 671, 1978.

488. **Kopin, I. J., Oliver, J. A., and Polinsky, R. J.,** Relationship between urinary excretion of homovanillic acid and norepinephrine metabolites in normal subjects and patients with orthostatic hypotension, *Life Sci.,* 43, 125, 1988.

489. **Kopin, I. J., Polinsky, R. J., Oliver, J. A., Oddershede, I. R., and Ebert, M. H.,** Urinary catecholamine metabolites distinguish different types of sympathetic neuronal dysfunction in patients with orthostatic hypotension, *J. Clin. Endocrinol. Metab.,* 57, 632, 1983.

490. **Korf, J., Ottema, S., and Vander Veen, I.,** Fluorometric determination of homovanillic acid in biological material after isolation on Sephadex G10, *Anal. Biochem.,* 40, 187, 1971.

491. **Korf, J., and Sebens, J. B.,** Determination of *O*-conjugates of 5-hydroxytryptamine in human urine, *Clin. Chim. Acta,* 27, 149, 1970.

492. **Korf, J., and Valkenburgh-Sikkema, T.,** Fluorimetric determination of 5-hydroxyindoleacetic acid in human urine and cerebrospinal fluid, *Clin. Chim. Acta,* 26, 301, 1969.

493. **Koslow, S. H., Maas, J. W., Bowden, C. L., Davis, J. M., Hanin, I., and Javaid, J.,** CSF and urinary biogenic amines and metabolites in depression and mania. A controlled univariate analysis, *Arch. Gen. Psychiatry,* 40, 999, 1983.

494. **Kotchen, T. A., Hartley, L. H., Rice, T. W., Mougey, E. H., Jones, L. G., and Mason, J. W.,** Renin, norepinephrine, and epinephrine responses to graded exercise, *J. Appl. Physiol.,* 31, 178, 1971.

495. **Koyama, E., Minegishi, A., and Ishizaki, T.,** Simultaneous determination of four monoamine metabolites and serotonin in cerebrospinal fluid by "high-performance" liquid chromatography with electrochemical detection; application for patients with Alzheimer's disease, *Clin. Chem.* (Winston-Salem, N. C.), 34, 680, 1988.

496. **Kozlowski, S., Brzezinska, Z., Nazar, K., Kowalski, W., and Franczyk, M.,** Plasma catecholamines during sustained isometric exercise, *Clin. Sci. Mol. Med.,* 45, 723, 1973.

497. **Krstulovic, A. M., Bertani-Dziedzic, L., Dziedzic, S. W., and Gitlow, S. E.,** Quantitative determination of 3-methoxy-4-hydroxyphenylethylene glycol and its sulfate conjugate in human lumbar cerebrospinal fluid using liquid chromatography with amperometric detection, *J. Chromatogr.,* 223, 305, 1981.

498. **Krstulovic, A. M., Matzura, C. T., Bertani-Dziedzic, L., Cerqueira, S., and Gitlow, S. E.,** Endogenous levels of free and conjugated urinary 3-methoxy-4-hydroxyphenylethyleneglycol in control subjects and patients with pheochromocytoma determined by reversed-phase liquid chromatography with electrochemical detection, *Clin. Chim. Acta,* 103, 109, 1980.

499.   **Kuchel, O., Buu, N. T., Unger, T., Lis, M., and Genest, J.,** Free and conjugated plasma and urinary dopamine in human hypertension, *J. Clin. Endocrinol. Metab.,* 48, 425, 1979.

500.   **Kuchel, O., Hausser, C., Buu, N. T., and Tenneson, S.,** CSF sulfoconjugated catecholamines in man: Their relationship with plasma catecholamines, *J. Neural Transm.,* 62, 91, 1985.

501.   **Kuehl, F. A., Ormond, R. E., and Vandenheuvel, W. J. A.,** Occurrence of 3,4-dimethoxyphenylacetic acid in urines of normal and schizophrenic individuals, *Nature,* 211, 606, 1966.

502.   **Kupfer, D. J., and Bowers, M. B.,** REM sleep and central monoamine oxidase inhibition, *Psychopharmacologia,* 27, 183, 1972.

503.   **La Brosse, E. H., Kopin, I. J., Felix, W. R., and Westlake, R. J.,** Urinary tryptamine and indole-3-acetic acid excretion by schizophrenic patients: Use of the tryptamine/ indole acetic acid ratio as an index of monoamine oxidase inhibition, *J. Psychiatr. Res.,* 2, 185, 1964.

504.   **Lake, C. R., Pickar, D., Ziegler, M. G., Lippes, S., Slater, S., and Murphy, D. L.,** High plasma norepinephrine levels in patients with major affective disorder, *Am. J. Psychiatry,* 139, 1315, 1982.

505.   **Lake, C. R., Sternberg, D. E., Van Kammen, D. P., Ballenger, J. C., Ziegler, M. G., Post, R. M., Kopin, I. J., and Bunney, W. E.,** Schizophrenia: Elevated cerebrospinal fluid norepinephrine, *Science,* 207, 331, 1980.

506.   **Lake, C. R., Ziegler, M. G., Coleman, M. D., and Kopin, I. J.,** Age-adjusted plasma norepinephrine levels are similar in normotensive and hypertensive subjects, *New Engl. J. Med.,* 296, 208, 1977.

507. **Lake, C. R., Ziegler, M. G., and Kopin, I. J.,** Use of plasma norepinephrine for evaluation of sympathetic neuronal function in man, *Life Sci.,* 18, 1315, 1976.

508. **Lakke, J. P. W. F., Korf, J., Van Praag, H. M., and Schut, T.,** Predictive value of the probenecid test for the effect of L-Dopa therapy in Parkinson's disease, *Nature* (London), *New Biology,* 236, 208, 1972.

509. **Lam, K.-C., Tall, A. R., Goldstein, G. B., and Mistilis, S. P.,** Role of a false neurotransmitter, octopamine, in the pathogenesis of hepatic and renal encephalopathy, *Scand. J. Gastroenterol.,* 8, 465, 1973.

510. **Lam, R. W., Artal, R., and Fisher, D. A.,** Radioimmunoassay for free and conjugated urinary metanephrine, *Clin. Chem.* (Winston-Salem, N. C.), 23, 1264, 1977.

511. **Lauber, J., and Waldmeier, P. C.,** Determination of 2-phenylethylamine in rat brain after MAO inhibitors, and in human CSF and urine by capillary GC and chemical ionization MS, *J. Neural Transm.,* 60, 247, 1984.

512. **Le Blanc, J., Coté, J., Jobin, M., and Labrie, A.,** Plasma catecholamines and cardiovascular responses to cold and mental activity, *J. Appl. Physiol.,* 47, 1207, 1979.

513. **Leckman, J. F., Maas, J. W., and Heninger, G. R.,** Covariance of plasma free 3-methoxy-4-hydroxyphenethyleneglycol and diastolic blood pressure, *Eur. J. Pharmacol.,* 70, 111, 1981.

514. **Leckman, J. F., Maas, J. W., Redmond, D. E., and Heninger, G. R.,** Effects of oral clonidine on plasma 3-methoxy-4-hydroxyphenethylene glycol (MHPG) in man: Preliminary report, *Life Sci.,* 26, 2179, 1980.

515. **Levine, R. J., Nirenberg, P. Z., Udenfriend, S., and Sjoerdsma, A.,** Urinary excretion of phenethylamine and tyramine in normal subjects and heterozygous carriers of phenylketonuria, *Life Sci.,* 3, 651, 1964.

516. **Lewy, A. J., and Markey, S. P.,** Analysis of melatonin in human plasma by gas chromatography negative chemical ionization mass spectrometry, *Science,* 201, 741, 1978.

517. **Lidberg, L., Tuck, J. R., Åsberg, M., Scalia-Tomba, G. P., and Bertilsson, L.,** Homicide, suicide and CSF-5-HIAA, *Acta Psychiatr. Scand.,* 71, 230, 1985.

518. **Liebowitz, M. R., Karoum, F., Quitkin, F. M., Davies, S. O., Schwartz, D., Levitt, M., and Linnoila, M.,** Biochemical effects of L-deprenyl in atypical depressives, *Biol. Psychiatry,* 20, 558, 1985.

519. **Lindgren, K., and Rodopoulos, N.,** Determination of vanillyl-mandelic acid with ion-pair chromatography and fluorescence detection, *Clin. Chem.* (Winston-Salem, N. C.), 32, 693, 1986.

520. **Lindstrom, L. H.,** Low HVA and normal 5HIAA CSF levels in drug free schizophrenic patients compared to healthy volunteers: Correlations to symptomatology and family history, *Psychiatry Res.,* 14, 265, 1985.

521. **Linnoila, M., Guthrie, S., Lane, E. A., Karoum, F., Rudorfer, M., and Potter, W. Z.,** Clinical studies on norepinephrine metabolism: How to interpret the numbers, *Psychiatry Res.,* 17, 229, 1986.

522. **Linnoila, M., Jacobson, K. A., Marshall, T. H., Miller, T. L., and Kirk, K. L.,** Liquid chromatographic assay for cerebrospinal fluid serotonin, *Life Sci.,* 38, 687, 1986.

523. **Linnoila, M., Karoum, F., Calil, H. M., Kopin, I. J. and Potter, W. Z.**, Alteration of norepinephrine metabolism with desipramine and zimelidine in depressed patients, *Arch. Gen. Psychiatry*, 39, 1025, 1982.

524. **Linnoila, M., Karoum, F., Miller, T., and Potter, W. Z.**, Reliability of urinary monoamine and metabolite output measurements in depressed patients, *Am. J. Psychiatry*, 140, 1055, 1983.

525. **Linnoila, M., Karoum, F., and Potter, W. Z.**, Effect of low-dose clorgyline on 24-hour urinary monoamine excretion in patients with rapidly cycling bipolar affective disorder, *Arch. Gen. Psychiatry*, 39, 513, 1982.

526. **Linnoila, M., Karoum, F., and Potter, W. Z.**, High correlation of norepinephrine and its major metabolite excretion rates, *Arch. Gen. Psychiatry*, 39, 521, 1982.

527. **Linnoila, M., Karoum, F., and Potter, W. Z.**, High positive correlation between urinary free tyramine excretion rate and "whole body" norepinephrine turnover in depressed patients, *Biol. Psychiatry*, 17, 1031, 1982.

528. **Linnoila, M., Karoum, F., and Potter, W. Z.**, Effects of antidepressant treatment on dopamine turnover in depressed patients, *Arch. Gen. Psychiatry*, 40, 1015, 1983.

529. **Linnoila, M., Litovitz, G., Scheinin, M., Chang, M.-D., and Cutler, N. R.**, Effects of electroconvulsive treatment on monoamine metabolites, growth hormone, and prolactin in plasma, *Biol. Psychiatry*, 19, 79, 1984.

530. **Linnoila, M., Ninan, P. T., Scheinin, M., Waters, R. N., Chang, W.-H., Bartko, J., and Van Kammen, D. P.,** Reliability of norepinephrine and major monoamine metabolite measurements in CSF of schizophrenic patients, *Arch. Gen. Psychiatry,* 40, 1290, 1983.

531. **Linnoila, M., Oliver, J., Adinoff, B., and Potter, W. Z.,** High correlations of norepinephrine, dopamine, and epinephrine and their major metabolite excretion rates, *Arch. Gen. Psychiatry,* 45, 701, 1988.

532. **Linnoila, M., Virkkunen, M., Scheinin, M., Nuutila, A., Rimon, R., and Goodwin, F. K.,** Low cerebrospinal fluid 5-hydroxyindoleacetic acid concentration differentiates impulsive from non-impulsive violent behavior, *Life Sci.,* 33, 2609, 1983.

533. **Lôo, H., Dennis, T., Vanelle, J.-M., Rouquier, L., Poirier-Littré, M.-F., Garreau, M., Benkelfat, C., Sechter, D., and Scatton, B.,** Lack of correlation between plasma DOPEG and urinary MOPEG levels in depressed patients, *Biol. Psychiatry,* 21, 900, 1986.

534. **Lôo, H., Poirier, M.-F., Dennis, T., Benkelfat, C., Vanelle, J.-M., Gay, C., Galinowski, A., Askienazy, S., and Scatton, B.,** Lack of correlation between DST results and urinary MHPG in depressed inpatients, *J. Neural Transm.,* 72, 121, 1988.

535. **Lopez-Ibor, J. J., Saiz-Ruiz, J., and Perez de los Cobos, J. C.,** Biological correlation of suicide and aggressivity in major depressions (with melancholia): 5-Hydroxyindoleacetic acid and cortisol in cerebral spinal fluid, dexamethasone suppression test and therapeutic response to 5-hydroxytryptophan, *Neuropsychobiology,* 14, 67, 1985.

536. **Lovegrove, T. D., Metcalfe, E. V., Hobbs, G. E., and Stevenson, J. A. F.**, The urinary excretion of adrenaline, noradrenaline, and 17-hydroxycorticosteroids in mental illness, *Can. Psychiatr. Assoc. J.*, 10, 170, 1965.

537. **Lundberg, U., Holmberg, L., and Frankenhaeuser, M.**, Urinary catecholamines: Comparison between HPLC with electrochemical detection and fluorophotometric assay, *Pharmacol. Biochem. Behav.*, 31, 287, 1988.

538. **Luthe, H., Ludwig-Köhn, H., and Langenbeck, U.**, Quantitative gas chromatographic mass spectrometric determination of mandelic acid in blood plasma. Comparison of deuterated and homologous internal standards, *Biomed. Mass Spectrom.*, 10, 183, 1983.

539. **Lykouras, E., Markianos, M., Malliaras, D., and Stefanis, C.**, Neurochemical variables in delusional depression, *Am. J. Psychiatry*, 145, 214, 1988.

540. **Lynch, H. J., Jimerson, D. C., Ozaki, Y., Post, R. M., Bunney, W. E., and Wurtman, R. J.**, Entrainment of rhythmic melatonin secretion in man to a 12-hour phase shift in the light/dark cycle, *Life Sci.*, 23, 1557, 1978.

541. **Maas, J. W.**, Biogenic amines and depression. Biochemical and pharmacological separation of two types of depression, *Arch. Gen. Psychiatry*, 32, 1357, 1975.

542. **Maas, J. W.**, Clinical and biochemical heterogeneity of depressive illness, *Ann. Int. Med.*, 88, 556, 1978.

543. **Maas, J. W., Contreras, S. A., Seleshi, E., and Bowden, C. L.**, Dopamine metabolism and disposition in schizophrenic patients, *Arch. Gen. Psychiatry*, 45, 553, 1988.

544.   **Maas, J. W., Fawcett, J., and Dekirmenjian, H.,** 3-Methoxy-4-hydroxyphenyl glycol (MHPG) excretion in depressive states, *Arch. Gen. Psychiatry,* 19, 129, 1968.

545.   **Maas, J. W., Hattox, S. E., Greene, N. M., and Landis, D. H.,** 3-Methoxy-4-hydroxyphenethyleneglycol production by human brain *in vivo. Science,* 205, 1025, 1979.

546.   **Maas, J. W., Kocsis, J. H., Bowden, C. L., Davis, J. M., Redmond, D. E., Hanin, L., and Robins, E.,** Pre-treatment neurotransmitter metabolites and response to imipramine or amitriptyline treatment, *Psychol. Med.,* 12, 37, 1982.

547.   **Maas, J. W., Koslow, S. H., Davis, J. M., Katz, M. M., Mendels, J., Robins, E., Stokes, P. E., and Bowden, C. L.,** Biological component of the NIMH clinical research branch collaborative program on the psychobiology of depression: I. Background and theoretical considerations, *Psychol. Med.,* 10, 759, 1980.

548.   **Maas, J. W., Koslow, S. H., Katz, M. M., Bowden, C. L., Gibbons, R. L., Stokes, P. E., Robins, E., and Davis, J. M.,** Pretreatment neurotransmitter metabolite levels and response to tricyclic antidepressant drugs, *Am. J. Psychiatry,* 141, 1159, 1984.

549.   **Mahler, D. J., and Humoller, F. L.,** A comparison of methods for determining catechol amines and 3-methoxy-4-hydroxymandelic acid in urine, *Clin. Chem.* (Winston-Salem, N. C.), 8, 47, 1962.

550.   **Major, L. F., Murphy, D. L., Lipper, S., and Gordon, E.,** Effects of clorgyline and pargyline on deaminated metabolites of norepinephrine, dopamine and serotonin in human cerebrospinal fluid, *J. Neurochem.,* 32, 229, 1979.

551. **Manger, W. H., Flock, E. V., Berkson, J., Bollman, J. L., Roth, G. M., Baldes, E. J., and Jacobs, M.,** Chemical quantitation of epinephrine and norepinephrine in thirteen patients with Pheochromocytoma, *Circulation,* 10, 641, 1954.

552. **Manghani, K. K., Lunzer, M. R., Billing, B. H., and Sherlock, S.,** Urinary and serum octopamine in patients with portal-systemic encephalopathy, *Lancet,* 2, 943, 1975.

553. **Markey, S. P., Lewy, A. J., Zavadil, A. P., Poppiti, J. A., and Hoveling, A. W.,** Quantitation of biogenic amines and metabolites using negative ion chemical ionization, *25th Annual Conference on Mass Spectrometry and Allied Topics,* 276, 1977.

554. **Markianos, E. S., Rüther, E., and Gluba, H.,** 3,4-Dihydroxyphenylacetic acid and homovanillic acid in serum and cerebrospinal fluid of psychotic patients estimated by a gas chromatographic method, *Neurosci. Lett.,* 3, 37, 1976.

555. **Markianos, M., Tripodianakis, J., and Garelis, E.,** Neurochemical studies on tardive dyskinesia. II. Urinary methoxyhydroxyphenylglycol and plasma dopamine-β-hydroxylase, *Biol. Psychiatry,* 18, 347, 1983.

556. **Martin, B. R., Timmons, M. C., and Prange, A. J.,** Enzymatic hydrolysis of 3-methoxy-4-hydroxyphenylethylene glycol conjugates, *Clin. Chim. Acta,* 38, 271, 1972.

557. **Martin, J. T., Barchas, J. D., and Faull, K. F.,** Fused silica capillary gas chromatography/negative chemical ionization mass spectrometry for determination of catecholamines and their *O*-methylated metabolites, *Anal. Chem.,* 54, 1806, 1982.

558.   **Martin, M. E., Karoum, F., and Wyatt, R. J.,** Phenylacetic acid excretion in man, *Anal. Biochem.,* 99, 283, 1979.

559.   **Martinez, E., Artigas, F., Suñol, C., Tusell, J. M., and Gelpi, E.,** Liquid chromatographic determination of indole-3-acetic acid and 5-hydroxyindole-3-acetic acid in human plasma, *Clin. Chem.* (Winston-Salem, N. C.), 29, 1354, 1983.

559a. **Maruta, K., Fujita, K., Ito, S., and Nagatsu, T.,** Liquid chromatography of plasma catecholamines with electrochemical detection after treatment with boric acid gel, *Clin. Chem.* (Winston-Salem, N. C.), 30, 1271, 1984.

560.   **Mathieu, P., Greffe, J., Lemoine, P., and Szestak, M.,** Determination of urinary homovanillic acid (HVA) using capillary gas chromatography, *Clin. Chim. Acta,* 139, 99, 1984.

561.   **Mattok, G. L., Wilson, D. L., and Hoffer, A.,** Catecholamine metabolism in schizophrenia, *Nature,* 213, 1189, 1967.

562.   **Mazure, C. M., Bowers, M. B., Hoffman, F., Miller, K. B., and Nelson, J. C.,** Plasma catecholamine metabolites in subtypes of major depression, *Biol. Psychiatry,* 22, 1469, 1987.

563.   **McCullough, H.,** Semi-automated method for the differential determination of plasma catecholamines, *J. Clin. Pathol.,* 21, 759, 1968.

564.   **McNamee, H. B., Moody, J. P., and Naylor, G. J.,** Indoleamine metabolism in affective disorders: Excretion of tryptamine, indoleacetic acid and 5-hydroxyindoleacetic acid in depressive states, *J. Psychosom. Res.,* 16, 63, 1972.

565. **Mefford, I. N., Ward, M. M., Miles, L., Taylor, B., Chesney, M. A., Keegan, D. L., and Barchas, J. D.,** Determination of plasma catecholamines and free 3,4-dihydroxyphenylacetic acid in continuously collected human plasma by high performance liquid chromatography with electrochemical detection, *Life Sci.,* 28, 477, 1981.

566. **Mell, L. D., and Gustafson, A. B.,** Urinary free norepinephrine and dopamine determined by reverse-phase high-pressure liquid chromatography, *Clin. Chem.* (Winston-Salem, N. C.), 23, 473, 1977.

567. **Mendels, J., Frazer, A., Fitzgerald, R. G., Ramsey, T. A., and Stokes, J. W.,** Biogenic amine metabolites in cerebrospinal fluid of depressed and manic patients, *Science,* 175, 1380, 1972.

568. **Mendlewicz, J., Vanderheyden, J. E., and Noel, G.,** Serotonin and dopamine disturbances in patients with unipolar depression and parkinsonism, *Adv. Exp. Med. Biol.,* 133, 753, 1981.

569. **Messiha, F. S., Agallianos, D., and Clower, C.,** Dopamine excretion in affective states and following Li_2CO_3 therapy, *Nature,* 225, 868, 1970.

570. **Messiha, F. S., Bakutis, E., and Frankos, V.,** Simultaneous separation of acid metabolites of catecholamines: Application to urine and tissue, *Clin. Chim. Acta,* 45, 159, 1973.

571. **Meyer, J. S., Stoica, E., Pascu, I., Shimazu, K., and Hartmann, A.,** Catecholamine concentrations in CSF and plasma of patients with cerebral infarction and haemorrhage, *Brain,* 96, 277, 1973.

572. **Michaels, R. R., Huber, M. J., and McCann, D. S.,** Evaluation of transcendental meditation as a method of reducing stress, *Science,* 192, 1242, 1976.

573.   **Midgley, J. M., Couch, M. W., Crowley, J. R., and Williams, C. M.,** Identification and quantitative determination of *o*- and *m*-hydroxymandelic acid in human urine, *Biomed. Mass Spectrom.,* 6, 485, 1979.

574.   **Miller, R. L., McCord, C., Sanda, M., Bourne, H. R., and Melmon, K. L.,** Application of the enzymatic double isotope dilution assay for the study of histamine in plasma, *J. Pharmacol. Exp. Ther.,* 175, 228, 1970.

575.   **Minegishi, A., and Ishizaki, T.,** Rapid and simple method for the simultaneous determination of 3,4-dihydroxyphenylacetic acid, 5-hydroxyindole-3-acetic acid and 4-hydroxy-3-methoxyphenylacetic acid in human plasma by high-performance liquid chromatography with electrochemical detection, *J. Chromatogr.,* 308, 55, 1984.

576.   **Minegishi, A., and Ishizaki, T.,** Determination of free 3-methoxy-4-hydroxyphenylglycol with several other monoamine metabolites in plasma by high-performance liquid chromatography with amperometric detection, *J. Chromatogr.,* 311, 51, 1984.

577.   **Mita, H., Yasueda, H., and Shida, T.,** Simultaneous determination of histamine and N^{τ}-methylhistamine in human plasma and urine by gas chromatography-mass spectrometry, *J. Chromatogr.,* 221, 1, 1980.

578.   **Mitchell, R. G., and Code, C. F.,** Effect of diet on urinary excretion of histamine, *J. Appl. Physiol.,* 6, 387, 1954.

579.   **Miyake, H., Yoshida, H., and Imaizumi, R.,** Determination methods for urinary 3-methoxy-4-hydroxymandelic acid and 3,4-dihydroxymandelic acid, *Jpn. J. Pharmacol.,* 12, 79, 1962.

580.   **Modai, I., Apter, A., Golomb, M., and Wijsenbeek, H.,** Response to amitriptyline and urinary MHPG in bipolar depressive patients, *Neuropsychobiology,* 5, 181, 1979.

581. **Moerman, E. J., Bogaert, M. G., and de Schaepdryver, A. F.,** Estimation of plasma catecholamines in man, *Clin. Chim. Acta,* 72, 89, 1976.

582. **Moir, A. T. B., Ashcroft, G. W., Crawford, T. B. B., Eccleston, D., Guldberg, H. C.,** Cerebral metabolites in cerebrospinal fluid as a biochemical approach to the brain, *Brain,* 93, 357, 1970.

583. **Moleman, P., and Borstrok, J. J. M.,** Determination of urinary vanillylmandelic acid by liquid chromatography with electrochemical detection, *Clin. Chem.* (Winston-Salem, N. C.), 29, 878, 1983.

584. **Molyneux, S. G., and Franklin, M.,** Routine determination of unconjugated 3-methoxy-4-hydroxyphenylglycol in plasma using high-performance liquid chromatography with electrochemical detection, *J. Chromatogr.,* 341, 160, 1985.

585. **Montplaisir, J., de Champlain, J., Young, S. N., Missala, K., Sourkes, T. L., Walsh, J., and Rémillard, G.,** Narcolepsy and idiopathic hypersomnia: Biogenic amines and related compounds in CSF, *Neurology,* 32, 1299, 1982.

586. **Mooney, J. J., Cole, J. O., Schatzberg, A. F., Gerson, B., and Schildkraut, J. J.,** Pretreatment urinary MHPG levels as predictors of antidepressant responses to alprazolam, *Am. J. Psychiatry,* 142, 366, 1985.

587. **Mooney, J. J., Schatzberg, A. F., Cole, J. O., Kizuka, P. P., Salomon, M., Lerbinger, J., Pappalardo, K. M., Gerson, B., and Schildkraut, J. J.,** Rapid antidepressant response to alprazolam in depressed patients with high catecholamine output and heterologous desensitization of platelet adenylate cyclase, *Biol. Psychiatry,* 23, 543, 1988.

588. **Moore, D. C., Glazer, W. M., Bowers, M. B., and Heninger, G. R.,** Tardive dyskinesia and plasma homovanillic acid, *Biol. Psychiatry,* 18, 1393, 1983.

589. **Mosnaim, A. D., Inwang, E. E., Sugerman, J. H., De Martini, W. J., and Sabelli, H. C.,** Ultraviolet spectrophotometric determination of 2-phenylethylamine in biological samples and its possible correlation with depression, *Biol. Psychiatry,* 6, 235, 1973.

590. **Moyer, T. P., Jiang, N.-S., Tyce, G. M., and Sheps, S. G.,** Analysis for urinary catecholamines by liquid chromatography with amperometric detection: Methodology and clinical interpretation of results, *Clin. Chem.* (Winston-Salem, N. C.), 25, 256, 1979.

591. **Mueser, K. T., Rosen, A. J., Dysken, M. W., and Javaid, J. I.,** Urinary MHPG and ward behavior in unmedicated psychiatric patients, *Psychiatry Res.,* 10, 275, 1983.

592. **Murphy, D. L., Brand, E., Goldman, T., Baker, M., Wright, C., Van Kammen, D., and Gordon, E.,** Platelet and plasma amine oxidase inhibition and urinary amine excretion changes during phenelzine treatment, *J. Nerv. Ment. Dis.,* 164, 129, 1977.

593. **Murphy, D. L., Goodwin, F. K., Brodie, H. K. H., and Bunney, W. E.,** L-Dopa, dopamine and hypomania, *Am. J. Psychiatry,* 130, 79, 1973.

594. **Murray, R. M., Oon, M. C. H., Rodnight, R., Birley, J. L. T., and Smith, A.,** Increased excretion of dimethyltryptamine and certain features of psychosis. A possible association, *Arch. Gen. Psychiatry,* 36, 644, 1979.

595. **Murray, S., Baillie, T. A., and Davies, D. S.,** A non-enzymatic procedure for the quantitative analysis of (3-methoxy-4-sulfoxyphenyl)ethylene glycol (MHPG sulfate) in human urine using stable isotope dilution and gas chromatography-mass spectrometry, *J. Chromatogr.,* 143, 541, 1977.

596. **Muscettola, G., Potter, W. Z., Gordon, E. K., and Goodwin, F. K.,** Methodological issues in the measurement of urinary MHPG, *Psychiatry Res.,* 4, 267, 1981.

597. **Muscettola, G., Potter, W. Z., Pickar, D., and Goodwin, F. K.,** Urinary 3-methoxy-4-hydroxyphenylglycol and major affective disorders. A replication and new findings, *Arch. Gen. Psychiatry,* 41, 337, 1984.

598. **Muskiet, F. A. J., Fremouw-Ottevangers, D. C., Nagel, G. T., Wolthers, B. G., and de Vries, J. A.,** Determination of 3-methoxy-4-hydroxyphenylpyruvic acid, 3,4-dihydroxyphenylethylene glycol and 3,4-dihydroxyphenylmandelic acid in urine by mass fragmentography with use of deuterium-labeled internal standards, *Clin. Chem.,* (Winston-Salem, N. C.), 24, 2001, 1978.

599. **Muskiet, F. A. J., Nagel, G. T., and Wolthers, B. G.,** Simultaneous determination of unconjugated homovanillic acid, vanilmandelic acid and 3-methoxy-4-hydroxyphenylethylene glycol in serum by mass fragmentography and deuterated internal standards, *Anal. Biochem.,* 109, 130, 1980.

600. **Muskiet, F. A. J., Thomasson, C. G., Gerding, A. M., Fremouw-Ottevangers, D. C., Nagel, G. T., and Wolthers, B. G.,** Determination of catecholamines and their 3-*O*-methylated metabolites in urine by mass fragmentography with use of deuterated internal standards, *Clin. Chem.,* (Winston-Salem, N. C.), 25, 453, 1979.

601. **Myers, G., Donlon, M., and Kaliner, M.,** Measurement of urinary histamine: Development of methodology and normal values, *J. Allergy Clin. Immunol.,* 67, 305, 1981.

602. **Naber, D., Finkbeiner, C., Fischer, B., Zander, K.-J., and Ackenheil, M.,** Effect of long-term neuroleptic treatment on prolactin and norepinephrine levels in serum of chronic schizophrenics: Relations to psychopathology and extrapyramidal symptoms, *Neuropsychobiology,* 6, 181, 1980.

603. **Naber, D., Pickar, D., Davis, G. C., Cohen, R. M., Jimerson, D. C., Elchisak, M. A., Defraites, E. G., Kalin, N. H., Risch, S. C., and Buchsbaum, M. S.,** Naloxone effects on β-endorphin, cortisol, prolactin, growth hormone, HVA and MHPG in plasma of normal volunteers, *Psychopharmacology,* 74, 125, 1981.

604. **Nagao, T., Ohshimo, T., Mitsunobu, K., Sato, M., and Otsuki, S.,** Cerebrospinal fluid monoamine metabolites and cyclic nucleotides in chronic schizophrenic patients with tardive dyskinesia or drug-induced tremor, *Biol. Psychiatry,* 14, 509, 1979.

605. **Nair, M. C., and Rama Rao, B. S. S.,** Tryptophan metabolites in cerebrospinal fluid and urine of patients with affective disorders, *Indian J. Med. Res.,* 75, 274, 1982.

606. **Narasimhachari, N., Baumann, P., Pak, H. S., Carpenter, W. T., Zocchi, A. F., Hokanson, L., Fujimori, M., and Himwich, H. E.,** Gas chromatographic-mass spectrometric identification of urinary bufotenin and dimethyltryptamine in drug-free chronic schizophrenic patients, *Biol. Psychiatry,* 8, 293, 1974.

607. **Narasimhachari, N., and Friedel, R. O.,** Quantitation of biologically important primary amines as their isothiocyanate derivatives by gas chromatography using nitrogen detector and validation by selected ion monitoring, *Clin. Chim. Acta,* 110, 235, 1981.

608. **Narasimhachari, N., and Himwich, H. E.,** The determination of bufotenin in urine of schizophrenic patients and normal controls, *J. Psychiatr. Res.,* 9, 113, 1972.

609. **Narasimhachari, N., and Himwich, H. E.,** Gas chromatographic-mass spectrometric identification of *N,N*-dimethyltryptamine in urine samples from drug-free chronic schizophrenic patients and its quantitation by the technique of single (selective) ion monitoring, *Biochem. Biophys. Res. Commun.,* 55, 1064, 1973.

610. **Narasimhachari, N., Leiner, K., and Brown, C.,** The simultaneous determination by selected ion monitoring of the levels of homovanillic, isohomovanillic, 3,4-dihydroxyphenylacetic and 3-methoxy-4-hydroxymandelic acids in single biological samples, *Clin. Chim. Acta,* 62, 245, 1975.

611. **Narasimhachari, N., Leiner, K., Plaut, J. M., and Lin, R.-L.,** Selective and specific gas-liquid chromatographic and gas-liquid chromatographic-mass spectrometric methods for the separation and quantitative determination of homovanillic and iso-homovanillic acids in urine samples, *Clin. Chim. Acta,* 50, 337, 1974.

612. **Nazarali, A. J., Baker, G. B., Coutts, R. T., Yeung, J. M., and Rao, T. S.,** Rapid analysis of β-phenylethylamine in tissues and body fluids utilizing pentafluorobenzoylation followed by electron-capture gas chromatography, *Prog. Neuropsychopharmacol. Biol. Psychiatry,* 11, 251, 1987.

613.   **Nelson, G. N., Masuda, M., and Holmes, T. H.,** Correlation of
       behavior and catecholamine metabolite excretion, *Psychosom. Med.,* 28,
       216, 1966.

614.   **Nelson, L. M., Bubb, F. A., Lax, P. M., Weg, M. W., and
       Sandler, M.,** An improved method for the differential assay of 3-*O*-
       methylated catecholamines in human urine using ion-pair extraction and
       gas chromatography electron capture detection, *Clin. Chim. Acta,* 92,
       235, 1979.

615.   **Nicholas, N. L., Brown, H., and Swander, A. M.,** An improved
       spectrophotometric method for determination of total 3-methoxy-4-
       hydroxyphenylglycol in urine, *Clin. Chem.* (Winston-Salem, N. C.), 15,
       884, 1969.

616.   **Nicoletti, F., Raffaele, R., Falsaperla, A., and Paci, R.,**
       Circadian variation in 5-hydroxyindoleacetic acid levels in human
       cerebrospinal fluid, *Eur. Neurol.,* 20, 9, 1981.

617.   **Ninan, P. T., Van Kammen, D. P., Scheinin, M., Linnoila, M.,
       Bunney, W. E., and Goodwin, F. K.,** CSF 5-hydroxyindoleacetic acid
       levels in suicidal schizophrenic patients, *Am. J. Psychiatry,* 141,
       566, 1984.

618.   **Noah, J. W., and Brand, A.,** Simplified micromethod of measuring
       histamine in human plasma, *J. Lab. Clin. Med.,* 62, 506, 1963.

619.   **Nordin, G., Ottosson, J.-O., and Roos, B.-E.,** Influence of
       convulsive therapy on 5-hydroxyindoleacetic acid and homovanillic acid
       in cerebrospinal fluid in endogenous depression, *Psychopharmacologia,*
       20, 315, 1971.

620. **Nybäck, H., Berggren, B.-M., Hindmarsh, T., Sedvall, G., and Wiesel, F.-A.,** Cerebroventricular size and cerebrospinal fluid monoamine metabolites in schizophrenic patients and healthy volunteers, *Psychiatry Res.,* 9, 301, 1983.

621. **Nybäck, H., Nyman, H., and Schalling, D.,** Neuropsychological test performance and CSF levels of monoamine metabolites in healthy volunteers and patients with Alzheimer's dementia, *Acta Psychiatr. Scand.,* 76, 648, 1987.

622. **Oates, J. A., Marsh, E., and Sjoerdsma, A.,** Studies on histamine in human urine using a fluorometric method of assay, *Clin. Chim. Acta,* 7, 488, 1962.

623. **Odink, J., Korthals, H., and Kniff, J. H.,** Simultaneous determination of the major acidic metabolites of catecholamines and serotonin in urine by liquid chromatography with electrochemical detection after a one-step sample clean-up on Sephadex G-10; influence of vanilla and banana ingestion, *J. Chromatogr.,* 424, 273, 1988.

624. **O'Hanlon, J. F., Campuzano, H. C., and Horvath, S. M.,** A fluorometric assay for subnanogram concentrations of adrenaline and noradrenaline in plasma, *Anal. Biochem.,* 34, 568, 1970.

625. **Oka, K., Sekiya, M., Osada, H., Fujita, K., Kato, T., and Nagatsu, T.,** Simultaneous fluorometry of urinary dopamine, norepinephrine, and epinephrine compared with liquid chromatography with electrochemical detection, *Clin. Chem. (Winston-Salem, N. C.),* 28, 646, 1982.

626. **O'Keeffe, R., and Brooksbank, B. W. L.,** Determination of 3-methoxy-4-hydroxyphenylethylene glycol, a noradrenaline metabolite, in cerebrospinal fluid and urine, *Clin. Chem. (Winston-Salem, N. C.),* 19, 1031, 1973.

627. **Olsson, R., and Roos, B.-E.,** Concentrations of 5-hydroxyindole-acetic acid and homovanillic acid in the cerebrospinal fluid after treatment with probenecid in patients with Parkinson's disease, *Nature,* 219, 502, 1968.

628. **Ong, C. N., Lee, B. L., Ong, H. Y., and Jaecob, E.,** Simple high-performance liquid chromatographic method for the simultaneous measurement of vanillylmandelic acid and homovanillic acid, *J. Chromatogr.,* 423, 278, 1987.

629. **Ong, H., Capet-Antonini, F., Yamaguchi, N., and Lamontagne, D.,** Simultaneous determination of free 3-methoxy-4-hydroxymandelic acid and free 3-methoxy-4-hydroxyphenylethylene glycol in plasma by liquid chromatography with electrochemical detection, *J. Chromatogr.,* 233, 97, 1982.

630. **Oon, M. C. H., Murray, R. M., Rodnight, R., Murphy, M. P., and Birley, J. L. T.,** Factors affecting the urinary excretion of endogenously formed dimethyltryptamine in normal human subjects, *Psychopharmacology,* 54, 171, 1977.

631. **Oon, M. C. H., and Rodnight, R.,** A gas chromatographic procedure for determining *N,N*-dimethyltryptamine and *N*-monomethyltryptamine in urine using a nitrogen detector, *Biochem. Med.,* 18, 410, 1977.

632. **O'Reilly, S., Loncin, M., and Cooksey, B.,** Dopamine and basal ganglia disorders, *Neurology,* 15, 980, 1965.

633. **Oreland, L., Wiberg, A., Åsberg, M., Träskman, L., Sjöstrand, L., Thorén, P., Bertilsson, L., and Tybring, G.,** Platelet MAO activity and monoamine metabolites in cerebrospinal fluid in depressed and suicidal patients and in healthy controls, *Psychiatry Res.,* 4, 21, 1981.

634. **Oxenstierna, G., Edman, G., Iselius, L., Oreland, L., Ross, S. B., and Sedvall, G.,** Concentrations of monoamine metabolites in the cerebrospinal fluid of twins and unrelated individuals - a genetic study, *J. Psychiatr. Res.,* 20, 19, 1986.

635. **Palmer, A. M., Sims, N. R., Bowen, D. M., Neary, D., Palo, J., Wikstrom, J., and Davison, A. N.,** Monoamine metabolite concentrations in lumbar cerebrospinal fluid of patients with histologically verified Alzheimer's disease, *J. Neurol. Neurosurg. Psychiatry,* 47, 481, 1984.

636. **Palmerini, C. A., Cantelmi, M. G., Minelli, A., Fini, C., Zampino, M., and Floridi, A.,** Determination of plasma serotonin by high-performance liquid chromatography with pre-column sample enrichment and fluorimetric detection, *J. Chromatogr.,* 417, 378, 1987.

637. **Papeschi, R., and McClure, D. J.,** Homovanillic and 5-hydroxy-indoleacetic acid in cerebrospinal fluid of depressed patients, *Arch. Gen. Psychiatry,* 25, 354, 1971.

638. **Papeschi, R., Molina-Negro, P., Sourkes, T. L., and Erba, G.,** The concentration of homovanillic and 5-hydroxyindoleacetic acids in ventricular and lumbar CSF, *Neurology,* 22, 1151, 1972.

639. **Papeschi, R., Molina-Negro, P., Sourkes, T. L., Hardy, J., and Bertrand, C.,** Concentration of homovanillic acid in the ventricular fluid of patients with Parkinson's disease and other dyskinesias, *Neurology,* 20, 991, 1970.

640. **Pare, C. M. B., and Sandler, M.,** A clinical and biochemical study of a trial of iproniazid in the treatment of depression, *J. Neurol. Neurosurg. Psychiatry,* 22, 247, 1959.

641. **Pare, C. M. B., Sandler, M., and Stacey, R. S.,** 5 - Hydroxyindoles in mental deficiency, *J. Neurol. Neurosurg. Psychiatry,* 23, 341, 1960.

642. **Parkes, J. D., Curzon, G., Knott, P. J., Tattersall, R., Baxter, R. C. H., Knill-Jones, R., Marsden, C. D., and Vollum, D.,** Treatment of Parkinson's disease with amantadine and levodopa. A one year study, *Lancet,* 1, 1083, 1971.

643. **Parkes, J. D., Marsden, C. D., Rees, J. E., Curzon, G., Kantamaneni, B. D., Knill-Jones, R., Akbar, A., Das, S., and Kataria, M.,** Parkinson's disease, cerebral arteriosclerosis, and senile dementia, *Q. J. Med.,* 43, 49, 1974.

644. **Parnetti, L., Gottfries, J., Karlsson, I., Langström, G., Gottfries, C.-G., and Svennerholm, L.,** Monoamines and their metabolites in cerebrospinal fluid of patients with senile dementia of Àlzheimer type using high-performance liquid chromatography and gas chromatography-mass spectrometry, *Acta Psychiatr. Scand.,* 75, 542, 1987.

645. **Pedersen, E. B., and Christensen, N. J.,** Catecholamines in plasma and urine in patients with essential hypertension determined by double-isotope derivative techniques, *Acta Med. Scand.,* 198, 373, 1975.

646. **Pennings, E. J. M., Verhagen, J. C. M., and Van Kempen, G. M. J.,** Assay of urinary phenylacetic acid by high-performance liquid chromatography, *J. Chromatogr.,* 341, 172, 1985.

647. **Perry, T. L., Hestrin, M., MacDougall, L., and Hansen, S.,** Urinary amines of intestinal bacterial origin, *Clin. Chim. Acta,* 14, 116, 1966.

648. **Persson, T., and Roos, B.-E.,** Acid metabolites from monoamines in cerebrospinal fluid of chronic schizophrenics, *Br. J. Psychiatry,* 115, 95, 1965.

649   **Persson, T., and Roos, B.-E.,** Clinical and pharmacological effects of monoamine precursors or haloperidol in chronic schizophrenia, *Nature,* 217, 854, 1968.

650. **Petruccelli, B., Bakris, G., Miller, T., Korpi, E. R., and Linnoila, M.,** A liquid chromatographic assay for 5-hydroxytryptophan, serotonin and 5-hydroxyindoleacetic acid in human body fluids, *Acta Pharmacol. Toxicol.,* 51, 421, 1982.

651. **Petty, F., Kramer, G., and Weed, J.,** Menstrual cycle affects plasma HVA, *Psychiatry Res.,* 17, 169, 1986.

652. **Petursson, H., Bond, P. A., Smith, B., and Lader, M. H.,** Monoamine metabolism during chronic benzodiazepine treatment and withdrawal, *Biol. Psychiatry,* 18, 207, 1983.

653. **Peuler, J. D., and Johnson, G. A.,** Simultaneous single isotope radioenzymatic assay of plasma norepinephrine, epinephrine and dopamine, *Life Sci.,* 21, 625, 1977.

654. **Peyrin, L., and Cottet-Emard, J. M.,** Automated specific fluorimetric methods for epinephrine and norepinephrine assay in a single biological extract, *Anal. Biochem.,* 56, 515, 1973.

655. **Peyrin, L., and Pequignot, J. M.,** Free and conjugated 3-methoxy-4-hydroxyphenylglycol in human urine: Peripheral origin of glucuronide, *Psychopharmacology,* 79, 16, 1983.

656. **Peyrin, L., Pequignot, J. M., Chauplannaz, G., Laurent, B., and Aimard, G.,** Sulfate and glucuronide conjugates of 3-methoxy-4-hydroxyphenylglycol (MHPG) in urine of depressed patients: Central and peripheral influences, *J. Neural Transm.,* 63, 255, 1985.

657. **Peyrin, L., Pequignot, J. M., Lacour, J. R., and Fourcade, J.,** Relationships between catecholamine or 3-methoxy-4-hydroxyphenylglycol changes and the mental performance under submaximal exercise in man, *Psychopharmacology,* 93, 188, 1987.

658. **Picard, M., Olichon, D., and Gombert, J.,** Determination of serotonin in plasma by liquid chromatography with electrochemical detection, *J. Chromatogr.,* 341, 445, 1985.

659. **Pickar, D., Labarca, R., Doran, A. R., Wolkowitz, O. M., Roy, A., Breier, A., Linnoila, M., and Paul, S. M.,** Longitudinal measurement of plasma homovanillic acid levels in schizophrenic patients: Correlation with psychosis and response to neuroleptic treatment, *Arch. Gen. Psychiatry,* 43, 669, 1986.

660. **Pickar, D., Labarca, R., Linnoila, M., Roy, A., Hommer, D., Everett, D., and Paul, S. M.,** Neuroleptic-induced decrease in plasma homovanillic acid and antipsychotic activity in schizophrenic patients, *Science,* 225, 954, 1984.

661. **Pickar, D., Sweeney, D. R., Maas, J. W., and Heninger, G. R.,** Primary affective disorder, clinical state change and MHPG excretion. A longitudinal study, *Arch. Gen. Psychiatry,* 35, 1378, 1978.

662. **Pind, K., and Faurbye, A.,** Concentration of homovanillic acid and 5-hydroxyindoleacetic acid in the cerebrospinal fluid after treatment with probenecid in patients with drug-induced tardive dyskinesia, *Acta Psychiatr. Scand.,* 46, 323, 1970.

663. **Pisano, J. J.,** A simple analysis for normetanephrine and metanephrine in urine, *Clin. Chim. Acta,* 5, 406, 1960.

664. **Pisano, J. J., Oates, J. A., Karmen, A., Sjoerdsma, A., and Udenfriend, S.,** Identification of *p*-hydroxy-α-(methylamino-methyl)benzyl alcohol (synephrine) in human urine, *J. Biol. Chem.,* 236, 898, 1961.

665. **Pohl, R., Ettedgui, E., Bridges, M., Lycaki, H., Jimerson, D., Kopin, I., and Rainey, J. M.,** Plasma MHPG levels in lactate and isoproterenol anxiety states, *Biol. Psychiatry,* 22, 1127, 1987.

666. **Pollin, W.,** A possible genetic factor related to psychosis, *Am. J. Psychiatry,* 128, 311, 1971.

667. **Post, R. M., Fink, E., Carpenter, W. T., and Goodwin, F. K.,** Cerebrospinal fluid amine metabolites in acute schizophrenia, *Arch. Gen. Psychiatry,* 32, 1063, 1975.

668. **Post, R. M., and Goodwin, F. K.,** Effects of amitriptyline and imipramine on amine metabolites in the cerebrospinal fluid of depressed patients, *Arch. Gen. Psychiatry,* 30, 234, 1974.

669. **Post, R. M., Goodwin, F. K., and Gordon, E.,** Amine metabolites in human cerebrospinal fluid: Effects of cord transection and spinal fluid block, *Science,* 179, 897, 1973.

670. **Post, R. M., Gordon, E. K., Goodwin, F. K., and Bunney, W. E.,** Central norepinephrine metabolism in affective illness: MHPG in cerebrospinal fluid, *Science,* 179, 1002, 1973.

671. **Post, R. M., Kotin, J., Goodwin, F. K., and Gordon, E. K.,** Psychomotor activity and cerebrospinal fluid amine metabolites in affective illness, *Am. J. Psychiatry,* 130, 67, 1973.

672. **Post, R. M., Lake, C. R., Jimerson, D. C., Bunney, W. E., Wood, J. H., Ziegler, M. G., and Goodwin, F. K.,** Cerebrospinal fluid norepinephrine in affective illness, *Am. J. Psychiatry,* 135, 907, 1978.

673. **Post, R. M., Stoddard, F. J., Gillin, J. C., Buchsbaum, M. S., Runkle, D. C., Black, K. E., and Bunney, W. E.,** Alterations in motor activity, sleep and biochemistry in a cycling manic-depressive patient, *Arch. Gen. Psychiatry,* 34, 470, 1977.

674. **Potkin, S. G., Karoum, F., Chuang, L.-W., Cannon-Spoor, H. E., Phillips, I., and Wyatt, R. J.,** Phenylethylamine in paranoid chronic schizophrenia, *Science,* 206, 470, 1979.

675. **Potkin, S. G., Weinberger, D. R., Linnoila, M., and Wyatt, R. J.,** Low CSF 5-hydroxyindoleacetic acid in schizophrenic patients with enlarged cerebral ventricles, *Am. J. Psychiatry,* 140, 21, 1983.

676. **Potkin, S. G., Wyatt, R. J., and Karoum, F.,** Phenylethylamine (PEA) and phenylacetic acid (PAA) in the urine of chronic schizophrenic patients and controls, *Psychopharmacol. Bull.,* 16, 52, 1980.

677. **Potter, W. Z., Calil, H. M., Extein, I., Gold, P. W., Wehr, T. A., and Goodwin, F. K.,** Specific norepinephrine and serotonin uptake inhibitors in man: A crossover study with pharmacokinetic, biochemical, neuroendocrine and behavioural parameters, *Acta Psychiatr. Scand.,* 63(Suppl. 290), 152, 1981.

678. **Potter, W. Z., Scheinin, M., Golden, R. N., Rudorfer, M. V., Cowdry, R. W., Calil, H. M., Ross, R. J., and Linnoila, M.,** Selective antidepressants and cerebrospinal fluid. Lack of specificity on norepinephrine and serotonin metabolites, *Arch. Gen. Psychiatry,* 42, 1171, 1985.

679. **Prange, A. J., Wilson, I. C., Knox, A. E., McClane, T. K., Breese, G. R., Martin, B. R., Alltop, L. B., and Lipton, M. A.**, Thyroid-imipramine clinical and chemical interaction: Evidence for a receptor deficit in depression, *J. Psychiatr. Res.*, 9, 187, 1972.

680. **Price, H. L., and Price, M. L.**, The chemical estimation of epinephrine and norepinephrine in human and canine plasma. II. A critique of the trihydroxyindole method, *J. Lab. Clin. Med.*, 50, 769, 1957.

681. **Pscheidt, G. R., Berlet, H. H., Bull, C., Spaide, J., and Himwich, H. E.**, Excretion of catecholamines and exacerbation of symptoms in schizophrenic patients, *J. Psychiatr. Res.*, 2, 163, 1964.

682. **Pullar, I. A., Weddell, J. M., Ahmed, R., and Gillingham, F. J.**, Phenolic acid concentrations in the lumbar cerebrospinal fluid of Parkinsonian patients treated with L-DOPA, *J. Neurol. Neurosurg. Psychiatry,* 33, 851, 1970.

683. **Räisänen, M. J.**, The presence of free and conjugated bufotenin in normal human urine, *Life Sci.,* 34, 2041, 1984.

684. **Räisänen, M. J., and Kärkkäinen, J.**, Mass fragmentographic quantification of urinary N,N-dimethyltryptamine and bufotenine, *J. Chromatogr.*, 162, 579, 1979.

685. **Raskind, M. A., Peskind, E. R., Halter, J. B., and Jimerson, D. C.**, Norepinephrine and MHPG levels in CSF and plasma in Alzheimer's disease, *Arch. Gen. Psychiatry,* 41, 343, 1984.

686. **Ratge, D., Bauersfeld, W., and Wisser, H.**, The relationship of free and conjugated catecholamines in plasma and cerebrospinal fluid in cerebral and meningeal disease, *J. Neural Transm.*, 62, 267, 1985.

687. **Raum, W. J., and Swerdloff, R. S.,** A radioimmunoassay for epinephrine and norepinephrine in tissues and plasma, *Life Sci.,* 28, 2819, 1981.

688. **Redmond, D. E., Katz, M. M., Maas, J. W., Swann, A., Casper, R., and Davis, J. M.,** Cerebrospinal fluid amine metabolites. Relationships with behavioral measurements in depressed, manic and healthy control subjects, *Arch. Gen. Psychiatry,* 43, 938, 1986.

689. **Reilly, J., and Regan, P. F.,** Plasma catechol amines in psychiatric patients, *Proc. Soc. Exp. Biol. Med.,* 95, 377, 1957.

690. **Reimherr, F. W., Wender, P. H., Ebert, M. H., and Wood, D. R.,** Cerebrospinal fluid homovanillic acid and 5-hydroxyindoleacetic acid in adults with attention deficit disorder, residual type, *Psychiatry Res.,* 11, 71, 1984.

691. **Renaud, B., Quenin, P., and Quincy, C.,** Determination fluorimetrique en flux continu de l'acide homovanillique. Application au liquide cephalorachidien, *Clin. Chim. Acta* 52, 179, 1974.

692. **Renzini, V., Brunori, C. A., and Valori, C.,** A sensitive and specific fluorimetric method for the determination of noradrenalin and adrenalin in human plasma, *Clin. Chim. Acta* 30, 587, 1970.

693. **Reynolds, G. P., and Gray, D. O.,** A method for the estimation of 2-phenylethylamine in human urine by gas chromatography, *Clin. Chim. Acta,* 70, 213, 1976.

694. **Reynolds, G. P., Rausch, W.-D., and Riederer, P.,** Effects of tranylcypromine stereoisomers on monoamine oxidation in man, *Br. J. Clin. Pharmacol.,* 9, 521, 1980.

695. **Reynolds, G. P., Seakins, J. W. T., and Gray, D. O.,** The urinary excretion of 2-phenylethylamine in phenylketonuria, *Clin. Chim. Acta,* 83, 33, 1978.

696. **Rimón, R., Roos, B.-E., Räkköläinen, V., and Alanen, Y.,** The content of 5-hydroxyindoleacetic acid and homovanillic acid in the cerebrospinal fluid of patients with acute schizophrenia, *J. Psychosom. Res.,* 15, 375, 1971.

697. **Rinne, U. K., and Sonninen, V.,** Urinary excretion of 3,4-dimethoxyphenylethylamine in Parkinson's disease, *Nature,* 216, 489, 1967.

698. **Rinne, U. K., and Sonninen, V.,** Homovanillic acid of the cerebrospinal fluid in Parkinson's disease, *Scand. J. Clin. Lab. Invest.,* 21(Suppl. 101), 22, 1968.

699. **Rinne, U. K., and Sonninen, V.,** Acid monoamine metabolites in the cerebrospinal fluid of patients with Parkinson's disease, *Neurology,* 22, 62, 1972.

700. **Rinne, U. K., Sonninen, V., and Siirtola, T.,** Acid monoamine metabolites in the cerebrospinal fluid of parkinsonian patients treated with levadopa alone or combined with a decarboxylase inhibitor, *Eur. Neurol.,* 9, 349, 1973.

701. **Risby, E. D., Hsiao, J. K., Sunderland, T., Ågren, H., Rudorfer, M. V., and Potter, W. Z.,** The effects of antidepressants on the cerebrospinal fluid homovanillic acid/5-hydroxyindoleacetic acid ratio, *Clin. Pharmacol. Ther.,* 42, 547, 1987.

702. **Rizzo, V., Melzi d'Eril, G. V.,** Determination of free 3-methoxy-4-hydroxyphenylethyleneglycol in plasma and in cerebrospinal fluid by liquid chromatography with coulometric detection, *Clin. Chem.,* (Winston-Salem, N. C.), 33, 844, 1987.

703. **Roberts, M., and Adam, H. M.,** New methods for the quantitative estimation of free and conjugated histamine in body fluids, *Br. J. Pharmacol.,* 5, 526, 1950.

704. **Robertson, D., Fröhlich, J. C., Carr, R. K., Watson, J. T., Hollifield, J. W., Shand, D. G., and Oates, J. A.,** Effects of caffeine on plasma renin activity, catecholamines and blood pressure, *New Engl. J. Med.,* 298, 181, 1978.

705. **Robertson, D., Heath, E. C., Falkner, F. C., Hill, R. E., Brilis, G. M., and Watson, J. T.,** A selective and sensitive assay for urinary metanephrine and normetanephrine using gas chromatography mass spectrometry with selected ion monitoring, *Biomed. Mass Spectrom.,* 5, 704, 1978.

706. **Robertson, D., Johnson, G. A., Robertson, R. M., Nies, A. S., Shand, D. G., and Oates, J. A.,** Comparative assessment of stimuli that release neuronal and adrenomedullary catecholamines in man, *Circulation,* 59, 637, 1979.

707. **Robinson, R. L., and Watts, D. T.,** An automated trihydroxyindole procedure for the differential analysis of catecholamines, *Clin. Chem. (Winston-Salem, N. C.),* 11, 986, 1965.

708. **Roccatagliata, G., Albano, C., and Abbruzzese, G.,** CSF-MHPG in depressive syndromes: Basal values and imipramine-induced modifications, *Neuropsychobiology,* 7, 169, 1981.

709. **Rodnight, R.,** Separation and characterization of urinary indoles resembling 5-hydroxytryptamine and tryptamine, *Biochem. J.,* 64, 621, 1956.

710. **Rodnight, R.,** Body fluid indoles in mental illness, Int. Rev. Neurobiol., 3, 251, 1961.

711. **Roginsky, M. S., Gordon, R. D., Bennett, M. J.,** A rapid and simple gas-liquid chromatographic procedure for homovanillic and vanillylmandelic acid in urine, *Clin. Chim. Acta,* 56, 261, 1974.

712. **Romoff, M. S., Keusch, G., Campese, V. M., Wang, M.-S., Friedler, R. M., Weidmann, P., and Massry, S. G.,** Effect of sodium intake on plasma catecholamines in normal subjects, *J. Clin. Endocrinol. Metab.,* 48, 26, 1979.

713. **Rosano, T. G., and Brown, H. H.,** Liquid-chromatographic assay for urinary 3-methoxy-4-hydroxymandelic acid, with use of a periodate oxidative monitor, *Clin. Chem.* (Winston-Salem, N. C.), 25, 550, 1979.

714. **Rosano, T. G., Brown, H. H., and Meola, J. M.,** Liquid-chromatographic assay for urinary homovanillic acid with fluorescent detection, *Clin. Chem.* (Winston-Salem, N. C.), 27, 228, 1981.

715. **Rosano, T. G., Meola, J. M., and Swift, T. A.,** Liquid-chromatographic determination of urinary 5-hydroxy-3-indoleacetic acid with fluorescence detection, *Clin. Chem.* (Winston-Salem, N. C.), 28, 207, 1982.

716. **Rosenbaum, A. H., Maruta, T., Schatzberg, A. F., Orsulak, P. J., Jiang, N.-S., Cole, J. O., and Schildkraut, J. J.,** Toward a biochemical classification of depressive disorders. VII. Urinary free cortisol and urinary MHPG in depressions, *Am. J. Psychiatry,* 140, 314, 1983.

717. **Rossi-Fanelli, F., Cangiano, C., Attili, A., Angelico, M., Cascino, A., Capocaccia, L., Strom, R., and Crifo, C.,** Octopamine plasma levels in hepatic encephalopathy: A re-appraisal of the problem, *Clin. Chim. Acta,* 67, 255, 1976.

718. **Rothschild, A. J., Langlais, P. J., Schatzberg, A. F., Walsh, F. X., Cole, J. O., and Bird, E. D.,** Dexamethasone increases plasma free dopamine in man, *J. Psychiatr. Res.,* 18, 217, 1984.

719. **Rothschild, A. J., Schatzberg, A. F., Langlais, P. J., Lerbinger, J. E., Miller, M. M., and Cole, J. O.,** Psychotic and nonpsychotic depressions: I. Comparison of plasma catecholamines and cortisol measures, *Psychiatry Res.,* 20, 143, 1987.

720. **Roy, A., Guthrie, S., Pickar, D., and Linnoila, M.,** Plasma norepinephrine responses to cold challenge in depressed patients and normal controls, *Psychiatry Res.,* 21, 161, 1987.

721. **Roy, A., Jimerson, D. C., and Pickar, D.,** Plasma MHPG in depressive disorders and relationship to the dexamethasone suppression test, *Am. J. Psychiatry,* 143, 846, 1986.

722. **Roy, A., Linnoila, M., Karoum, F., and Pickar, D.,** Urinary excretion of free tyramine and of norepinephrine and its metabolites in unipolar depressed patients, *Biol. Psychiatry,* 21, 221, 1986.

723. **Roy, A., Pickar, D., De Jong, J., Karoum, F., and Linnoila, M.,** Norepinephrine and its metabolites in cerebrospinal fluid, plasma and urine. Relationship to hypothalamic pituitary-adrenal axis function in depression, *Arch. Gen. Psychiatry,* 45, 849, 1988.

724. **Roy, A., Pickar, D., Douillet, P., Karoum, F., and Linnoila, M.,** Urinary monoamines and monoamine metabolites in subtypes of unipolar depressive disorder and normal controls, *Psychol. Med.* 16, 541, 1986.

725. **Roy, A., Pickar, D., Linnoila, M., and Potter, W. Z.,** Plasma norepinephrine levels in affective disorders. Relationship to melancholia, *Arch. Gen. Psychiatry,* 42, 1181, 1985.

726. **Roy, A., Pickar, D., Linnoila, M., Doran, A. R., Ninan, P., and Paul, S. M.,** Cerebrospinal fluid monoamine and monoamine metabolite concentrations in melancholia, *Psychiatry Res.,* 15, 281, 1985.

727. **Rubin, A. L., Price, L. H., Charney, D. S., and Heninger, G. R.**, Noradrenergic function and the cortisol response to dexamethasone in depression, *Psychiatry Res.,* 15, 5, 1985.

728. **Rudorfer, M. V., Ross, R. J., Linnoila, M., Sherer, M. A., and Potter, W. Z.**, Exaggerated orthostatic responsivity of plasma norepinephrine in depression, *Arch. Gen. Psychiatry,* 42, 1186, 1985.

729. **Ruthven, C. R. J., and Sandler, M.**, The estimation of homovanillic acid in urine, *Biochem. J.,* 83, 30P, 1962.

730. **Ruthven, C. R. J., and Sandler, M.**, The estimation of 4-hydroxy-3-methoxyphenylglycol and total metadrenalines in human urine, *Clin. Chim. Acta,* 12, 318, 1965.

731. **Ruthven, C. R. J., and Sandler, M.**, An improved method for the estimation of homovanillic acid in human urine, *Clin. Chim. Acta,* 14, 511, 1966.

732. **Rydin, E., Schalling, D., and Åsberg, M.**, Rorschach ratings in depressed and suicidal patients with low levels of 5-hydroxyindole-acetic acid in cerebrospinal fluid, *Psychiatry Res.,* 7, 229, 1982.

733. **Sabelli, H. C., Fawcett, J., Gusovsky, F., Javaid, J., Edwards, J., and Jeffriess, H.**, Urinary phenyl acetate: A diagnostic test for depression? *Science,* 220, 1187, 1983.

734. **Sacchetti, E., Allaria, E., Negri, F., Biondi, P. A., Smeraldi, E., and Cazzullo, C. L.**, 3-Methoxy-4-hydroxyphenyl-glycol and primary depression: Clinical and pharmacological considerations, *Biol. Psychiatry,* 14, 473, 1979.

735. **Saito, T., Ishizawa, H., Tsuchiya, F., Ozawa, H., and Takahata, N.**, Neurochemical findings in the cerebrospinal fluid of schizophrenic patients with tardive dyskinesia and neuroleptic-induced parkinsonism, *Jpn. J. Psychiatr. Neurol.,* 40, 189, 1986.

736. **Sakai, T., Ozawa, M., Aonuma, K., Shimojo, E.,** and **Umeda, N.,** Determination of indole-3-acetic acid in human serum by mass fragmentography, *Koenshu-Iyo Masu Kenkyukai,* 3, 231, 1978; *Chem. Abstr.,* 92, 193778r, 1980.

737. **Sandler, M.,** and **Ruthven, C. R. J.,** Quantitative colorimetric method for estimation of 3-methoxy-4-hydroxymandelic acid in urine. Value in diagnosis of pheochromocytoma, *Lancet,* 2, 114, 1959.

738. **Sandler, M.,** and **Ruthven, C. R. J.,** Colorimetric estimation of 3-methoxy-4-hydroxymandelic acid in urine, *Lancet,* 2, 1034, 1959.

739. **Sandler, M.,** and **Ruthven, C. R. J.,** The estimation of 4-hydroxy-3-methoxymandelic acid in urine, *Biochem. J.,* 80, 78, 1961.

740. **Sandler, M., Ruthven, C. R. J., Goodwin, B. L.,** and **Coppen, A.,** Decreased cerebrospinal fluid concentration of free phenylacetic acid in depressive illness, *Clin. Chim. Acta,* 93, 169, 1979.

741. **Sandler, M., Ruthven, C. R. J., Goodwin, B. L., Field, H., and Matthews, R.,** Phenylethylamine overproduction in aggressive psychopaths, *Lancet,* 2, 1269, 1978.

742. **Sandler, M., Ruthven, C. R. J., Goodwin, B. L., King, G. S., Pettit, B. R., Reynolds, G. P., Tyrer, S. P., Weller, M. P., and Hirsch, S. R.,** Raised cerebrospinal fluid phenylacetic acid concentration: Preliminary support for the phenylethylamine hypothesis of schizophrenia? *Commun. Psychopharmacol.,* 2, 199, 1978.

743. **Sandler, M., Ruthven, C. R. J., Goodwin, B. L., Lees, A., and Stern, G. M.,** Phenylacetic acid in human body fluids: High correlation between plasma and cerebrospinal fluid concentration values, *J. Neurol. Neurosurg. Psychiatry,* 45, 366, 1982.

744. **Sandler, M., Ruthven, C. R. J., Goodwin, B. L., Reynolds, G. P., Rao, V. A. R., and Coppen, A.,** Deficient production of tyramine and octopamine in cases of depression, *Nature,* 278, 357, 1979.

745. **Sankoff, I., and Sourkes, T. L.,** Determination by thin-layer chromatography of urinary homovanillic acid in normal and disease states, *Can. J. Biochem. Physiol.,* 41, 1381, 1963.

746. **Santagostino, G., Frattini, P., Schinelli, S., Cucchi, M. L., and Corona, G. L.,** Urinary 3-methoxy-4-hydroxyphenylglycol determination using reversed-phase chromatography with amperometric detection, *J. Chromatogr.,* 233, 89, 1982.

747. **Sapira, J. D.,** The determination of urinary 3-methoxy-4-hydroxy-mandelic acid and free 3-methoxy-4-hydroxyphenylglycol, *Clin. Chim. Acta,* 20, 139, 1968.

748. **Saran, R. K., Sahuja, R. C., Gupta, N. N., Hasan, M., Bhargava, K. P., Shanker, K., and Kishor, K.,** 3-methoxy-4-hydroxyphenylglycol in cerebrospinal fluid and vanillylmandelic acid in urine of humans with hypertension, *Science,* 200, 317, 1978.

749. **Sarrias, M. J., Artigas, F., Martinez, E., Gelpi, E., Alvarez, E., Udina, C., and Casas, M.,** Decreased plasma serotonin in melancholic patients: A study with clomipramine, *Biol. Psychiatry,* 22, 1429, 1987.

750. **Sasa, S., Blank, C. L., Wenke, D. C., and Sczupak, C. A.,** Liquid-chromatographic determination of serotonin in serum and plasma, *Clin. Chem.* (Winston-Salem, N. C.), 24, 1509, 1978.

751. **Sato, T. L.,** The quantitative determination of 3-methoxy-4-hydroxyphenylacetic acid (homovanillic acid) in urine, *J. Lab. Clin. Med.,* 66, 517, 1965.

752.   **Sato, T., and De Quattro, V.**, Enzymatic assay for 3,4-dihydroxymandelic acid (DOMA) in human urine, plasma and tissues, *J. Lab. Clin. Med.*, 74, 672, 1969.

753.   **Scatton, B., Lôo, H., Dennis, T., Benkelfat, C., Gay, C., Poirier-Littre, M.-F.**, Decrease in plasma levels of 3,4-dihydroxyphenylethyleneglycol in major depression, *Psychopharmacology*, 88, 220, 1986.

754.   **Schatzberg, A. F., Orsulak, P. J., Rosenbaum, A. H., Maruta, T., Kruger, E. R., Cole, J. O., and Schildkraut, J. J.**, Toward a biochemical classification of depressive disorders.   V. Heterogeneity of unipolar depressions, *Am. J. Psychiatry*, 139, 471, 1982.

755.   **Scheinin, M., Seppala, T., Koulu, M., Linnoila, M.**, Determination of conjugated dopamine in cerebrospinal fluid from humans and non-human primates with high performance liquid chromatography using electrochemical detection, *Acta Pharmacol. Toxicol.*, 55, 88, 1984.

756.   **Schildkraut, J. J., Gordon, E. K., and Durell, J.**, Catecholamine metabolism in affective disorders.   I. Normetanephrine and VMA excretion in depressed patients treated with imipramine, *J. Psychiatr. Res.*, 3, 213, 1965.

757.   **Schildkraut, J. J., Green, J., Gordon, E. K., and Durell, J.**, Normetanephrine excretion and affective state in depressed patients treated with imipramine, *Am. J. Psychiatry*, 123, 690, 1966.

758.   **Schildkraut, J. J., Keeler, B. A., Papousek, M., and Hartmann, E.**, MHPG excretion in depressive disorders: Relation to clinical subtypes and desynchronized sleep, *Science*, 181, 762, 1973.

759. **Schildkraut, J. J., Klerman, G. L., Hammond, R., and Friend, D. G.,** Excretion of 3-methoxy-4-hydroxymandelic acid (VMA) in depressed patients treated with antidepressant drugs, *J. Psychiatr. Res.,* 2, 257, 1964.

760. **Schildkraut, J. J., Orsulak, P. J., La Brie, R. A., Schatzberg, A. F., Gudeman, J. E., Cole, J. O., and Rohde, W. A.,** Towards a biochemical classification of depressive disorders. II. Application of multivariate discriminant function analysis to data on urinary catecholamines and metabolites, *Arch. Gen. Psychiatry,* 35, 1436, 1978.

761. **Schildkraut, J. J., Orsulak, P. J., Schatzberg, A. F., Gudeman, J. E., Cole, J. O., Rohde, W. A., and La Brie, R. A.,** Toward a biochemical classification of depressive disorders. I. Differences in urinary excretion of MHPG and other catecholamine metabolites in clinically defined subtypes of depression, *Arch. Gen. Psychiatry,* 35, 1427, 1978.

762. **Schinelli, S., Frattini, P., Cucchi, M. L., Peroni, A. E., and Santagostino, G.,** Determination of vanillylmandelic acid in plasma by high-performance liquid chromatography with electrochemical detection, *J. Chromatogr.,* 431, 150, 1988.

763. **Schinelli, S., Santagostino, G., Frattini, P., Cucchi, M. L., and Corona, G. L.,** Assay of 3-methoxy-4-hydroxyphenylglycol in human plasma using high-performance liquid chromatography with amperometric detection, *J. Chromatogr.,* 338, 396, 1985.

764. **Schweitzer, J. W., Friedhoff, A. J., and Schwartz, R.,** Phenethylamine in normal urine: Failure to verify high values, *Biol. Psychiatry,* 10, 277, 1975.

765. **Scott, M. C., and Elchisak, M. A.,** Direct measurement of dopamine-O-sulfate in plasma and cerebrospinal fluid, *J. Chromatogr.,* 413, 17, 1987.

766. **Seakins, J. W. T.,** The determination of urinary phenylacetylglutamine as phenylacetic acid. Studies on its origin in normal subjects and children with cystic fibrosis, *Clin. Chim. Acta,* 35, 121, 1971.

767. **Sedvall, G.,** Concentrations of monoamine metabolites and chlorpromazine in cerebrospinal fluid for prediction of therapeutic response in psychotic patients treated with neuroleptic drugs, *Prog. Biochem. Pharmacol.,* 16, 133, 1980.

768. **Sedvall, G., Fyrö, B., Gullberg, B., Nybäck, H., Wiesel, F. A., and Wode-Helgodt, B.,** Relationships in healthy volunteers between concentrations of monoamine metabolites in cerebrospinal fluid and family history of psychiatric morbidity, *Br. J. Psychiatry,* 136, 366, 1980.

769. **Sedvall, G., Fyrö, B., Nybäck, H., Wiesel, F. A., and Wode-Helgodt, B.,** Mass fragmentographic determination of homovanillic acid in lumbar cerebrospinal fluid of schizophrenic patients during treatment with antipsychotic drugs, *J. Psychiatr. Res.,* 11, 75, 1974.

770. **Sedvall, G., and Wode-Helgodt, B.,** Aberrant monoamine metabolite levels in CSF and family history of schizophrenia. Their relationships in schizophrenic patients, *Arch. Gen. Psychiatry,* 37, 1113, 1980.

771. **Seki, T., and Hamaji, M.,** Method for the fluorimetric estimation of dopamine, *J. Chromatogr.,* 162, 388, 1979.

772.   **Semba, J. I., Watanabe, A., and Takahashi, R.,** Determination of plasma homovanillic acid by two-step solid-phase extraction and high-performance liquid chromatography with electrochemical detection, *J. Chromatogr.,* 430, 118, 1988.

773.   **Seppala, T., Scheinin, M., Capone, A., and Linnoila, M.,** Liquid chromatographic assay for CSF catecholamines using electro-chemical detection, *Acta Pharmacol. Toxicol.,* 55, 81, 1984.

774.   **Sever, P. S., Birch, M., Osikowska, B., and Tunbridge, R. D. G.,** Plasma-noradrenalin in essential hypertension, *Lancet,* 1, 1078, 1977.

775.   **Sevy, S., Papadimitriou, G. N., Surmont, D. W., Goldman, S., and Mendlewicz, J.,** Noradrenergic function in generalized anxiety disorder, major depressive disorder, and healthy subjects, *Biol. Psychiatry,* 25, 141, 1989.

776.   **Shaff, R. E., and Beaven, M. A.,** Increased sensitivity of the enzymatic isotopic assay of histamine: Measurement of histamine in plasma and serum, *Anal. Biochem.,* 94, 425, 1979.

777.   **Sharma, M., Palacios-Bois, J., Schwartz, G., Iskandar, H., Thakur, M., Quirion, R., and Nair, N. P. V.,** Circadian rhythms of melatonin and cortisol in aging, *Biol. Psychiatry,* 25, 305, 1989.

778.   **Sharpless, N. S.,** Determination of 3-methoxy-4-hydroxyphenylglycol in urine and the effect of diet on its excretion, *Res. Commun. Chem. Pathol. Pharmacol.,* 18, 257, 1977.

779.   **Sharpless, N. S., Halbreich, U., and Feldfogel, B.,** Determination of total 3-methoxy-4-hydroxyphenylglycol in plasma using reversed-phase liquid chromatography with electrochemical detection, *J. Chromatogr.,* 377, 101, 1986.

780.   **Shaw, D. M., O'Keeffe, R., MacSweeney, D. A., Brooksbank, B. W. L., Noguera, R., and Coppen, A.,** 3-Methoxy-4-hydroxyphenyl-glycol in depression, *Psychol. Med.,* 3, 333, 1973.

781.   **Shea, P. A., and Howell, J. B.,** High-performance liquid chromatographic method for determining plasma and urine 3-methoxy-4-hydroxyphenylglycol by amperometric detection, *J. Chromatogr.,* 306, 358, 1984.

782.   **Shen, Y., and Zhang, W.,** 5-Hydroxytryptamine metabolism in schizophrenics, *Chin. Med. J.,* 92, 817, 1979.

783.   **Shimizu, H., and La Brosse, E. H.,** Metabolism of catecholamines. Identification and quantification of 3-methoxy-4-hydroxyphenylglycol glucuronide in human urine, *Biochem. Pharmacol.,* 18, 1643, 1969.

784.   **Shopsin, B., Wilk, S., Gershon, S., Davis, K., and Suhl, M.,** Cerebrospinal fluid MHPG. An assessment of norepinephrine metabolism in affective disorders, *Arch. Gen. Psychiatry,* 28, 230, 1973.

785.   **Shopsin, B., Wilk, S., Sathananthan, G., Gershon, S., and Davis, K.,** Catecholamines and affective disorders revised: A critical assessment, *J. Nerv. Ment. Dis.,* 158, 369, 1974.

786.   **Shoup, R. E., and Kissinger, P. T.,** Determination of urinary normetanephrine, metanephrine and 3-methoxytyramine by liquid chromatography with amperometric detection, *Clin. Chem.* (Winston-Salem, N. C.), 23, 1268, 1977.

787.   **Siegel, M., and Tefft, H.,** "Pink spot" and its components in normal and schizophrenic urine, *J. Nerv. Ment. Dis.,* 152, 412, 1971.

788.   **Sieghart, W., Ronca, E., Drexler, G., and Karall, S.,** Improved radioimmunoassay of melatonin in serum, *Clin. Chem.* (Winston-Salem, N. C.), 33, 604, 1987.

789.   **Siever, L. J., Uhde, T. W., Jimerson, D. C., Lake, C. R., Silberman, E. R., Post, R. M., and Murphy, D. L.,** Differential inhibitory noradrenergic responses to clonidine in 25 depressed patients and 25 normal control subjects, *Am. J. Psychiatry,* 141, 733, 1984.

790.   **Siever, L. J., Uhde, T. W., Jimerson, D. C., Lake, C. R., Kopin, I. J., and Murphy, D. L.,** Indices of noradrenergic output in depression, *Psychiatry Res.,* 19, 59, 1986.

791.   **Siggers, D. C., Salter, C., and Toseland, P. A.,** A double isotope dilution method for differential determination of adrenaline and noradrenaline in plasma, *Clin. Chim. Acta,* 30, 373, 1970.

792.   **Sireix, D. W., and Marini, F. A.,** Studies on the elimination of bufotenin in urine, *Behav. Neuropsychiatry,* 1(5), 29, 1969.

793.   **Sisak, M. E., Markey, S. P., Colburn, R. W., Zavadil, A. P., and Kopin, I. J.,** Identification of 6-hydroxymelatonin in normal human urine by gas chromatography-mass spectrometry, *Life Sci.,* 25, 803, 1979.

794.   **Siwers, B., Ringberger, V.-A., Tuck, J. R., and Sjöqvist, F.,** Initial clinical trial based on biochemical methodology of zimelidine (a serotonin uptake inhibitor) in depressed patients, *Clin. Pharmacol. Ther.,* 21, 194, 1977.

795.   **Sjaastad, O.,** Urinary excretion of free and conjugated histamine in healthy individuals, *Scand. J. Clin. Lab. Invest.,* 18, 617, 1966.

796.   **Sjoerdsma, A., Lovenberg, W., Oates, J. A., Crout, J. R., and Udenfriend, S.,** Alterations in the pattern of amine excretion in man produced by a monoamine oxidase inhibitor, *Science,* 130, 225, 1959.

797. **Sjoerdsma, A., Oates, J. A., Zaltzman, P., and Udenfriend, S.,** Identification and assay of urinary tryptamine: Application as an index of monoamine oxidase inhibition in man, *J. Pharmacol. Exp. Ther.,* 126, 217, 1959.

798. **Sjöquist, B.,** Mass fragmentographic determination of 4-hydroxy-3-methoxymandelic acid in human urine, cerebrospinal fluid, brain and serum using a deuterium-labelled internal standard, *J. Neurochem.,* 24, 199, 1975.

799. **Sjöquist, B., and Ånggård, E.,** Gas chromatographic determination of homovanillic acid in human cerebrospinal fluid by electrochemical detection and by mass spectrometry with a deuterated internal standard, *Anal. Chem.,* 44, 2297, 1972.

800. **Sjöquist, B., and Johansson, B.,** A comparison between fluorometric and mass fragmentographic determinations of homovanillic acid and 5-hydroxyindoleacetic acid in human cerebrospinal fluid, *J. Neurochem.,* 31, 621, 1978.

801. **Sjöquist, B., Lindström, B., and Ånggård, E.,** Mass fragmentographic determination of homovanillic acid in tissues and body fluids using the deuterium-labeled species as internal standard, *Life Sci.,* 13, 1655, 1973.

802. **Sjöquist, B., Lindström, B., and Ånggård, E.,** Mass fragmentographic determination of 4-hydroxy-3-methoxyphenylglycol (HMPG) in urine, cerebrospinal fluid, plasma and tissues using a deuterium-labelled internal standard, *J. Chromatogr.,* 105, 309, 1975.

803. **Sjöstrom, R., Ekstedt, J., and Ånggård, E.,** Concentration gradients of monoamine metabolites in human cerebrospinal fluid, *J. Neurol. Neurosurg. Psychiatry,* 38, 666, 1975.

804. **Skrinska, V., and Hahn, S.,** High-performance liquid chromatography of 5-hydroxyindole-3-acetic acid in urine with direct sample injection, *J. Chromatogr.,* 311, 380, 1984.

805. **Slingsby, J. M., and Boulton, A. A.,** Separation and quantitation of some urinary arylalkylamines, *J. Chromatogr.,* 123, 51, 1976.

806. **Sloane, R. B., Hughes, W., and Haust, H. L.,** Catecholamine excretion in manic depressive and schizophrenic psychosis and its relationship to symptomatology, *Can. Psychiatr. Assoc. J.,* 11, 6, 1966.

807. **Smith, E. R. B., and Weil-Malherbe, H.,** Metanephrine and normetanephrine in human urine: Method and results, *J. Clin. Lab. Med.,* 60, 212, 1962.

808. **Smith, E. R. B., and Weil-Malherbe, H.,** On the occurrence of glusulase-hydrolyzable conjugates of 3,4-dihydroxyphenylacetic and homovanillic acids in human urine, *Clin. Chim. Acta,* 35, 505, 1971.

809. **Smith, I., and Kellow, A. H.,** Aromatic amines and Parkinson's disease, *Nature,* 221, 1261, 1969.

810. **Smith, I., and Kellow, A. H.,** The estimation of true urinary tyramine in man, *Clin. Chim. Acta,* 40, 353, 1972.

811. **Smith, I., Kellow, A. H., Mullen, P. E., and Hanington, E.,** Dietary migraine and tyramine metabolism, *Nature,* 230, 246, 1971.

812. **Smith, J. A., Padwick, D., Mee, T. J. X., Minneman, K. P., and Bird, E. D.,** Synchronous nyctohemeral rhythms in human blood melatonin and in human post mortem pineal enzyme, *Clin. Endocrinol.,* 6, 219, 1977.

813. **Smythies, J. R., Morin, R. D., and Brown, G. B.,** Identification of dimethyltryptamine and *O*-methylbuftenin in human cerebrospinal fluid by combined gas chromatography/mass spectrometry, *Biol. Psychiatry,* 14, 549, 1979.

814. **Soininen, H., MacDonald, E., Rekonen, M., and Riekkinen, P. J.,** Homovanillic acid and 5-hydroxyindoleacetic acid levels in cerebrospinal fluid of patients with senile dementia of Alzheimer type, *Acta Neurol. Scand.,* 64, 101, 1981.

815. **Sole, M. J., and Hussani, M. N.,** A simple specific radioenzymatic assay for the simultaneous measurement of picogram quantities of norepinephrine, epinephrine, and dopamine in plasma and tissues, *Biochem. Med.,* 18, 301, 1977.

816. **Sparks, D. L., and Slevin, J. T.,** Determination of tyrosine, tryptophan and their metabolic derivatives by liquid chromatography-electrochemical detection: Application to post mortem samples from patients with Parkinson's and Alzheimer's disease, *Life Sci.,* 36, 449, 1985.

817. **Spatz, H., and Spatz, N.,** Spectrophotofluorometric determination of *beta*-phenylethylamine in blood and urine, *Biochem. Med.,* 6, 1, 1972.

818. **Spiker, D. G., Edwards, D., Hanin, I., Neil, J. F., and Kupfer, D. J.,** Urinary MHPG and clinical response to amitriptyline in depressed patients, *Am. J. Psychiatry,* 137, 1183, 1980.

819. **Sprince, H.,** Biochemical aspects of indole metabolism in normal and schizophrenic subjects, *Ann. N. Y. Acad. Sci.,* 96, 399, 1962.

820. **Stabenau, J. R., Creveling, C. R., and Daly, J.,** The "pink spot", 3,4-dimethoxyphenylethylamine, common tea, and schizophrenia, *Am. J. Psychiatry,* 127, 611, 1970.

821. **Stachow, A., Bousquet, B., and Dreux, C.,** Variation du rapport tryptamine/acide indolylacetique urinaire dans divers cas pathologiques affectant le metabolisme du tryptophanne, *Clin. Chim. Acta,* 50, 329, 1974.

822. **Stahl, S. M., Faull, K. F., Barchas, J. D., and Berger, P. A.,** CSF monoamine metabolites in movement disorders and normal aging, *Arch. Neurol.,* 42, 166, 1985.

823. **Standish-Barry, H. M. A. S., Bouras, N., Hale, A. S., Bridges, P. K., and Bartlett, J. R.,** Ventricular size and CSF transmitter metabolite concentrations in severe endogenous depression, *Br. J. Psychiatry,* 148, 386, 1986.

824. **Stanley, M., Träskman-Bendz, L., Dorovini-Zis, K.,** Correlations between aminergic metabolites simultaneously obtained from human CSF and brain, *Life Sci.,* 37, 1279, 1985.

825. **Stene, M., Panagiotis, N., Tuck, M. L., Sowers, J. R., Mayes, D., and Berg, G.,** Plasma norepinephrine levels are influenced by sodium intake, glucocorticoid administration and circadian changes in normal man, *J. Clin. Endocrinol. Metab.,* 51, 1340, 1980.

826. **Sternberg, D. E., Charney, D. S., Heninger, G. R., Leckman, J. F., Hafstad, K. M., and Landis, D. H.,** Impaired presynaptic regulation of norepinephrine in schizophrenia. Effects of clonidine in schizophrenic patients and normal controls, *Arch. Gen. Psychiatry,* 39, 285, 1982.

827. **Sternberg, D. E., Van Kammen, D. P., Lake, C. R., Ballenger, J. C., Marder, S. R., and Bunney, W. E.,** The effect of pimozide on CSF norepinephrine in schizophrenia, *Am. J. Psychiatry,* 138, 1045, 1981.

828. **Stewart, J. W., and Halbreich, U.,** Plasma melatonin levels in depressed patients before and after treatment with antidepressant medication, *Biol. Psychiatry,* 25, 33, 1989.

829. **Stokes, P. E., Maas, J. W., Davis, J. M., Koslow, S. H., Casper, R. C., and Stoll, P. M.,** Biogenic amine and metabolite levels in depressed patients with high versus normal hypothalamic-pituitary-adrenocortical activity, *Am. J. Psychiatry,* 144, 868, 1987.

830. **Stott, A. W., Lindsay Smith, J. R., Hanson, P., and Robinson, R.,** A simple chromatographic procedure for the concurrent estimation of urinary 4-hydroxy-3-methoxymandelic acid (HMMA) and homovanillic acid (HVA) using a scanning technique, *Clin. Chim. Acta,* 63, 7, 1975.

831. **Ström-Olsen, R., Weil-Malherbe, H.,** Humoral changes in manic-depressive psychosis with particular reference to the excretion of catechol amines in urine, *J. Ment. Sci.,* 104, 696, 1958.

832. **Subrahmanyam, S.,** Role of biogenic amines in certain pathological conditions, *Brain Res.,* 87, 355, 1975.

833. **Sullivan, J. L., Coffey, C. E., Basuk, B., Cavenar, J. O., Maltbie, A. A., and Zung, W. W. K.,** Urinary tryptamine excretion in chronic schizophrenics with low platelet MAO activity, *Biol. Psychiatry,* 15, 113, 1980.

834. **Sunderland, T., Tariot, P. N., Cohen, R. M., Newhouse, P. A., Mellow, A. M., and Mueller, E. A.,** Dose-dependent effects of deprenyl on CSF monoamine metabolites in patients with Alzheimer's disease, *Psychopharmacology,* 91, 293, 1987.

835. **Sunderman, Jr., F. W., Cleveland, P. D., Law, N. C., and Sunderman, F. W.,** A method for the determination of 3-methoxy-4-hydroxymandelic acid (vanilmandelic acid) for the diagnosis of pheochromocytoma, *Am. J. Clin. Pathol.,* 34, 293, 1960.

836. **Suñol, C., Tusell, J. M., Artigas, F., Martinez, E., Adell, A., and Gelpi, E.,** Studies on tryptamine metabolism by GC-MS and HPLC techniques, in *Neurobiology of the Trace Amines: Analytical, Physiological, Pharmacological, Behavioral, and Clinical Aspects,* Boulton, A. A., Baker, G. B., Dewhurst, W. G., and Sandler, M., Eds., Humana Press Inc., Clifton, New Jersey, 1984, 71.

837. **Suzuki, O., and Hattori, H.,** Determination of β-phenylethylamine as its isothiocyanate derivative in biological samples by gas chromatography mass spectrometry, *Biomed. Mass Spectrom.,* 10, 430, 1983.

838. **Suzuki, O., and Yagi, K.,** A fluorometric assay for β-phenyl-ethylamine in human urine, *Clin. Chim. Acta,* 78, 401, 1977.

839. **Swahn, C.-G., Sandgärde, B., Wiesel, F.-A., and Sedvall, G.,** Simultaneous determination of the three major monoamine metabolites in brain tissue and body fluids by a mass fragmentographic method, *Psychopharmacology,* 48, 147, 1976.

840. **Swahn, C.-G., and Sedvall, G.,** Identification and determination of tele-methyl-histamine in cerebrospinal fluid by gas chromatography-mass spectrometry, *J. Neurochem.,* 37, 461, 1981.

841. **Swahn, C.-G., and Sedvall, G.,** Identification and determination of 1-methyl-imidazole-4-acetic acid in human cerebrospinal fluid by gas chromatography-mass spectrometry, *J. Neurochem.,* 40, 688, 1983.

842. **Swann, A. C., Maas, J. W., Hattox, S. E., and Landis, H.,** Catecholamine metabolites in human plasma as indices of brain function: Effects of debrisoquin, *Life Sci.,* 27, 1857, 1980.

843. **Swann, A. C., Secunda, S., Davis, J. M., Robins, E., Hanin, I., Koslow, S. H., and Maas, J. W.,** CSF monoamine metabolites in mania, *Am. J. Psychiatry,* 140, 396, 1983.

844. **Swann, P. G., and Elchisak, M.-A.,** Sample preparation procedure for determination of dopamine sulfate isomers in human urine by high-performance liquid chromatography with dual-electrode electrochemical detection, *J. Chromatogr.,* 381, 241, 1986.

845. **Sweeney, D. R., Leckman, J. F., Maas, J. W., Hattox, S., and Heninger, G. R.,** Plasma free and conjugated MHPG in psychiatric patients. A pilot study, *Arch. Gen. Psychiatry,* 37, 1100, 1980.

846. **Sweeney, D. R., Maas, J. W., and Heninger, G. R.,** State anxiety, physical activity, and urinary 3-methoxy-4-hydroxyphenethylene glycol excretion, *Arch. Gen. Psychiatry,* 35, 1418, 1978.

847. **Sweeney, D., Nelson, C., Bowers, M., Maas, J., and Heninger, G.,** Delusional vs. non-delusional depression: Neurochemical differences, *Lancet,* 2, 100, 1978.

848. **Szymanski, H. V., Naylor, E. W., and Karoum, F.,** Plasma phenylethylamine and phenylalanine in chronic schizophrenic patients, *Biol. Psychiatry,* 22, 194, 1987.

849. **Takahashi, R., Nagao, Y., Tsuchiya, K., Takamizawa, M., Kobayashi, T., Toru, M., Kobayashi, K., and Kariya, T.,** Catecholamine metabolism of manic-depressive illness, *J. Psychiatr. Res.,* 6, 185, 1968.

850. **Takahashi, S., and Gjessing, L. R.,** A fluorometric method combined with thin layer chromatography for the determination of norepinephrine, epinephrine and dopamine in human urine, *Clin. Chim. Acta,* 36, 369, 1972.

851. **Takahashi, S., Godse, D. D., Warsh, J. J., and Stancer, H. C.,** A gas chromatographic-mass spectrometric (GC-MS) assay for 3-methoxy-4-hydroxyphenethyleneglycol and vanilmandelic acid in human serum, *Clin. Chim. Acta,* 81, 183, 1977.

852. **Takahashi, S., Godse, D. D., Naqvi, A., Warsh, J. J., and Stancer, H. C.,** 5-Hydroxytryptophol in human cerebrospinal fluid: Quantitative determination by gas chromatography-mass spectrometry using a deuterated internal standard, *Clin. Chim. Acta,* 84, 55, 1978.

853. **Takahashi, S., Yoshioka, M., Yoshiue, S., and Tamura, Z.,** Mass fragmentographic determination of vanilmandelic acid, homovanillic acid and isohomovanillic acid in human body fluids, *J. Chromatogr.,* 145, 1, 1978.

854. **Tamarkin, N. R., Goodwin, F. K., and Axelrod, J.,** Rapid elevation of biogenic amine metabolites in human CSF following probenecid, *Life Sci.,* 9, 1397, 1970.

855. **Taniguchi, K., Kakimoto, Y., and Armstrong, M. D.,** Quantitative determination of metanephrine and normetanephrine in urine, *J. Lab. Clin. Med.,* 64, 469, 1964.

856. **Taube, S. L., Kirstein, L. S., Sweeney, D. R., Heninger, G. R., and Maas, J. W.,** Urinary 3-methoxy-4-hydroxyphenylglycol and psychiatric diagnosis, *Am. J. Psychiatry,* 135, 78, 1978.

857. **Tetsuo, M., Markey, S. P., Colburn, R. W., and Kopin, I. J.,** Quantitative analysis of 6-hydroxymelatonin in human urine by gas chromatography-negative chemical ionization mass spectrometry, *Anal. Biochem.,* 110, 208, 1981.

858. **Tetsuo, M., Markey, S. P., and Kopin, I. J.,** Measurement of 6-hydroxymelatonin in human urine and its diurnal variations, *Life Sci.,* 27, 105, 1980.

859. **Tham, R.,** Gas chromatographic analysis of histamine metabolites in urine. Quantitative determination of ring methylated imidazole acetic acids in healthy man, *J. Chromatogr.,* 23, 207, 1966.

860.   **Thiede, H.-M., and Kehr, W.,** Conjoint radioenzymatic measurement of catecholamines, their catechol metabolites and DOPA in biological samples, *Naunyn Schmiedeberg's Arch. Pharmacol.,* 318, 19, 1981.

861.   **Toth, L. A., Scott, M. C., and Elchisak, M. A.,** Dopamine sulfate formation and phenol sulfotransferase activity in dog and human platelets, *Life Sci.,* 39, 519, 1986.

862.   **Townshend, M. M., and Smith, A. J.,** Factors influencing the urinary excretion of free catecholamines in man, *Clin. Sci.,* 44, 253, 1973.

863.   **Tracy, R. P., Wold, L. E., Jones, J. D., and Burritt, M. F.,** Colorimetric vs. liquid-chromatographic determination of urinary 5-hydroxyindole-3-acetic acid, *Clin. Chem.* (Winston-Salem, N. C.), 27, 160, 1981.

864.   **Träskman, L., Åsberg, M., Bertilsson, L., Cronholm, B., Mellström, B., Neckers, L. M., Sjöqvist, F., Thorén, P., and Tybring, G.,** Plasma levels of chlorimipramine and its demethyl metabolite during treatment of depression, *Clin. Pharmacol. Ther.,* 26, 600, 1979.

865.   **Träskman, L., Åsberg, M., Bertilsson, L., and Sjöstrand, L.,** Monoamine metabolites in CSF and suicidal behavior, *Arch. Gen. Psychiatry,* 38, 631, 1981.

866.   **Tsuchiya, H., Tatsumi, M., Takagi, N., Koike, T., Yamaguchi, H., and Hayashi, T.,** High-performance liquid chromatographic determination of urinary catecholamines by pre-column solid-phase dansylation on alumina, *Anal. Biochem.,* 155, 28, 1986.

867. **Tsuji, M., Ohi, K., Taga, C., Myojin, T., and Takahashi, S.,** Determination of β-phenylethylamine concentrations in human plasma, platelets, and urine and in animal tissues by high-performance liquid chromatography with fluorometric detection, *Anal. Biochem.*, 153, 116, 1986.

868. **Tsuruta, Y., Kohashi, K., and Ohkura, Y.,** Determination of histamine in plasma by high-speed liquid chromatography, *J. Chromatogr.*, 146, 490, 1978.

869. **Tsuruta, Y., Kohashi, K., and Ohkura, Y.,** Simultaneous determination of histamine and N^τ-methylhistamine in human urine and rat brain by high performance liquid chromatography with fluorescence detection, *J. Chromatogr.*, 224, 105, 1981.

870. **Tsuruta, Y., Tomida, H., Kohashi, K., and Ohkura, Y.,** Simultaneous determination of imidazoleacetic acid and N^τ- and N^π-methylimidazoleacetic acids in human urine by high-performance liquid chromatography with fluorescence detection, *J. Chromatogr.*, 416, 63, 1987.

871. **Turnbull, M. J., and Kelvin, A. S.,** Cigarette dependence, *Br. Med. J.*, 3, 115, 1971.

872. **Turton, M. B., and Deegan, T.,** Circadian variations of plasma catecholamine, cortisol and immunoreactive insulin concentrations in supine subjects, *Clin. Chim. Acta,* 55, 389, 1974.

872a. **Tyce, G. M., Van Dyke, R. A., Rettge, S. R., Atchison, S. R., Wiesner, R. H., Dickson, E. R., and Krom, R. A.,** Human liver and conjugation of catecholamines, *J. Lab. Clin. Med.*, 109, 532, 1987.

873. **Uchikura, K., Horikawa, R., Tanimura, T., Kabasawa, Y.,** Determination of catecholamines by radioenzymatic assay using ion-pair liquid chromatography, *J. Chromatogr.*, 223, 41, 1981.

874. **Ueda, E., Yoshida, N., Nishimura, K., Joh, T., Antoku, S., Tsukada, K., Ganno, S., and Kokubu, T.,** A semi-automated measurement of urinary catecholamines using high-speed ion-exchange column chromatography, *Clin. Chim. Acta,* 80, 447, 1977.

875. **Uhde, T. W., Joffe, R. T., Jimerson, D. C., and Post, R. M.,** Normal urinary free cortisol and plasma MHPG in panic disorder: Clinical and theoretical considerations, *Biol. Psychiatry,* 23, 575, 1988.

876. **Vahidi, A., Roberts, H. R., San Filippo, J., Siva Sankar, D. V.,** Paper-chromatographic quantitation of 4-hydroxy-3-methoxymandelic acid (VMA) in urine, *Clin. Chem.* (Winston-Salem, N. C.), 17, 903, 1971.

877. **Van Bemmel, A. L., Smeets, E. H. J., and Van Diest, R.,** The 24-hour pattern of urinary MHPG excretion in depressives and normals, *Acta Psychiatr. Scand.,* 78, 298, 1988.

878. **Van Bockstaele, M., Dillen, L., Claeys, M., and de Potter, W. P.,** Simultaneous determination of the three major monoamine metabolites in cerebrospinal fluid by high-performance liquid chromatography with electrochemical detection, *J. Chromatogr.,* 275, 11, 1983.

879. **Van de Calseyde, J. F., Scholtis, R. J. H., Schmidt, N. A., and Leyton, C. J. J. A.,** Gas chromatography in the estimation of urinary metanephrines and VMA, *Clin. Chim. Acta,* 32, 361, 1971.

880. **Van Kammen, D. P., Mann, L. S., Sternberg, D. E., Scheinin, M., Ninan, P. T., Marder, S. R., Van Kammen, W. B., Rieder, R. O., and Linnoila, M.,** Dopamine-β-hydroxylase activity and homovanillic acid in spinal fluid of schizophrenics with brain atrophy, *Science,* 220, 974, 1983.

881. **Van Loon, G. R., Schwartz, L., and Sole, M. J.,** Plasma dopamine responses to standing and exercise in man, *Life Sci.,* 24, 2273, 1979.

882. **Van Praag, H. M.,** New evidence of serotonin deficient depressions, *Neuropsychobiology,* 3, 56, 1977.

883. **Van Praag, H. M., Flentge, F., Korf, J., Dols, L. C. W., and Schut, T.,** The influence of probenecid on the metabolism of serotonin, dopamine and their precursors in man, *Psychopharmacologia,* 33, 141, 1973.

884. **Van Praag, H. M., and Korf, J.,** A pilot study of some kinetic aspects of the metabolism of 5-hydroxytrypamine in depressive patients, *Biol. Psychiatry,* 3, 105, 1971.

885. **Van Praag, H. M., and Korf, J.,** Endogenous depressions with and without disturbances in the 5-hydroxytryptamine metabolism: A biochemical classificastion? *Psychopharmacologia,* 19, 148, 1971.

886. **Van Praag, H. M., and Korf, J.,** Retarded depression and the dopamine metabolism, *Psychopharmacologia,* 19, 199, 1971.

887. **Van Praag, H. M., and Korf, J.,** Cerebral monoamines and depression: An investigation with the probenecid technique, *Arch. Gen. Psychiatry,* 28, 827, 1973.

888. **Van Praag, H. M., Korf, J., Dols, L. C. W., and Schut, T.,** A pilot study of the predictive value of the probenecid test in application of 5-hydroxytryptophan as antidepressant, *Psychopharmacologia,* 25, 14, 1972.

889. **Van Praag, H. M., Korf, J., Lakke, J. P. W. F., and Schut, T.,** Dopamine metabolism in depression, psychoses, and Parkinson's disease: The problem of the specificity of biological variables in behaviour disorders, *Psychol. Med.,* 5, 138, 1975.

890. **Van Praag, H. M., Korf, J., Van Woudenberg, F., and Kits, T. P.,** Influencing the human indoleamine metabolism by means of a chlorinated amphetamine derivative with antidepressive action (*p*-chloro-N-methylamphetamine), *Psychopharmacologia,* 13, 145, 1968.

891. **Van Praag, H. M., and Leijnse, B.,** Die Bedeutung der Monoaminoxydasehemmung als antidepressives Prinzip, *Psychopharmacologia,* 4, 1, 1963.

892. **Van Woert, M. H., and Bowers, M. B.,** The effect of L-dopa on monoamine metabolites in Parkinson's disease, *Experientia,* 26, 161, 1970.

893. **Verburg, K. M., Bowsher, R. R., and Henry, D. P.,** A new radioenzymatic assay for histamine using purified histamine *N*-methyltransferase, *Life Sci.,* 32, 2855, 1983.

894. **Vestergaard, P., Sorensen, T., Hoppe, E., Rafaelsen, O. J., Yates, C. M., and Nicolaou, N.,** Biogenic amine metabolites in cerebrospinal fluid of patients with affective disorders, *Acta Psychiatr. Scand.,* 58, 88, 1978.

895. **Vidi, A., and Bonardi, G.,** Simple quantitative method for determining 3-methoxy-4-hydroxyphenylacetic acid and 3,4-dihydroxyphenylacetic acid in urine, *Clin. Chim. Acta,* 38, 463, 1972.

896. **Viktora, J. K., Baukal, A., and Wolff, F. W.,** New automated fluorometric methods for estimation of small amounts of adrenaline and noradrenaline, *Anal. Biochem.,* 23, 513, 1968.

897. **Virkkunen, M., Nuutila, A., Goodwin, F. K., and Linnoila, M.,** Cerebrospinal fluid monoamine metabolite levels in male arsonists, *Arch. Gen. Psychiatry,* 44, 241, 1987.

898. **Vlachakis, N. D., Alexander, N., Velasquez, M. T., and Maronde, R. F.,** A radioenzymatic microassay for simultaneous measurement of catecholamines and their deaminated metabolites, *Biochem. Med.,* 22, 323, 1979.

899. **Vlachakis, N. D., and De Quattro, V.,** A simple and specific radioenzymatic assay for measurement of urinary normetanephrine, *Biochem. Med.,* 20, 107, 1978.

900. **Vlachakis, N. D., Kogosov, E., Yoneda, S., Alexander, N., and Maronde, R. F.,** Plasma levels of free and total catecholamines and two deaminated metabolites in man - rapid deconjugation by heat in acid, *Clin. Chim. Acta,* 137, 199, 1984.

901. **Vlachakis, N. D., Lampano, C., Alexander, N., and Maronde, R. F.,** Catecholamines and their major metabolites in plasma and cerebrospinal fluid of man, *Brain Res.,* 229, 67, 1981.

902. **Vlachakis, N. D., and Niarchos, A.,** Plasma normetanephrine measurements for detection of pheochromocytoma in patients with hypertension, *Clin. Chim. Acta,* 99, 283, 1979.

903. **Vogel, W. H., Ahlberg, C. D., Di Carlo, V., and Horwitt, M. K.,** Pink spot, *p*-tyramine and schizophrenia, *Nature,* 216, 1038, 1967.

904. **Vogel, W. H., Ahlberg, C. D., and Horwitt, M. K.,** Time study of the urinary excretion of 3,4-dimethoxyphenylethylamine and 3,4-dimethoxyphenylacetic acid by schizophrenic and normal individuals, *Int. J. Neuropsychiatry,* 3, 292, 1967.

905. **Vogt, W., Jacob, K., Ohnesorge, A.-B., and Schwertfeger, G.,** Highly sensitive method for the quantitation of homovanillic acid in cerebrospinal fluid, *J. Chromatogr.,* 199, 191, 1980.

906. **Volicer, L., Direnfeld, L. K., Freedman, M., Albert, M. L., Langlais, P. J., and Bird, E. D.,** Serotonin and 5-hydroxyindoleacetic acid in CSF. Difference in Parkinson's disease and dementia of the Alzheimer's type, *Arch. Neurol.,* 42, 127, 1985.

907. **Volicer, L., Langlais, P. J., Matson, W. R., Mark, K. A., and Gamache, P. H.,** Serotoninergic system in dementia of the Alzheimer type. Abnormal forms of 5-hydroxytryptophan and serotonin in cerebrospinal fluid, *Arch. Neurol.* 42, 1158, 1985.

908. **Von Studnitz, W.,** Methodische und klinische Untersuchungen über die Ausscheidung der 3-Methoxy-4-hydroxymandelsäure im Urin, *Scand. J. Clin. Lab. Invest.,* 12(Suppl. 48), 1, 1960.

909. **Von Studnitz, W., and Hanson, A.,** Determination of 3-methoxy-4-hydroxymandelic acid in urine by high-voltage paper electrophoresis, *Scand. J. Clin. Lab. Invest.,* 11, 101, 1959.

910. **Wadman, S. K., Ketting, D., and Voûte, P. A.,** Gas chromatographic determination of urinary vanilglycolic acid, vanilglycol, vanilacetic acid and vanillactic acid - chemical parameters for the diagnosis of neurogenic tumors and the evaluation of their treatment, *Clin. Chim. Acta,* 72, 49, 1976.

911. **Waldmeier, P. C., Antonin, K.-H., Feldtrauer, J.-J., Grunenwald, C., Paul, E., Lauber, J., and Bieck, P.,** Urinary excretion of *O*-methylated catecholamines, tyramine and phenylethylamine by volunteers treated with tranylcypromine and CGP 11305A, *Eur. J. Clin. Pharmacol.,* 25, 361, 1983.

912. **Walker, R. W., Ahn, H. S., Albers-Schönberg, G., Mandel, L. R., and Vandenheuvel, W. J. A.,** Gas chromatographic-mass spectrometric isotope dilution assay for *N,N*-dimethyltryptamine in human plasma, *Biochem. Med.,* 8, 105, 1973.

913. **Walker, R. W., Mandel, L. R., Kleinman, J. E., Gillin, J. C., Wyatt, R. J., and Vandenheuvel, W. J. A.,** Improved selective ion monitoring mass spectrometric assay for the determination of N,N-dimethyltryptamine in human blood utilizing capillary column gas chromatography, *J. Chromatogr.,* 162, 539, 1979.

914. **Wang, M.-T., Imai, K., Yoshioka, M., and Tamura, Z.,** Gas-liquid chromatographic and mass fragmentographic determination of catecholamines in human plasma, *Clin. Chim. Acta,* 63, 13, 1975.

915. **Wang, M.-T., Yoshioka, M., Imai, K., and Tamura, Z.,** Gas-liquid chromatographic and mass fragmentographic determination of 3-*O*-methylated catecholamines in human plasma, *Clin. Chim. Acta,* 63, 21, 1975.

916. **Wang, P. C., Buu, N. T., Kuchel, O., and Genest, J.,** Conjugation patterns of endogenous plasma catecholamines in human and rat. A new specific method for analysis of glucuronide-conjugated catecholamines, *J. Lab. Clin. Med.,* 101, 141, 1983.

917. **Ward, M. M., Mefford, I. N., Parker, S. D., Chesney, M. A., Taylor, C. B., Keegan, D. L., and Barchas, J. D.,** Epinephrine and norepinephrine responses in continuously collected human plasma to a series of stressors, *Psychosom. Med.,* 45, 471, 1983.

918. **Warsh, J. J., Hasey, G., Cooke, R. G., Stancer, H. C., Persad, E., Jorna, T., and Godse, D. D.,** Elevated 3,4-dihydroxyphenylethyleneglycol (DHPG) excretion in dexamethasone resistant depressed patients, *Prog. Neuropsychopharmacol. Biol. Psychiatry,* 9, 661, 1985.

919. **Watson, E., and Wilk, S.,** Assessment of cerebrospinal fluid levels of dopamine metabolites by gas chromatography, *Psychopharmacologia,* 42, 57, 1975.

920.   **Watson, R. D. S., Hamilton, C. A., Jones, D. H., Reid, J. L., Stallard, T. J., and Littler, W. A.,** Sequential changes in plasma noradrenaline during bicycle exercise, *Clin. Sci.,* 58, 37, 1980.

921.   **Watts, D. T., and Bragg, A. D.,** Effect of smoking on the urinary output of epinephrine and norepinephrine in man, *J. Appl. Physiol.,* 9, 275, 1956.

922.   **Weg, M. W., Ruthven, C. R. J., Goodwin, B. L., and Sandler, M.,** Specific gas chromatographic measurement of urinary 3,4-dihydroxyphenylacetic acid, *Clin. Chim. Acta,* 59, 249, 1975.

923.   **Weidmann, P., de Chatel, R., Schiffmann, A., Bachmann, E., Beretta-Piccoli, C., Reubi, F. C., Ziegler, W. H., and Vetter, W.,** Interrelations between age and plasma renin, aldosterone and cortisol, urinary catecholamines, and the body sodium/volume state in normal man, *Klin. Wschr.,* 55, 725, 1977.

924.   **Weil-Malherbe, H.,** The estimation of 3,4-dihydroxymandelic acid in urine and its excretion by man, *J. Lab. Clin. Med.,* 69, 1025, 1967.

925.   **Weil-Malherbe, H., and Bone, A. D.,** The adrenergic amines of human blood, *Lancet,* 1, 974, 1953.

926.   **Weil-Malherbe, H., and Liddell, D. W.,** Adrenaline and noradrenaline in cerebrospinal fluid, *J. Neurol. Neurosurg. Psychiatry,* 17, 247, 1954.

927.   **Weil-Malherbe, H., and Van Buren, J. M.,** The excretion of dopamine and dopamine metabolites in Parkinson's disease and the effect of diet thereon, *J. Lab. Clin. Med.,* 74, 305, 1969.

928.   **Weiner, W., Harrison, W., and Klawans, H.,** L-Dopa and cerebrospinal fluid homovanillic acid in Parkinsonism, *Life Sci.,* 8, 971, 1969.

929. **Weise, V. K., and Kopin, I. J.,** Assay of catecholamines in human plasma: Studies of a single isotope radioenzymatic procedure, *Life Sci.,* 19, 1673, 1976.

930. **Weise, V. K., McDonald, R. K., and La Brosse, E. H.,** Determination of urinary 3-methoxy-4-hydroxymandelic acid in man, *Clin. Chim. Acta,* 6, 79, 1961.

931. **Weissbach, H., King, W., Sjoerdsma, A., and Udenfriend, S.,** Formation of indole-3-acetic acid and tryptamine in animals, *J. Biol. Chem.,* 234, 81, 1959.

932. **Westenberg, H. G. M., and Verhoeven, W. M. A.,** CSF monoamine metabolites in patients and controls: Support for a bimodal distribution in major affective disorders, *Acta Psychiatr. Scand.,* 78, 541, 1988.

933. **Westerink, B. H. C., Bosker, F. J., and O'Hanlon, J. F.,** Use of alumina, Sephadex G10, and ion-exchange columns to purify samples for determination of epinephrine, norepinephrine, dopamine, homovanillic acid and 5-hydroxyindoleacetic acid in urine, *Clin. Chem.* (Winston-Salem, N. C.), 28, 1745, 1982.

934. **Wetterberg, L., Eriksson, O., Friberg, Y., and Vangbo, B.,** A simplified radioimmunoassay for melatonin and its application to biological fluids. Preliminary observations on the half-life of plasma melatonin in man, *Clin. Chim. Acta,* 86, 169, 1978.

935. **Wiesel, F.-A., Fyrö, B., Nybäck, H., Sedvall, G., Wode-Helgodt, B.,** Relationships in healthy volunteers between secretion of monoamine metabolites in urine, and family history of psychiatric morbidity, *Biol. Psychiatry,* 17, 1403, 1982.

936. **Wilk, E. K., Gitlow, S. E., and Bertani, L. M.,** Modification of the Taniguchi Method for the determination of normetanephrine and metanephrine, *Clin. Chim. Acta,* 20, 147, 1968.

937. **Wilk, S., Davis, K. L., and Thacker, S. B.,** Determination of 3-methoxy-4-hydroxyphenylethylene glycol (MHPG) in cerebrospinal fluid, *Anal. Biochem.,* 39, 498, 1971.

938. **Wilk, S., Gitlow, S. E., Clarke, D. D., and Paley, D. H.,** Determination of urinary 3-methoxy-4-hydroxyphenylethylene glycol by gas-liquid chromatography and electron capture detection, *Clin. Chim. Acta,* 16, 403, 1967.

939. **Wilk, S., Gitlow, S. E., Mendlowitz, M., Franklin, M. J., Carr, H. E., and Clarke, D. D.,** A quantitative assay for vanillylmandelic acid (VMA) by gas-liquid chromatography, *Anal. Biochem.,* 13, 544, 1965.

940. **Wilk, S., and Mones, R.,** Cerebrospinal fluid levels of 3-methoxy-4-hydroxyphenylethylene glycol in Parkinsonism before and after treatment with L-DOPA, *J. Neurochem.,* 18, 1771, 1971.

941. **Wilkes, M. M., Babaknia, A., Hoff, J. D., Quigley, M. E., Kraus, P. F., and Yen, S. S. C.,** Circadian rhythm in circulating concentration of dihydroxyphenylacetic acid in normal women, *J. Clin. Endocrinol. Metab.,* 52, 608, 1981.

942. **Williams, C. M., Maury, S., and Kibler, R. F.,** Normal excretion of homovanillic acid in the urine of patients with Huntington's Chorea, *J. Neurochem.,* 6, 254, 1960.

943. **Williams, C. M., and Sweeley, C. C.,** A new method for the determination of urinary aromatic acids by gas chromatography, *J. Clin. Endocrinol. Metab.,* 21, 1500, 1961.

944. **Wilson, B. W., and Snedden, W.,** Capillary column GCMS detection of 5-methoxytryptamine in human plasma using selected ion monitoring, *J. Neurochem.,* 33, 939, 1979.

945. **Wilson, B. W., Snedden, W., Silman, R. E., Smith, I., and Mullen, P.,** A gas chromatography-mass spectrometry method for the quantitative analysis of melatonin in plasma and cerebrospinal fluid, *Anal. Biochem.,* 81, 283, 1977.

946. **Winer, N., and Carter, C.,** Effect of cold pressor stimulation on plasma norepinephrine, dopamine-β-hydroxylase, and renin activity, *Life Sci.,* 20, 887, 1977.

947. **Woiwod, A. J., and Knight, R.,** The determination of 3-methoxy-4-hydroxymandelic acid in urine, *J. Clin. Pathol.,* 14, 502, 1961.

948. **Wolkowitz, O. M., Breier, A., Doran, A., Kelsoe, J., Lucas, P., Paul, S. M., and Pickar, D.,** Alprazolam augmentation of the antipsychotic effects of fluphenazine in schizophrenic patients, *Arch. Gen. Psychiatry,* 45, 664, 1988.

949. **Wolkowitz, O. M., Doran, A., Breier, A., Roy, A., Jimerson, D. C., Sutton, M. E., Golden, R. N., Paul, S. M., and Pickar, D.,** The effects of dexamethasone on plasma homovanillic acid and 3-methoxy-4-hydroxyphenylglycol. Evidence for abnormal corticosteroid-catecholamine interactions in major depression, *Arch. Gen. Psychiatry,* 44, 782, 1987.

950. **Wolkowitz, O. M., Sutton, M. E., Doran, A. R., Labarca, R., Roy, A., Thomas, J. M., Pickar, D., and Paul, S. M.,** Dexamethasone increases plasma HVA but not MHPG in normal humans, *Psychiatry Res.,* 16, 101, 1985.

951. **Wollin, A., and Navert, H.,** Quantitation of histamine and some of its basic methylated metabolites in biological materials by gas-liquid chromatography, *Anal. Biochem.,* 145, 73, 1985.

952. **Wong, J. T. F., Baker, G. B., and Coutts, R. T.,** Rapid and simple procedure for the determination of urinary phenylacetic acid using derivatization in aqueous medium followed by electron-capture gas chromatography, *J. Chromatogr.,* 428, 140, 1988.

953. **Wong, K. P., Ruthven, C. R. J., and Sandler, M.,** Gas chromatographic measurement of urinary catecholamines by an electron capture detection procedure, *Clin. Chim. Acta,* 47, 215, 1973.

954. **Wood, P. L., Etienne, P., Lal, S., Gauthier, S., Cajal, S., Nair, N. P. V.,** Reduced lumbar CSF somatostatin levels in Alzheimer's disease, *Life Sci.,* 31, 2073, 1982.

955. **Wyatt, R. J., Mandel, L. R., Ahn, H. S., Walker, R. W., Vanden Heuvel, W. J. A.,** Gas chromatographic-mass spectrometric isotope dilution determination of *N,N*-dimethyltryptamine concentrations in normals and psychiatric patients, *Psychopharmacologia,* 31, 265, 1973.

956. **Wybenga, D., and Pileggi, V. J.,** Quantitative determination of 3-methoxy-4-hydroxymandelic acid (VMA) in urine, *Clin. Chim. Acta,* 16, 147, 1967.

957. **Yamada, K., Kayama, E., and Aizawa, Y.,** Determination of vanillylmandelic acid in urine by pre-column dansylation using micro high-performance liquid chromatography with fluorescence detection, *J. Chromatogr.,* 223, 176, 1981.

958. **Yamaguchi, Y., and Hayashi, C.,** Simple determination of high urinary excretion of 5-hydroxyindole-3-acetic acid with ferric chloride, *Clin. Chem.* (Winston-Salem, N. C.), 24, 149, 1978.

959. **Yamamoto, T., Yamatodani, A., Nishimura, M., and Wada, H.,** Determination of dopamine-3- and -4-O-sulfate in human plasma and urine by anion-exchange high-performance liquid chromatography with fluorometric detection. *J. Chromatogr.,* 342, 261, 1985.

960. **Yamatodani, A., and Wada, H.,** Automated analysis for plasma epinephrine and norepinephrine by liquid chromatography, including a sample clean-up procedure, *Clin. Chem.* (Winston-Salem, N. C.), 27, 1983, 1981.

961. **Yoneda, S., Alexander, N., and Vlachakis, N. D.,** Enzymatic deconjugation of catecholamines in human and rat plasma and red blood cell lysate, *Life Sci.,* 33, 935, 1983.

962. **Yoshida, A., Yamazaki, T., and Sakai, T.,** Determination of urinary 5-hydroxyindole-3-acetic acid by high-speed liquid chromatography, *Clin. Chim. Acta,* 77, 95, 1977.

963. **Yoshida, A., Yoshioka, M., Yamazaki, T., Sakai, T., and Tamura, Z.,** Urinary levels of vanilmandelic acid and homovanillic acid determined by high-speed liquid chromatography, *Clin. Chim. Acta,* 73, 315, 1976.

964. **Yoshida, J. I., Yoshino, K., Matsunaga, T., Higa, S., Suzuki, T., Hayashi, A., and Yamamura, Y.,** An improved method for determination of plasma norepinephrine: Isolation by boric acid gel and assay by selected ion monitoring, *Biomed. Mass. Spectrom.,* 7, 396, 1980.

965. **Yoshimoto, S., Kaku, H., Shimogawa, S., Watanabe, A., Nakagawara, M., and Takahashi, R.,** Urinary trace amine excretion and platelet monoamine oxidase activity in schizophrenia, *Psychiatry Res.,* 21, 229, 1987.

966. **Yoshinaga, K., Itoh, C., Ishida, N., Sato, N., and Wada, Y.,** Quantitative determination of metadrenaline and normetadrenaline in normal human urine, *Nature,* 191, 599, 1961.

967. **Youdim, M. B. H., Bonham Carter, S., Sandler, M., Hanington, E., and Wilkinson, M.,** Conjugation defect in tyramine-sensitive migraine, *Nature,* 230, 127, 1971.

968. **Young, S. N., Anderson, G. M., Gauthier, S., and Purdy, W. C.,** The origin of indoleacetic acid and indolepropionic acid in rat and human cerebrospinal fluid, *J. Neurochem.,* 34, 1087, 1980.

969. **Young, S. N., Davis, B. A., and Gauthier, S.,** Precursors and metabolites of phenylethylamine, *m-* and *p-*tyramine and tryptamine in human lumbar and cisternal cerebrospinal fluid, *J. Neurol. Neurosurg. Psychiatry,* 45, 633, 1982.

970. **Young, S. N., Gauthier, S., Anderson, G. M., and Purdy, W. C.,** Tryptophan, 5-hydroxyindoleacetic acid and indoleacetic acid in human cerebrospinal fluid: Interrelationships and the influence of age, sex, epilepsy and anticonvulsant drugs, *J. Neurol. Neurosurg. Psychiatry,* 43, 438, 1980.

971. **Young, S. N., Lal, S., Sourkes, T. L., Feldmuller, F., Aronoff, A., and Martin, J. B.,** Relationship between tryptophan in serum and CSF, and 5-hydroxyindoleacetic acid in CSF of man: Effect of cirrhosis of liver and probenecid administration, *J. Neurol. Neurosurg. Psychiatry,* 38, 322, 1975.

972. **Yu, P. H., Bowen, R. C., Davis, B. A., and Boulton, A. A.,** Platelet monoamine oxidase activity and trace acid levels in plasma of agoraphobic patients, *Acta Psychiatr. Scand.,* 67, 188, 1983.

973. **Yu, P. H., Davis, B. A., Bowen, R. C., Wormith, S., Addington, D., and Boulton, A. A.,** The catabolism of trace amines in some psychiatric disorders, in *Neurobiology of the Trace Amines,* Boulton, A. A., Baker, G. B., Dewhurst, W. G., and Sandler, M., Eds., Humana Press Inc., Clifton, New Jersey, 1984, 475.

974. **Yu, P. H., Davis, B. A., Durden, D. A., Gordon, A., Greene, C., Reid, D. M., Quinn, D., Matthews, P., D'Arcy, C., and Boulton, A. A.,** Further studies on platelet monoamine oxidase and phenolsulfotransferase and plasma levels of acid metabolites in aggressive and non-aggressive prisoners and children with attention deficit disorders, in *Neuropsychopharmacology of the Trace Amines,* Boulton, A. A., Maitre, L., Bieck, P. R., and Reiderer, P., Eds., Humana Press Inc., Clifton, New Jersey, 1985, 329.

975. **Yui, Y., Fujita, T., Yamamoto, T., Itokawa, Y., and Kawai, C.,** Liquid-chromatographic determination of norepinephrine and epinephrine in human plasma, *Clin. Chem.* (Winston-Salem, N. C.), 26, 194, 1980.

976. **Zander, K. J., Fischer, B., Zimmer, R., and Ackenheil, M.,** Long-term neuroleptic treatment of chronic schizophrenic patients: Clinical and biochemical effects of withdrawal, *Psychopharmacology,* 73, 43, 1981.

977. **Zhou, D., Shen, Y., Shu, L., Lo, H.,** Dexamethasone suppression test and urinary MHPG·SO_4 determination in depressive disorders, *Biol. Psychiatry,* 22, 883, 1987.

978. **Ziegler, M. G., Lake, C. R., and Kopin, I. J.,** Plasma noradrenaline increases with age, *Nature,* 261, 333, 1976.

979.   **Ziegler, M. G., Wood, J. H., Lake, C. R., and Kopin, I. J.,** Norepinephrine and 3-methoxy-4-hydroxyphenyl glycol gradients in human cerebrospinal fluid, *Am. J. Psychiatry,* 134, 565, 1977.